Clinical Costing Techniques and Analysis in Modern Healthcare Systems

Ronald Ma
Austin Health, Australia

A volume in the Advances in Medical Technologies and Clinical Practice (AMTCP) Book Series

IGI Global
DISSEMINATOR OF KNOWLEDGE

Published in the United States of America by
IGI Global
Medical Information Science Reference (an imprint of IGI Global)
701 E. Chocolate Avenue
Hershey PA, USA 17033
Tel: 717-533-8845
Fax: 717-533-8661
E-mail: cust@igi-global.com
Web site: http://www.igi-global.com

Library of Congress Cataloging-in-Publication Data

Names: Ma, Ronald, 1961- editor.
Title: Clinical costing techniques and analysis in modern healthcare systems / Ronald Ma, editor.
Description: Hershey, PA : Medical Information Science Reference/IGI Global, [2018] | Includes bibliographical references.
Identifiers: LCCN 2017035092| ISBN 9781522550822 (h/c) | ISBN 9781522550839 (eISBN)
Subjects: | MESH: Health Care Costs | Delivery of Health Care--economics | Costs and Cost Analysis | Australia
Classification: LCC RA971.3 | NLM W 74 KA8 | DDC 362.1068/1--dc23 LC record available at https://lccn.loc.gov/2017035092

This book is published in the IGI Global book series Advances in Medical Technologies and Clinical Practice (AMTCP) (ISSN: 2327-9354; eISSN: 2327-9370)

British Cataloguing in Publication Data
A Cataloguing in Publication record for this book is available from the British Library.

All work contributed to this book is new, previously-unpublished material.
The views expressed in this book are those of the authors, but not necessarily of the publisher.

For electronic access to this publication, please contact: eresources@igi-global.com.

Advances in Medical Technologies and Clinical Practice (AMTCP) Book Series

ISSN:2327-9354
EISSN:2327-9370

Editor-in-Chief: Srikanta Patnaik, SOA University, India & Priti Das, S.C.B. Medical College, India

MISSION

Medical technological innovation continues to provide avenues of research for faster and safer diagnosis and treatments for patients. Practitioners must stay up to date with these latest advancements to provide the best care for nursing and clinical practices.

The **Advances in Medical Technologies and Clinical Practice (AMTCP) Book Series** brings together the most recent research on the latest technology used in areas of nursing informatics, clinical technology, biomedicine, diagnostic technologies, and more. Researchers, students, and practitioners in this field will benefit from this fundamental coverage on the use of technology in clinical practices.

COVERAGE

- Telemedicine
- Medical informatics
- Nursing Informatics
- Biomechanics
- Diagnostic Technologies
- Medical Imaging
- Biomedical Applications
- Clinical Studies
- Clinical Data Mining
- Biometrics

IGI Global is currently accepting manuscripts for publication within this series. To submit a proposal for a volume in this series, please contact our Acquisition Editors at Acquisitions@igi-global.com or visit: http://www.igi-global.com/publish/.

The Advances in Medical Technologies and Clinical Practice (AMTCP) Book Series (ISSN 2327-9354) is published by IGI Global, 701 E. Chocolate Avenue, Hershey, PA 17033-1240, USA, www.igi-global.com. This series is composed of titles available for purchase individually; each title is edited to be contextually exclusive from any other title within the series. For pricing and ordering information please visit http://www.igi-global.com/book-series/advances-medical-technologies-clinical-practice/73682. Postmaster: Send all address changes to above address.

Titles in this Series

For a list of additional titles in this series, please visit:
https://www.igi-global.com/book-series/advances-medical-technologies-clinical-practice/73682

Electrocardiogram Signal Classification and Machine Learning Emerging Research ...
Sara Moein (Mount Sinai School of Medicine, USA)
Medical Information Science Reference • ©2018 • 196pp • H/C (ISBN: 9781522555803) • US $160.00

Research Advancements in Pharmaceutical, Nutritional, and Industrial Enzymology
Shashi Lata Bharati (North Eastern Regional Institute of Science and Technology, India) and Pankaj Kumar Chaurasia (Babasaheb Bhimrao Ambedkar Bihar University, India)
Medical Information Science Reference • ©2018 • 549pp • H/C (ISBN: 9781522552376) • US $255.00

Microbial Cultures and Enzymes in Dairy Technology
Şebnem Öztürkoğlu Budak (Ankara University, Turkey) and H. Ceren Akal (Ankara University, Turkey)
Medical Information Science Reference • ©2018 • 413pp • H/C (ISBN: 9781522553632) • US $265.00

Multifunctional Nanocarriers for Contemporary Healthcare Applications
Md. Abul Barkat (K.R. Mangalam University, India) Harshita A.B. (K.R. Mangalam University, India) Sarwar Beg (Jubilant Generics, India) and Farhan J. Ahmad (Jamia Hamdard, India)
Medical Information Science Reference • ©2018 • 602pp • H/C (ISBN: 9781522547815) • US $265.00

Biomedical Signal and Image Processing in Patient Care
Maheshkumar H. Kolekar (Indian Institute of Technology Patna, India) and Vinod Kumar (Indian Institute of Technology Roorkee, India)
Medical Information Science Reference • ©2018 • 312pp • H/C (ISBN: 9781522528296) • US $265.00

For an entire list of titles in this series, please visit:
https://www.igi-global.com/book-series/advances-medical-technologies-clinical-practice/73682

IGI Global
DISSEMINATOR OF KNOWLEDGE

701 East Chocolate Avenue, Hershey, PA 17033, USA
Tel: 717-533-8845 x100 • Fax: 717-533-8661
E-Mail: cust@igi-global.com • www.igi-global.com

Editorial Advisory Board

Table of Contents

Detailed Table of Contents

Standards are part of our lives. Clinical costing is no exception in this regard. Clinical costing standards are published documents comprising specifications and procedures to build consistent datasets for statutory purposes. The Independent Hospital Pricing Authority publishes and updates Australian Hospital Patient Costing Standards. The standards ensure compatibility and credibility. The standards formulate a consistent and transparent way to process costing. Compliance represents the production of reliable information which could be compared locally, nationally, and internationally. Health professionals could utilize these standards-compliant datasets for testing clinical guidelines for patient safety, developing patient classification systems for counting clinical services, and setting national efficient price for public hospital funding. The ultimate goal is to improve healthcare delivery in an equitable way and reduce human suffering.

Until now, the revenue allocation of a hospital service has not received sufficient attention. Previous research done on this subject overlooked the details of revenue streams in the activity-based funding environment and has not introduced any technical dimension faced by new clinical costers. On the other hand, clinical costers (who manage clinical costing database) have a strong aversion to talking about revenue, because of the exclusion of revenue data collection and submission for most funding authorities. Clinical costing also tries to prevent revenue information from influencing on cost allocation methods. That makes research on this subject extremely difficult. However, the chapter uses a language called "revenue is an integral part of clinical costing" as an alternative way to explore this subject, including fine technical details. The benefits of investing in the revenue allocation process seem to exceed its cost, since the cost, revenue, and clinical outcomes could be analyzed in toto for delivering information on safety and quality of care.

Most healthcare organizations would like to provide actionable information to the managers of their various service lines. Bringing administrative, clinical, and financial data together is critical to operating the service lines efficiently. It also presents a strategic advantage, as the applications of funding are more closely monitored, and regulatory reporting requirements increase. With a clearer picture of their financial and clinical performance together, organizations are better prepared to put efficient strategies in place to meet their goals and demonstrate value. However, that requires thorough planning and forward-thinking leadership. This chapter discusses approaches to how organizations can empower their stakeholders by providing them with integrated clinical and costing data. It addresses how business intelligence supports the management and reporting of clinical costing data, the utilization of data visualization and advanced analytics, the importance of data governance, and the role of a BI strategy, illustrated throughout with a case study.

The physician often spends far more time gazing at the screen than at the person who has made the appointment. The patient has booked with the expectation their illness or accident will receive undivided attention. Immediately there is a problem, both for the doctor and the patient. Careful medical record-keeping is one of the most important duties of a clinician. How else can a patient's history be documented, the clinical findings recorded, the provisional diagnosis entered, and the chosen treatment pathway defined? But how does the doctor maintain confidence-giving eye contact whilst doing all this? The 19th century physician, as exemplified by the famous painting of "The Doctor" by Luke Fildes in 1891, typifies the devotion to care exhibited by the committed physician. The actuality is that today's physicians display equal amounts of dedication to their work; the difference in 1891 was that there was very little available to treat the great majority of illnesses. EHR, if used to its potential, is the means of pulling all this data together and getting it right every time!

Activity-based funding (ABF) is a way of funding hospitals whereby they get paid for the number and mix of patients they treat. In order for governments to fund hospitals using ABF, hospitals use costing to inform the development of classification systems which provide valuable information for pricing purposes. Hospital patient costing is essential for understanding the total costs involved in treating a patient including the services or products used. This chapter outlines a methodology using simple statistics to prepare a budget for an inpatient ward using costing data. This method can be extended to other clinical areas (e.g., residential aged care or non-admitted).

This chapter will show how detailed information from an activity-based costing (ABC) system can be used to support activity-based funding (ABF) by providing management with a detailed perspective of the activity and how it can be used to internally model the allocation of target activity to build an activity-based budget (ABB). By building a set of internal cost weights based on ABC data, this chapter will show how activity forecast in a funding agreement can be broken up and applied to the individual cost centers that contributed to the activity in the current year. Building an ABB provides an evidence base for the overarching hospital budget and encourages the adoption of a focus on efficiency by hospital departments.

Clinical costing is a powerful tool to bridge the disconnect between financial and clinical information, and is an ideal platform to conduct research aimed at informing value-based clinical decision making. This chapter will provide an example of the

Foreword

There is an oft-used phrase in health care that states that when it comes to patient care, "better has no limits." This book captures the essence of this philosophy. It delves into clinical costing. With the proliferation of electronic health records and extensive data collection systems, there is a wealth of information that is collected, but not comprehensively analysed. To this end, clinical costing is becoming an area in healthcare services that is becoming increasingly quintessentially important.

A recent global initiative called Choosing Wisely aims to change clinicians' practice to align with best practice by encouraging them to stop using unnecessary investigations and interventions that are not supported by evidence. The Choosing Wisely Australia campaign (www.choosingwisely.org.au) was launched in January 2015 by the National Prescribing Service to engage clinicians and patients in meaningful conversation about tests, treatments and procedures that are unnecessary and that may, in fact, cause harm. It is a clinician led movement to articulate the right investigations and treatments for the right patient, through the creation of evidence-based lists of investigations and treatments. An important part of that evidence is to wisely utilise the stewardship that has been bestowed upon us. As a Choosing Wisely clinical lead for our health service, I understand the major motivation behind such an initiative is in providing the best in patient care, rather than saving money. The same ethos applies in this book where we discover that clinical costing is not all about cost containment. It is about our responsibility as health care providers. It is about always striving to be better than ourselves in our healthcare systems. In essence, it is about ensuring equity in quality healthcare delivery and the generation of new lean hospitals where efficiency and safety coincides with exceptional patient care.

I met the editor of this book, Ronald Ma, during a retreat in our health service known as the "Meeting of the Minds." This inspirational weekend brings together the greatest minds, both junior and senior, across the many disciplines in our health service. I discovered that Ronald's background as a surgeon ensures he thinks translationally in clinical costing. As a clinician, researcher, educator and administrator, I found his book inspirational in the breadth and depth in which it covers domains critical in healthcare systems. Utilising holistic, multifaceted methodologies, clinical costing complements pioneering in healthcare delivery. This is reflected in this Ronald's constant links to real models of care in his chapters. The translatability of this book is in actionable items and real-world case studies that allow readers from various backgrounds to capitalise on clinical costing data. As an educator, I understand the power of such practical examples and this book utilises these in multiple chapters to translationally bring concept to clinical practice.

In addition, as a researcher overseeing the University of Melbourne, Doctor of Medicine Research Program at our health service's clinical school, I understand the importance of driving clinical outcomes with data and research. Inherent in this is the ability to critically study current practice to drive innovation in future care. And with the dissemination of such research, clinical costing considerations can truly contribute to improving the overall health of a nation. True to his roots in clinical practice, Ronald engages and equips the reader with the practical tools to implement such research and apply business intelligence, big data and analytics to clinical costing data. As a clinician, I see first-hand how such evidence-based practice based on sound data analysis can transform the lives of patients who have been entrusted in our care.

Ultimately, this book represents the tantalising benefits of embracing analysis in clinical costing to transform health care delivery. Enjoy, discuss and reflect how the following chapters can revolutionise your workplace!

Christopher Leung
University of Melbourne, Australia & Austin Health, Australia
For patients, staff and students, always

Preface

INTRODUCTION

This book is about clinical costing, the discipline which studies the cost of resources used to deliver patient care. The costing of healthcare services has not received the attention it deserves (Ma, 2016) and the following pages seek to redress this issue. No apology is made for presenting the accurate costing of health care services as important as the delivery of healthcare itself.

Perhaps the main reason for this is that if there is no effective cost-containment and present expenditure trends continue, public expenditure on health and long-term care in OECD countries is set to increase from around 6% of GDP in 2015 to almost 9% of GDP in 2030 (OECD, 2015) and 14% by 2060 (De La Maisoneuve & Martins, 2013). Unless the cost of care delivery is sustainable in terms of a nation's economy, services currently provided will, over the course of time, be reduced.

Fortunately, there are many avenues available to contain costs. In every health system areas of significant waste can be identified, including unnecessary service duplication, "trial and error" decision-making, rampant cost shifting and focusing too broadly on hospital care when outpatient and "in the home" therapies provide the same or better outcomes at lesser cost. Accurate costing systems, in conjunction with suitable analytics, with petabyte storage capabilities for average sized economies, are required to examine clinical decision-making in terms of its value relative to its cost. The clinical pathways followed for each individual patient, using suitable algorithms, are benchmarked against best practice protocols in terms of the quality of service delivery, the safety and the cost. Insights from large volumes of patient data are utilised to improve clinical decision-making. With the appropriate strategy, cost containment is achieved as well as improvement in service quality. Costs are lowered, not by reducing services, but preserving them where cost-effective and, where necessary, expanding existing and introducing new ones, always ensuring that chosen interventions are likely to produce healthcare of the highest possible quality and be delivered in the safest possible setting.

Despite the many and varied types of health care systems globally, all consuming a considerable portion of a nation's wealth, there are large numbers of patients in every nation who do not receive optimal health care. Effective cost-containment should be accompanied by strategies to improve the overall health of a nation. Socio-economic differences in health exist in every country and produce a diverse range of health outcomes. Poor households are more likely to have sick children (Hernandez & Blazer, 2006) but, despite the many known determinants affecting health there are as many unanswered questions about the mechanisms underlying their effects (Braveman & Gottlieb, 2014) (Cutler & Lleras-Muney, 2006). Universal access to high-quality healthcare is one factor in significantly improving a nation's health but must be combined with universal health affordability so people can obtain the health services they require without risking financial hardship from unaffordable out-of-pocket expenses (Evans, Hsu, & Boerma, 2013).

With accurate costing systems projections can be made as to the fiscal sustainability of various policy initiatives. The lack of such costing systems is partly responsible for many OECD countries, whilst professing to have universal access, to have de facto rationing, with long waiting lists and closure of public hospital beds to reduce expenditure (Hurst & Siciliani, 2003). Throughout the world various strategies have been invoked to deliver health care to their peoples, with varying degrees of success, as evidenced by the very large differences in healthcare access, affordability, quality and expenditure, as a proportion of GDP, in various nations. Leaving aside the developing countries where high quality health care is simply not available to all its citizens and expenditure per capita is consequently low, there is a large range in health expenditure in the 24 OECD countries, from 5.1% in Turkey to 16.4% in the U.S. (OECD, 2016).

To ensure the ability of a nation to continue to provide the type of healthcare it considers reasonable for its citizens, all funders, whether government, health insurers or individual patients paying out-of-pocket expenses, they all should be striving to obtain value from the money spent. Many treatment regimens give little or no benefit to patients, there is considerable duplication of services and care is often provided in high-cost facilities when it could have been carried out in community settings (Glennie, 1992). Wachter notes that "uncertainty is endemic in medical diagnosis; the correct answer is a surprisingly probabilistic notion" (Wachter, 2015). Instead of "best guess" modes of therapy, analysis of sufficiently large databases is required to provide insights into optimal care, analysing the response to one treatment regime for a particular set of clinical symptoms with alternative clinical pathways.

Using computational tools to construct and evaluate a combined anatomico-physiologic model to predict the outcome of alternative treatment plans for individual patients in the treatment of cardiovascular disease (Taylor, et al., 1999), an integrated set of tools to test hypotheses on blood flow in the cardiovascular system was utilised. This combined an internet-based user interface developed using Java and VRML, image segmentation, geometric solid modelling, automatic finite element mesh generation, computational fluid dynamics and scientific visualisation techniques. Similar predictive insights into the efficacy of different treatment regimens are likely to become standard, with available computational power being harnessed in various clinical situations, particularly with the increasing utilisation of genomic data (Stephens, et al., 2015).

The accurate costing of all the clinical services provided in a nation and the benchmarking of this information against best practice pathways for each condition treated, matched for case-complexity and demographics, should be a nation's objective. Precision medicine, where health care is individually tailored on the basis of a person's genes, lifestyle and environment (Hodson, 2016), is in its infancy but is beginning to provide the means to transform diagnostic and therapeutic pathways, markedly reducing intuitive decision making. 70% of total healthcare costs are spent on 8% of the population (Bertsimas, et al., 2008); most of this on patients with chronic or complex conditions. The cost of care for Type I and type II diabetes in the U.S. in 2012 was estimated at $245 billion, with direct medical costs at $176 billion and reduced productivity costing an additional $69 billion (Yang, et al., 2013). Maintaining blood glucose levels within a narrow range significantly reduces the complications of this condition. Sensors measuring glucose levels, which direct pumps to administer insulin in its correct dose, are being developed. These will be one of many mobile devices custom-designed to maintain people with chronic illness in their optimal state of health. Population health will be enhanced and productivity will be increased. Overall social and cost benefit will result from the improvement in the quality of life from these interventions.

Unfortunately, healthcare has not yet embraced the potential benefit of analysis and effective decision-making which has transformed the banking sector, the airline industry, retail shopping, to name a few (Manyika, et al., 2012). Though huge amounts of data are collected in the health sector analysis has been very limited in terms of its potential value. Sophisticated clinical costing systems, accurately measuring the cost of care to the individual patient level, are commonly employed in hospitals throughout the world. Obtaining the same information in community settings has also been possible, particularly in the U.S. with the Veterans Administration, with 6 million enrolled patients a good example (Oliver, 2007). However, both in hospital and community settings, very little costing information has been matched with outcome data.

What is needed is the matching of input costs with clinical outcomes so that valid comparisons can be made as to the effectiveness of one treatment compared with another and whether this outcome could be achieved at lesser cost. In the following chapters the means by which accurate costings for hospitals and community health care settings are achieved are discussed, together with the means by which these costs can be compared with those hospitals and individual clinicians treating patients with similar conditions in different locations. The goal is to always deliver the right treatment at the right time, in the right place and at the right cost to all those who require it.

For some, this happens. For others, it doesn't. The right diagnosis is not made, the wrong treatment is given, and complications occur, a sub-optimal outcome is obtained. In other cases long delays occur because of limited resources. All these happenings need to be costed, including the opportunity cost to the patient if the treatment had been carried out sooner, with faster return to productive activity. These analyses should be benchmarked against costs when optimal care is provided for the same or similar conditions. There is a complex relationship between quality and cost. In some conditions higher costs provide better outcomes (Silber, Kaestner, Even-Shoshan, Wang, & Bressler, 2010) and in other conditions no benefits ensue (Burke & Ryan, 2014). Comprehensive costings throughout the health sector at the individual patient level, combined with reliable data on outcomes of care, is the means by which the quality of care will improve and be delivered within sustainable levels of expenditure.

Any such strategy has to be carefully executed, as demonstrated by the Blair government's data analytics strategy in the U.K. in the late 1990s. The Blair NHS vision was a system which was fully integrated with all stakeholders; patients, carers, doctors, whether community- or hospital-based, nurses, allied health workers, administrators and funders. The objective was to bring about better care, better health and lesser cost. The result was that the status quo, with occasional notable exceptions, continued; inputs (revenue streams) were still predetermined on historic data, outputs measured in terms of numbers of patients treated and little or no analysis of outcomes relative to resources employed (Triggle, 2007).

Regrettably this situation still persists throughout the world, masses of data is collected within the health sector but very little is used to improve the delivery of optimal healthcare at a sustainable cost. The data which is collected and analysed is almost irrelevant in terms of providing the very best care at the lowest possible cost. Generally, performance levels in the hospitals throughout Australia and other Western nations are benchmarked in terms of the number of patients admitted and outpatients treated, the lengths of hospital stay, the number of unplanned readmissions, the length of time in emergency rooms, infection rates, and length of waiting lists for surgical procedures etc. At the general practice (primary care) level performance levels are measured against a number of outcome measurements such as immunisation rates and chronic care initiatives.

These measurements are not sufficient. What is required is comprehensive data matching of the resources employed by every primary care physician (GP) and every hospital doctor in a community in the treatment of similar conditions and the outcomes achieved in terms of return to productive activity, restoration of function, alleviation of pain and suffering. A large part of the problem is the fact that health systems been far too selective in choosing which data to collect and analyse. This has led to the situation where data collection in terms of the outcomes of treatment and the cost to provide that outcome have been shamefully ignored. In sharp contrast, big data giants like Tesco, Walmart or Amazon have realised that every piece of collected data could be valuable to some extent or other; they mine massive datasets to deliver insights.

Health care requires the same strategy and the means to achieve this is the universal adoption, at least amongst OECD nations, to establish comprehensive electronic health records which are interoperable (see Chapter 9), with all privacy and security measures in place to ensure data is appropriately de-identified and utilised solely for outcome research. This is particularly important when the ability to find the right treatment may only be evident from comprehensive analysis of data obtained from very large patient populations. Human Longevity Inc. is a company aiming to scan the genomes of 100,000 people a year and complement this with proteomic, metabolomics and microbionic analyses. It is expected that this data, matched for age and the presence or absence of overt disease, will lead to new tests and therapies to extend healthy human life (Langreth, 2014). Most likely, because of the great social and economic potential personalized medicine has, within five years similar companies will be operating in all Western nations, their rationale being to prolong the quality of life. Data is the fuel of the future as well as the rich soil in which everything will grow (Eggleton, 2017).

In terms of cost containment and quality of care it is the monitoring of the decisions made by doctors that is imperative. They are the cost drivers of health expenditure, responsible for up to 80% of total costs (Norbeck, 2012). Nurses and allied health workers work under the supervision; compared with doctors they do not make resource decisions to any significant extent. And the health systems in which they work, the world over, are beset with inefficient practices. Revenue streams to hospitals and community care facilities are too often inefficiently managed and, almost universally the results of care provision, the outcomes of treatment, inadequately collected and poorly analysed. The result, but for a few notable exceptions which will be examined in succeeding chapters, is the survival of inefficient health systems which governments have either chosen not to overhaul or have failed in their attempts!

To sum up, masses of information is collected in the health sector but very little of it is analysed in terms of its value relative to the costs incurred. Appropriate analysis of these very large databases provides the opportunity to obtain the very best value from every healthcare dollar and mechanisms to achieve this are herewith examined. In order to do this the book is arranged into a series of chapters written by acknowledged experts in their respective fields. Chapter 1 discusses clinical costing standards development. Electronic health records and their potential to transform the delivery of healthcare is Chapter 2. Chapter 3 is about business intelligence (BI) and big data analytics applied to clinical costing, and this chapter includes a case study on an unplanned readmission. Chapter 4 examines activity-based budgeting versus traditional budgeting using clinical costing data. Statistical inference to develop budgets from activity based funding by costing data is discussed in Chapter 5. Revenue allocation under activity-based funding environments is in Chapter 6, and Chapter 7 is based around a case study, focussing on an ECMO business case writing using clinical costing data. Chapter 8 introduces clinical costing of a major abdominal operation, beset by complications, and discusses the opportunities created to effect clinical improvement.

Henry Glennie
Medilink Australia, Australia

REFERENCES

Bertsimas, D., Bjarnadottir, M. V., Kane, M. A., Kryder, J. C., Pandey, R., Vempala, S., & Wang, G. (2008). Algorithmic prediction of health-care costs. *Operations Research*, *56*(6), 1382–1392. doi:10.1287/opre.1080.0619

Braveman, P., & Gottlieb, L. (2014). *The social determinants of health: It's time to consider the causes of the causes* (Vol. 129). Public Health Reports. Retrieved from https://www.ncbi.nlm.nih.gov/pmc/articles/PMC3863696/

Burke, L. A., & Ryan, A. M. (2014). The complex relationship between cost and quality in US health care. *AMA Journal of Ethics*, *16*(2), 124–130. Retrieved from http://journalofethics.ama-assn.org/2014/02/pfor1-1402.html PMID:24553333

Cutler, D. M., & Lleras-Muney, A. (2006). *Education and health: evaluating theories and evidence*. National Bureau of Economic Research Working Paper. Retrieved from http://www.scirp.org/reference/ReferencesPapers.aspx?ReferenceID=1244315

De La Maisoneuve, C., & Martins, J. O. (2013). *Public spending on health and long-term care: A new set of projections* (OECD Economic Policy Papers. No.6. ed.). OECD Publishing. Retrieved from https://www.oecd.org/eco/growth/Health%20 FINAL.pdf

Eggleton, M. (2017). *Data as the fuel of the future*. Retrieved from The Australian Financial Review: http://www.afr.com/news/special-reports/future-now-series/data-as-the-fuel-of-the-future-20170716-gxc4u1

Evans, D. B., Hsu, J., & Boerma, T. (2013). Universal health coverage and universal access. *Bulletin of the World Health Organization*, *91*(8), 546–546A. doi:10.2471/BLT.13.125450 PMID:23940398

Glennie, H. (1992). Downsizing of Hospitals with Effective Community Care. *The New Zealand Medical Journal*, *105*, 202–203. PMID:1625828

Hernandez, L. M., & Blazer, D. G. (2006). *Genes, behavior and the social environment: Moving beyond the nature/nurture debate*. National Academies Press (US). Retrieved from https://www.ncbi.nlm.nih.gov/books/NBK19929/

Hodson, R. (2016). Precision medicine. *Nature Outlook*, *537*(49). doi:10.1038/537S49a PMID:27602738

Hurst, J., & Siciliani, L. (2003). Tackling excessive waiting times for elective surgery: A comparison of policies in twelve OECD countries. In *OECD Health Working Papers* (Vol. 6). Paris: OECD Publishing. 10.1787/108471127058

Langreth, R. (2014). *Venter starts DNA-scanning company to boost longevity*. Retrieved from Health Freedom Alliance: http://www.healthfreedoms.org/venter-starts-dna-scanning-company-to-boost-longevity/

Ma, R. (2016). *From the margins to the mainstream: Clinical costing for clinical improvement. In J. Moon & M. P. Galea (Eds.), Improving Health Management through Clinical Decision Support Systems*. IGI Global. doi:10.4018/978-1-4666-9432-3.ch009

Manyika, J., Chui, M., Brown, B., Bughin, J., Dodds, R., Roxburgh, C., & Byers, A. H. (2012). *Big data: the next frontier for innovation, competition and productivity*. Retrieved from McKinsey & Company: http://www.mckinsey.com/business-functions/digital-mckinsey/our-insights/big-data-the-next-frontier-for-innovation

Norbeck, T. (2012). Drivers of health care costs; A physicians foundation white paper. *The Physicians Foundation, Empowering Physicians, Improving Healthcare*. Retrieved from http://www.physiciansfoundation.org/uploads/default/Drivers_of_Health_Care_Costs_-_November_2012.pdf

OECD. (2015). *Fiscal sustainability of health systems: Bridging health and finance perspectives*. Paris: OECD Publishing. doi:10.1787/9789264233386-

OECD. (2016). *Health at a Glance: Europe 2016; State of Health in the EU Cycle*. Paris: OECD Publishing. doi:10.1787/9789264265592-

Oliver, A. (2007). *The Veterans Health Administration: An American success story?* doi:10.1111/j.1468-0009.2007.00475.x

Silber, J. H., Kaestner, R., Even-Shoshan, O., Wang, Y., & Bressler, L. J. (2010). Aggressive treatment style and surgical outcomes. *Health Services Research*, *45*(6), 1872–1892. doi:10.1111/j.1475-6773.2010.01180.x PMID:20880043

Stephens, Z. D., Lee, S. V., Faghri, F., Campbell, R. H., Zhai, C., Efron, M. J., . . . Robinson, G. E. (2015). Big data: Astronomical or genomical? doi: 10.1371/journal.pbio.1002195

Taylor, C. A., Draney, M. T., Ku, J. P., Parker, D., Steele, B. N., Wang, K., & Zarins, C. K. (1999). Predictive pedicine: Computational techniques in therapeutic decision-making. *Computer Aided Surgery*, *4*(5), 231–247. doi:10.3109/10929089909148176 PMID:10581521

Triggle, N. (2007). Blair's legacy: Health. *BBC News*. Retrieved from http://news.bbc.co.uk/2/hi/health/4555344.stm

Wachter, R. (2015). *The digital doctor: Hope, hype, and harm at the dawn of medicine's computer age (business books)*. Amazon. Retrieved from https://www.amazon.com/Digital-Doctor-Hope-Medicines-Computer/dp/0071849467

Yang, W., Dall, T. M., Halder, P., Gallo, P., Kowal, S. L., & Hogan, P. F. (2013). Economic costs of diabetes in the U.S. in 2012. *Diabetes Care*, *36*(4), 1033–1046. doi:10.2337/dc12-2625 PMID:23468086

Acknowledgment

I thank Stephen Cole for his guidance on many aspects of the activity-based budgeting and clinical costing interfaces

I am grateful to all reviewers for their thoughtful comments, especially Patrick Horan (Auckland District Health Board) for his comments on the revenue dataset approach, Dean Athan (Peninsula Health) for his editing work on the Clinical Costing Standards Association of Australia section, and Peter Carty (Austin Health) for his comments on Business Intelligence chapter.

Chapter 1
Clinical Costing Standards

Ronald Ma
Austin Health, Australia

ABSTRACT

Standards are part of our lives. Clinical costing is no exception in this regard. Clinical costing standards are published documents comprising specifications and procedures to build consistent datasets for statutory purposes. The Independent Hospital Pricing Authority publishes and updates Australian Hospital Patient Costing Standards. The standards ensure compatibility and credibility. The standards formulate a consistent and transparent way to process costing. Compliance represents the production of reliable information which could be compared locally, nationally, and internationally. Health professionals could utilize these standards-compliant datasets for testing clinical guidelines for patient safety, developing patient classification systems for counting clinical services, and setting national efficient price for public hospital funding. The ultimate goal is to improve healthcare delivery in an equitable way and reduce human suffering.

DOI: 10.4018/978-1-5225-5082-2.ch001

INTRODUCTION

We use standards every day in our lives such as in computing, healthcare, transport and measurements. The main purpose is to ensure quality, safety, reliability and consistency in performing an intended purpose.

Definition

Standards are published documents forming specifications and procedures to follow. They address a range of issues and institute protocols that help ensure compatibility and credibility.

Why It Is Important?

Clinical costing standards (CCS) are no exception. They are developed to provide a common language and set of expectations enabling interoperability, comparability and consistency between different systems and health services. They are best-practice principles to costing hospital services. They provide a safety net and remove anxiety for users by assuring the fitness for purpose.

The application of CCS usually generates reliable and comparable datasets. Health professionals could utilise the standards-compliant datasets for testing clinical guidelines for safety, developing classification systems for counting services, and setting the National Efficient Price (NEP) for funding. The ultimate goal is to improve healthcare delivery and reduce human sufferings. CCS are similar to other healthcare informatics standards such as data exchange and system standards, and pharmacy and terminology standards, and medical device standards and public health reporting standards.

Who Develops Them?

Clinical costing community members and clinical costers (practitioners) are the driving force behind the development of standards providing their expertise and innovation, and promoting new concepts of 'clinico-financial' data interface and research.

A good quality clinical costing information is vital to day-to-day healthcare management. It is able to guide clinical services to understand clinical variation and patient-level costs. Therefore, it enhances quality clinical outcomes and eliminates waste. Clinician participation in clinical costing is central to this quality enhancement process since clinicians are key resource decision makers and quality pathway designers. However, the foundation for this participation is the standardised clinical cost data that is accurate, meaningful and comparable across peer hospitals. The standards help clinicians to see how best practice in clinical costing is embedded in the data.

THE OBJECTIVES OF THE PAPER

This paper is aiming to provide the description of the standards development and analyses of significant issues with real-world examples and case studies. The paper does not just stop at the issues around the standards but also moves a step further, and explores a possible association between the development of the standards and the value-based care (maximal clinical benefit at minimum unit cost after removing avoidable costs for inefficiency and poor quality).

HOW MANY SETS OF STANDARDS IN AUSTRALIA?

For Victoria, there are two: the Clinical Costing Standards Association of Australia (CCSAA) Standards (1996 – 2013), which precede AHPCS (2011 – present).

BACKGROUND

Victorian clinical costers usually follow both CCSAA Standards and AHPCS. The following section will describe briefly about how the CCSAA came into existence and finally scaled down to its current form.

CCSAA STANDARDS

The CCSAA was incorporated in 1998 at the time when there was a proliferation of the use of clinical costing systems in Australia, namely, Transition, Trendstar, PowerPerformance Management (PowerHealth) and CostPro. The CCSAA took up a role to standardise costing methodologies in a software-neutral way for comparability and benchmarking across hospitals. It was born out of Clinical Costing Standards Committee (CCSC) of 1997. The committee comprises clinical costers from Victorian healthcare networks and interstate hospitals. Therefore, CCSAA Standards are fully compliant with Queensland's standards (The Clinical Costing Standards Association of Australia, 2013). Two New Zealand hospitals, the Department of Health and Children in Dublin (Ireland), the Kyoto University (Japan), Norway, Belgium, United Kingdom and Turkey were also members of the committee. In 2007, New South Wales Department of Health became a CCSAA member. The Clinical Costing Standards of England (CCSAE) was permitted to use CCSAA standards.

A significant milestone for CCSAA was in 2010 when it supported the National Activity Based Funding (ABF) initiatives. It sent a representative to the national ABF Working Group and Hospital Cost Data Collection Technical Reference Group for participating in the initiative at a national level.

Protocol

A protocol is adopted in the CCSAA to ensure consistency across all standards development. The costing industry will identify the need for development of a new standard or refinement of existing standard. Priorities will be given to emerging key issues in cost data collection and reporting. For example, costing and reporting of radiotherapy cancer services was a priority in 2013, and the CCSG4 was specifically developed to meet that demand. The CCSC seeks industry inputs to leverage its key resources. A draft is issued to the industry for comments and necessary changes are made on consensus. A revised draft is issued for further discussion. If all issues are rectified then the CCSC will ratify the completed standards and publish as a formal document.

Contents

CCSAA Standards are comprehensive and contain two main components: standards and guidelines. The latest version 5.1.17 (2013) holds fifteen standards and five guidelines.

The structure is consistent across all entries. It starts with the name of the standard, for example, CCS1: Assignment of direct and indirect/overhead departmental costs, version 1.9.7, Date: 24/09/2007. The body of the standard includes the purpose, definition and relevant guidelines. It concludes with important notes. For example, in CCS1 mentioned above, one of the notes mentions about cross-charging which could create 'direct' cost (which can be exclusively and specifically traced back to patient care) when charged to a direct cost centre or 'indirect' when charged to an indirect cost centre. The last entry to the notes under CCS1 is that this standard is Queensland State compliant.

Current Form

A restructure was implemented in 2012 to form a new "CCSAA – Victorian Clinical Costing User Group" bringing in new members such as rural health services and software system vendors. The emphasis was given to the implementation of AHPCS and ABF requirements, and the development of costing methodology for Victorian Cost Data Collection. The new group is currently developing standards on mental health costing, revenue allocation, palliative care, radiotherapy service and subacute non-admitted patient costing. The latest version of the CCSAA Standards was 5.1.17 published in April, 2013 with the contribution from nearly 70 experts.

MAIN FOCUS OF THE CHAPTER

The Standards Development

Internationally, there are different costing standards set out in different countries. For example, in England, Hospital Financial Management Association (HFMA) works on CCS for National Health Service to drive the quality and cost-effectiveness of public health services. Health Financing & Insurance Department Qatar develops costing standards for the Supreme Council of Health based on AHPCS (Health Financing & Insurance Department, 2013). For this chapter, the Australian standards development process will be used as an example.

Australian Hospital Patient Costing Standards (AHPCS) are developed to meet the demands of a significant health reform in Australia. The National Health Reform Agreement (2011) defines public hospital funding for services based on the activity level (activity-based funding or ABF model) (Council of Australian Governments, 2011). The AHPCS is part of the work to establish equitable funding for public hospitals across Australia. An independent organisation called "Independent Hospital Pricing Authority or IHPA" was established under Commonwealth legislation in 2011 to determine the National Efficient Price (NEP) to allow for the introduction of ABF. The determination of NEP is based on the National Hospital Cost Data Collection (NHCDC). Therefore, the NHCDC needs standards which can report a consistent, reliable and timely clinical costing information.

The AHPCS incorporates a standards governance structure and works with the NHCDC Advisory Committee (NAC) to develop and refine the standards by drawing on a wide array of sources including international professional bodies. The task of NAC is to advise new and revised standards to the Pricing Authority. The top of the hierarchy in the governance structure is the Minister for Health and Ageing, Clinical Advisory Committee, Pricing Authority, IHPA Chief Executive and Executive Committee. The next level comprises three significant groups such as NHCDC Advisory Committee, ABF Technical Advisory Committee and Finance Committee. The lowest in the hierarchy is composed of different working groups such as Subacute Care Working Group and Mental Health Working Group.

The standards development process is an ongoing in nature and constant evaluation is carried out based on the feedback from various organisations and consultations. For example, IHPA is aware of a need for a new standards or revision to an existing one. Then, it passes onto one of IHPA committees and working groups. The NHCDC Advisory Committee/Standards Subgroup will draft a new or revised standard and provide recommendations to the Pricing Authority. If the Pricing Authority accepted the recommendation then IHPA would update the AHPCS and issue to Ministers for 45-day comment period. After settling all issues around the newly developed or amended standards IHPA will publish the new AHPCS.

IHPA produces 37 standards based on the best available evidence and practice in the version 3.1 (2014). For overhead allocation statistics, there are two categories: financial and non-financial statistics. Financial statistics consist of salaries such as nursing salaries for allocating nursing administration costs to all relevant patient care areas. Non-financial statistics involve the length of hospital stay in days for allocating allied health management costs or the area of floor space for cleaning and energy supplies. For both categories, there are 31 statistics with the provision of three-tier order of preference (The Independent Hospital Pricing Authority, 2014). For example, the computer department's overheads could be allocated by the number of personal computers (first order) followed by total full-time equivalent amount of all staff (second order) and then followed by the headcount of all staff (the last order). The order of preference provides both flexibility and consistency to find an appropriate measure suitable for individual hospitals. This is one of the examples of CCS accommodating a "globally-consistent and locally-relevant" approach.

The structure of the standards is consistent across all 37 standards. It is described in a tabular format starting with the name of the standard, status of approval, implementation date, revision date, the purpose, the relevant standard to be met, the definition, guidelines to explain how to comply and the sources of definition and classification systems. For example, the COST 2.004 – Overhead Allocation Statistics include the status as approved, July 2004 as the implementation date and February 2014 as the revision date. The purpose is to ensure that hospitals are using the most appropriate statistic to allocate overheads, thereby improving quality and comparability of clinical costing datasets. The guidelines proposes that each patient service attracts its fair share of overheads and each hospital needs to document which allocation statistic is used for which overhead cost centre as part of clinical costing process. In the end, the COST 2.004 concludes with the NHCDC Hospital Reference Manual as the source of reference.

Issues

The major difficulty for health services is the building of the allocation statistic standards locally. For example, the accurate floor space measure for each cost centre seems to be impossible for many health services and the overhead allocation likely ends up with using readily-available statistics such as total full-time equivalent (FTE) and total expenses. Therefore, the standards developers need to consider which measures would be consistently and accurately available at local levels by weighing global significance against local relevance. It is noted that no matter how detailed costing standards and methodologies are, if the source activity data informing them is inaccurate, this will lead to inaccurate cost outputs. The benefits of Investing in source data quality usually exceeds the cost of doing so, because the quality data improves overall information consistency in the clinical costing system.

Case Study 1: Overhead Allocation

Background

Overhead allocation is one of the most important clinical costing functions and needs thorough investigation to allocate accurately. The indirect costs are costs which cannot be specifically and exclusively traced back to patient care activities such as utility and administrative costs. Inappropriate allocations can affect management decision makings in terms of resource investment and terminating services (Kaplan & Porter, 2011). For example, the Schon Klinik in Germany had reduced the capacity of its knee replacement rehabilitation unit in the past because of the faulty overhead allocation based on length of stay. The journey of these knee replacement patients was mainly in the rehabilitation unit (75% of their stay) and therefore, attracted the majority of overheads. The Schon Klinik began to see better financial performance in these units after introducing an appropriate allocation statistic, and re-expanded the rehabilitation unit.

The costs of support services are allocated as indirect costs by using weights such as direct costs, head count, floor space and the number of patients. The indirect costs are distributed to all patient care areas or final cost centres based on an allocation statistic. The allocation statistic is a relative value unit (RVU) or weight reflecting the level of consumption such as floor space area for allocating overheads of energy supplies and cleaning services. The purpose is to ensure a consistent and appropriate overhead allocation.

The standards are created to allow a certain degree of flexibility in implementing consistent allocations by having an order of preference. For example, some hospitals do not hold an accurate and timely floor space measurement at the time of allocation. In this case, these hospitals could use the next order of statistics such as full time equivalent figures of all staff.

Issues

Clinical costing processes could be lengthy when arguments on the accuracy of cost-drivers deriving from individuals' subjective beliefs rather than solutions on the deficiencies of the costing model such as unprofitable products and inefficient processes (Kaplan & Anderson, 2004). One of those lengthy processes may be overhead allocation statistics. Many arguments arise from a misunderstanding of the basic concept of overhead allocation.

For example, the CCSAA Standard CCS5 (2006) on overhead allocations specifies that total cost (first priority) or the full time equivalent (FTE) could be used as allocation statistics (weights) for finance department whereas the AHPCS proposes three alternatives for the same department: TransGL (the total number of transactions by cost centre), ExpAll (the total expenses of the hospital) and FteTotalAll (the value of the total hospital FTE).

While the allocation statistics of the CCSAA and AHPCS may look different the underlying principle for overhead allocation is identical. Both standards acknowledge that patient care areas should get a fair share of overheads based on the level of consumption. They agree on the method of simultaneous equation which is the most commonly used and the most accurate cost outputs. The simultaneous equation is a series of mathematical formulae allocating costs back and forth between cost areas to honour that a cost centre consumes its own services. Both CCSAA and AHPCS reflect the "non-stepdown" allocation principle that both overhead and final cost centres consume the outputs of overhead cost centres. This principle can only realistically be done in a specialist software package, which performs an infinite number of distribution iterations on each iteration of removing expenses from the overhead cost centre until all expenses have been totally absorbed into the direct patient care cost centre while also allocating back both to the originating and other overhead cost centres (The Independent Hospital Pricing Authority, 2014, p. 42).

The quality of allocated overhead cost outputs depends on the integrity, accuracy, completeness, consistency and timeliness of the overhead allocation statistics rather than their preference level of alternatives. No matter how detailed and sophisticated overhead allocation methods are, if the source data creating these allocation statistics are inaccurate and unreliable the whole clinical costing dataset will lack credibility. For example, the FTE and headcount statistics usually provided by human resources department need to be updated at least annually, because these statistics may change significantly from year to year, especially when a hospital goes through a restructuring process which affects both cost centre codes and the statistics.

Validating Allocation Statistics

Clinical costers are responsible for acquiring allocation statistics from various departments. All statistics are validated against the business model to assess the level of consistency, reliability, availability, timeliness, accuracy and completeness. For example, floor space is usually owned by the estate department and used to allocate significant volumes of cost according to the AHPCS standards, but it may not qualify as an allocation statistic if it fails the test. Since the standards recommend three alternatives for each department the resultant cost outputs provided by different allocation statistics need to be compared to see which statistic is superior based on the intended proportion reflecting the actual consumption of overheads.

Clinical costing systems are able to report the details of overhead allocation by tracking the cost movement from the original overhead cost area to the destination patient care area. For example, finance department is an overhead area and ExpAll is its allocation statistic. The overhead details show that 30% of the finance department are allocated to pharmacy, radiology, intensive care unit, anaesthetics, emergency, mental health clinical area and operating theatres. This baseline proportion must be evaluated with another recommended statistic such as TransGL (the number of transactions by cost centre). The final choice of the statistic must be justified by the following Rule of Two Principle.

A report showing indirect cost to total cost ratio by cost area or indirect cost to direct cost ratio would help justify the chosen statistic objectively. For example, a cost area has 96% of indirect cost or 25:1 for indirect to direct cost ratio will usually be investigated for its overhead allocation system configuration. The overhead allocation problem is a systemic issue, and a local solution generally fails to rectify the problem and can potentially cause collateral damage to other area setups.

Rule of Two

The "Rule of Two (ROT)" from the principle of ordering orthopaedic radiographs in suspicion of fracture could be adapted for the triangulation of cost outputs created with different allocation statistics such as:

- Two datasets (two views: Antero-posterior and lateral) with different statistics
- Two sources (two limbs: including the normal side) with pre- (baseline) and post-allocations
- Two groups (study and control) (two joints: above and below the suspected fracture), for example, two cost areas with the same statistics
- Two independent 'blinded' researchers whose only involvement is to assess the outcome measure (Webb & Bain, 2011)

This ROT test is performed to adopt an optimal performing statistic in comparison to other alternatives. For example, if the FTE is performing better than TransGL in terms of cost outputs reflecting the actual overhead consumption then the FTE would be adopted to allocate overheads from Financial Administration regardless of its third position of preference in AHPCS (The Independent Hospital Pricing Authority, 2014).

It is important that the validity test and principle of triangulation are included within the clinical costing department's information policies and guidelines. The information used to allocate costs are subject to data quality checks and rigour as other information in the hospital.

The allocation statistics are usually sourced from account codes, FTE and headcount, and system-generated figures.

Source 1: Account Codes

Expense accounts could be used as an allocation statistic for allocating overheads. They are general ledger expenses for total hospital or a specific service. The advantages of using accounts are that they are accurate, consistent, reliable and readily available from the system. The first step is to define an account or a range of accounts as an allocation statistic. For example, in Victoria, "Basic Pay – Nursing" account 10010 could be defined as "nursing FTE" to allocate nursing administration overheads. Since this common chart of account code is consistent the nursing FTE statistic reliably represents the level of consumption from the nursing administration resources.

Source 2: FTE and Headcount From Human Resources Department (HR)

HR holds FTE and headcount statistics by cost centre and reflects any organisational restructure. For example, cost centre code and associated FTE volumes are constantly updated in HR systems. Therefore, "Extract, Transform, Validate and Load (ETVL)" process for HR data is usually positive. The FTE and headcount statistics are the principal allocation statistics in overhead allocation. They are generally applied in many management and administration areas since they meet the validity test fully.

Source 3: System-Generated Figures

Recently, Improvements in systems programming and technologies have made "in-system" generation of allocation statistics instead of relying only on the external data provided by various staff from different departments. Staff who usually provide allocation statistics might leave the hospital or move on to other positions and also healthcare industry itself is in a constant time of change. Skilled and stable source for the statistics is impossible in volatile healthcare environment where staff turnover is high. The in-system generation could be a solution to ensure the statistics are up to date and relevant.

For example, PowerHealth has introduced an in-system generation function called "Built Data Postback (BDPB)" since 2013. This function provides statistics of hospital admissions, patent counts and other aggregated figures from any field in the source system by cost centre in the general ledger. The BDPB utilises the service building (intermediate product) and mapping steps to generate specified statistics. The Postback data processing is simple, convenient, fast and reliable. The BDPB statistics could be updated regularly with the costing database annual update.

The first step to set up BDPB is defining the parameters of the statistic. If "all admissions" is designated as the statistic to allocate overheads from Clinical Information Department then its BDPB configuration will include the name of the statistic, which field of the service file to aggregate (e.g. adding the attendances of the admission ward from the ward transfer quantity field built), the account type to populate (e.g. unit account) and the account code (e.g. 500). The BDPB process for all admission is now ready to generate the sum of attendances to the specified account by cost centre in the loaded general ledger.

There are some exceptions to usual overhead allocations. These exceptions will be described in the next section.

Allocating Overheads to Services Provided to Other Hospitals

When a hospital provides a service to another hospital the recipient side usually records the service and costs in its production volumes. Therefore, the service provision hospital needs to stop allocating its overheads to the service recipient cost centre. It is important that the system is configured properly to stop allocating overheads to the cost centre concerned for complying with the AHPCS SCP 3E.001 Matching Production and Cost – Offsets and Recoveries (The Independent Hospital Pricing Authority, 2014).

One of the easiest ways is creating a Boolean data type field (Yes/No) for receiving overheads in each cost centre setup. For example, if A1234 is the recipient hospital cost centre with "No" to overheads in the configuration then the overhead allocation process will omit this cost centre. The resultant cost outputs must still need to be verified with the relevant clinical director or service manager.

A Special Case of Reporting Requirements: Business Rules for Blood and Medical Indemnity

The Victoria State in Australia has set specific business rules of reporting on blood and medical indemnity expenditure since 2013. The general ledger of Victorian public hospitals lacks the National Blood Authority expenses. The Department of Health Victoria (DHV) provides blood expenses at the end of each financial year for cost data collections. A specific cost centre/account combination (Y0398/24101) is designated to report the expenses of blood and blood products without any overheads (indirect costs). The method of Boolean data type configuration for the blood cost centre would be beneficial to divert incoming overheads.

The DHV specifies medical indemnity allocation statistics to distribute indemnity expenses in its cost data collection. The statistics are the proportion of insurance premium for each specialty calculated by the Victorian Managed Insurance Authority (VMIA) (Department of Health Victoria, 2016). The VMIA has reduced the number of specialties from 29 to 8 and aggregated them at 8 specialty groups in recent years. This apparent lack of detailed information has left many hospitals at a loss as to how to formulate an appropriate allocation algorithm for each individual specialty or even how to rationalise the principle of specialty groupings (neurosurgery and gynaecology are grouped together). One of the solutions would be the actual individual premium contribution. Neurosurgery, thoracic/cardiovascular surgery and general surgery are reported as high risk areas (Jena, Seabury, Lakdawalla, & Chandra, 2011).

Summary

In summary, the overhead allocation is an important clinical costing function and needs a thorough investigation to allocate correctly, because improper allocations could impact management decisions. AHPCS has three orders of allocation alternatives for most hospital overhead areas. The primary data which builds the allocation statistic is as important as the order of the allocation statistic selected, and this primary data must be consistent, tested and constantly updated on a timely basis.

Case Study 2: Developing Mental Health Costing Guidelines in Victoria

Background

The Parliament of Victoria has enacted a new Mental Health Act 2014, which came into effect on July 1st, 2014. The act reforms Victoria's mental healthcare system to place people with mental health issues at the centre of their treatment decision makings. It provides the appointment of new professionals and institutions including chief psychiatrist, Mental Health Tribunal, Mental Health Complaints Commissioner and the Victorian Institute of Forensic Mental Health (The Parliament of Victoria, 2014). The appointment and functions of community visitors, and bodily restraint and capacity to give informed consent are important definitions for clinical costing in terms of counting services and identifying cost drivers. The Victorian Clinical Costing User Group (VCCUG) reached a consensus that a new set of mental health clinical costing guidelines was needed to deliver a consistent, accurate and reliable mental health dataset submission to the State Department of Health, and in the same year, IHPA was also developing and refining a new mental health classification and phase of care concept. The purpose of the Victorian mental health costing guidelines is to investigate and document the most appropriate method of costing mental health services.

Step 1: Identifying the Data Source

The development of the guidelines starts with the investigation of the data sources which record mental health services. The data source for clinical costing must meet certain criteria, which include consistency, completeness, reliability, electronic-format availability and reporting feasibility.

In Victoria, the principal data source for public mental health services is Client Management Interface/Operational Data Store (CMI/ODS). This data source meets most of the above criteria and holds two components. The CMI component is the local system for each public mental health service and the ODS provides the subset of data elements from the CMI for reporting to the state health department, chief psychiatrist and Mental Health Review Board.

However, eligible data sources for clinical costing may not be able to record all mental health services. For example, in Victoria, inpatient consultation liaison services may be recorded in an in-house, specialty-specific database. In this situation, the Department of Health Victoria could not be able to find liaison services in the CMI activity dataset, because the in-house database lacks CMI unique identifiers and mental health program code 'M'. A potential danger of recording in a separate in-house database is that patient identifiers could not be verified and validated through the official hospital patient management systems. This danger might lead to 'unlinked' services in the clinical costing system. Mental health services need to ensure that all their mental health activities are recorded in an appropriate electronic database to facilitate clinical data linkage (CDL).

The CDL is a statistical tool which allows linking of different datasets kept in different locations that relate to the same individual breaking down the usual *ghettoised* information, and therefore, an appropriate economic evaluation can be performed on various clinical settings to choose the most-preferred value-based option for the patients (Ma, 2015).

When an eligible database is selected for clinical costing a special attention is given to investigate the number of fields and their values, and how their relationships with the service provisions. For example, a single or multiple entries may be recorded for a service provided by multiple healthcare professionals at the same point of care. In the same way, a service location may represent a single or multiple cost centres with different proportions of resource utilisation (one-to-many relationships). Therefore, clinical costing needs to consider suitable methodologies for cost area and service mappings to cope with these different service entries, and the clinical costing process takes priority over reporting requirements. However, classifying and counting of a service at appropriate levels (service contacts or episodic levels) for reporting are important steps in developing guidelines.

Step 2: Defining the Service

This step involves defining what constitutes a mental health service from clinical costing perspectives. A "mental health service by type" involves acute, subacute, specialist, residential and community services based on clinical settings. Mental health service recipients include patients and consumers. Mental health consumers are the ones who receive services from a mental health service provider, and assessed by an authorised a psychiatrist and not provided with treatment (The Parliament of Victoria, 2014). The IHPA specifies the mental health care as a service delivered under the management of a clinician with specialised expertise in mental health and evidenced by an individualised formal mental health assessment and documented by a mental health plan, and may include psychosocial components such as family and carer support (HealthConsult, 2016, p. 6).

Acute clinical settings have two categories: admitted and non-admitted. Acute admitted services deliver inpatient care which is reimbursed on a single unit price irrespective of the bed setting or patient characteristics in 2016-17 (The Victorian Government, 2016). For example, AUD646 per available bed day is funded for an acute admitted specialist service.

Acute non-admitted service encompasses clinical community care and non-admitted bed-based treatment services focusing on prevention and recovery. Clinical community care comprises community-based bed substitution programs for people with a mental illness. For example, an adult bed-based service would attract AUD482 per available bed day, and ambulatory care AUD390 per community service hour.

In-scope mental health services also include forensic community service which provides community-based assessment and multidisciplinary treatment services to high-risk clients from criminal justice systems.

In summary, this step consists of understanding the various aspects of the mental health service, which include information storage, finance, performance measures and targets. Clinical costing specific tasks include organising an Extract-Transform-Verify-Load (ETVL) process, linking services to the patient, and defining the cost driver and allocation rule. The science and art of clinical costing is to explain cost variations or resource consumption levels for different services. Clinical costers are, therefore, usually seen as "mini" health ministers, because every costing guideline development process involves a thorough mastery of multiple subject areas (Ma, 2015).

Step 3: The Development Process

The VCCUG meets every month in the State Department of Health to develop a new set of mental health costing standards (MHCS). A new sub-committee called "Mental Health Sub-committee (MHSC)" was formed in 2014 with fifteen core members to formulate guidelines for costing mental health services. The MHSC has continued its predecessor CCSAA's work on the mental health guidelines, and invited information managers from major mental health services for their expert advice. In the same year, the IHPA also conducted a mental health costing study at the national level where most Australian states participated.

The core members come from the VCCUG itself and are willing to contribute their expertise for the group. A chairperson is nominated to organise the meeting and document the development process. A Google Drive is set up to store and share necessary information among members.

The first step is defining the function of the MHSC. Its role is to document costing methodologies, develop guidelines and provide benchmarking opportunities among members. The sharing of the data is only allowed within the group.

The second step is defining the terms of reference. It is an open group welcoming any interested participant from the main VCCUG. The role of individual participants includes the provision of any necessary input to achieve the group's objectives.

The third step is to reach agreements on the frequency of meetings. The MHSC usually meets once a month on the same day as the parent VCCUG meetings. The Victorian Department of Health provides the meeting venue. A minimum of five hospital representatives are required as the quorum requirement. The committee members must all be hospital representatives from the main VCCUG.

The fourth step is establishing the governance structure. The MHSC is responsible for reporting back to the main VCCUG and the Department of Health Victoria.

The first task for the MHSC is to investigate how Victorian hospitals are costing mental health services. A structured survey method with pre-defined format in a spreadsheet is used to speed up the investigation process on the current costing methodology. The survey topics include: the scope of activity, data sources, linking of services to patients, cost area mappings, service building, allocation rules and cost drivers, validation and issues. About ten major mental health service providers participated in the survey and the survey results were shared in the committee meeting.

The second task is documenting the mental health costing process and assumptions. For example, a standardised Structured Query Language (SQL) script is distributed among members to extract data from CMI. Therefore, the clinical costing process is standardised at the stage of data extraction (ETVL process). Linking of consultation liaison services (CL) to patients is also standardised with a set of business rules and included in the Victorian Cost Data Collection (VCDC) business rules and file specifications. This linking business rule specifies how to count consultation liaison services. For example, the first priority to link CL could be emergency episodes, followed by admitted episodes based on patient unique identifiers and service date. Unlinked contacts become "occasions of service", which is a technical term for any examination, consultation or treatment provided to a patient. All electroconvulsive therapy (ECT) services could be linked to admitted patients. If admitted patients are on leave then their leave days will be excluded from the length of stay calculation and costing. One of the challenges is the recording of travel time for visiting patients in the community. Travel services are built from the time taken to travel between the hub and the destination postcodes, and the number of clients seen in the same trip. A consensus is reached to add the travel time to the clinician contact time as the total consultation time to be costed.

The third task is standardising cost drivers and allocation rules. The survey shows that many mental health services use clinician contact time as a relative value unit (RVU) to allocate costs. An issue has arisen for identifying the duration of a group session with a single or multiple healthcare professionals. The time must be apportioned to reflect the actual clinician contact time received by a patient. For example, the duration is divided by the number of clients in a group session or multiplied by the number of professionals in a multidisciplinary treatment session.

The fourth task is to define all key terms and abbreviations. For example, the definition of mental health service must include services provided to patients with mental illness, mental health consumers, and their carers and families. A sub-centre or a service location created in the CMI is defined as a physical or virtual location from which mental health treatment programs are delivered. The definition must be accurate, consistent and reliable taking into accounts of all possible scenarios. From the clinical costing perspective, the definition of a service contact includes a statement pointing to a service contact between a client and an ambulatory care unit with a dated entry in a specified database. Contact types are defined further with Type A registered clients, Type B unregistered clients and Type C community contacts. The contribution from the mental health information managers is expansive and valuable for addressing technical requirements of standards within their specific area of expertise.

Therefore, the mental health costing standards development process ensures openness, balance, consensus and collaboration. The hallmarks of this process include: firstly, consensus must be reached by all representatives; secondly, standards are required to undergo member reviews; and thirdly, any feedback must be responded truthfully. In summary, MHSC continues to be fully involved in its support of the goals of setting a new set of mental health costing standards and remains committed to enhancing of the quality of AHPCS.

Case Study 3: Costing Frequency

What Is the Standard for Costing Frequency in Australia?

The AHPCS 3.1, COST 4.002 suggests that regular interim costing improves data quality and usefulness to end users (The Independent Hospital Pricing Authority, 2014, p. 55). The standard came into effect in July, 2014 and encourages hospitals to review cost outputs for reasonableness, and use these cost outputs to refine costing methods for subsequent costing periods. However, the standard fails to provide the definition and optimal frequency of cost update, and the sources of justification underpinning the standard, and its references, case studies, and the relevant international standards and the exceptions to the standard. It also omits any discussion on necessary resources to comply with this particular standard. The standard that in itself would cause controversy. Compliance with this standard poses a resource challenge for many hospitals.

Cost Update Process

Many Australian public hospitals go through a cost updating process annually at the end of each financial year, typically in July. The Australian public hospital financial year starts from July to June next year. The main purpose of the timing is to bring cost outputs closely in alignment with actual costs since the general ledger is usually finalised between July and August. Victorian public hospitals are required to report patient level costs for all operational funded activity, and expected to maintain patient costing systems to monitor service provisions. Therefore, the July update enables Victorian hospitals to prepare the annual VCDC submissions in October. The update process incorporates new business rules and file specifications, which are usually received in September. The submission conformity processes usually span six months from October to March. The conformity includes a set of quality assurance checks that may need re-submission.

Challenges

ETVL

Each cost update involves an end-to-end data management from ETVL to cost outputs and consumes staff time from various departments. It is a resource-intensive process and involves data gathering from the entire hospital. The data gathering may take several months based on the number of extracts, the availability of database owners and the status of existing information systems. For example, a delay is expected when database owners are on leave or a new information system is commissioned and therefore, a new extract is needed.

Clinical costing data extracts usually have two kinds: automated and manual extracts. Automated extracts are the ones that retrieve and configure source information systems directly and usually ready to load into the costing system via SQL Server Integration Services Package (SSIS). It is usually a seamless procedure without any user inputs, but an evaluation of the incoming data still needs a considerable amount of time from clinical costing team members. For example, interpreter services failed to link to any encounter within the current costing period. A thorough audit discovered that the values for the date range parameters were wrongly coded. A new interpreter service file was recreated, verified and loaded after correcting the coding errors.

The manual extracts comprises spreadsheets prepared by the data owners and dummy files prepared by clinical costers. Dummy files include three files: a patient file, an encounter file and a service file. The dummy services are those services, which lack patient-level data, and therefore, costing those dummy encounters enables clinical costers to reconcile the entire operational costs with the general ledger in the financial reconciliation report (Department of Health Victoria, 2016, p. 63).

The number of extracts vary from hospital to hospital. For example, one of the Victorian public hospitals gathers forty data extracts over two months with a full-time clinical coster. A quarterly cost data update means that the annual update process is repeated four times. A more frequent cost update schedule would put a great pressure on the unprepared, yet already strained, Victorian clinical costing workforce.

The time and cost demands of clinical costing update work is a major barrier to comply with the standard COST 4.002. An example from the banking sector demonstrates the actual workload of activity-based costing, in comparison to the individual's perception of the workload. A bank needs 70,000 employees from a hundred facilities for providing monthly time allocation reports and fourteen full-time staff for data gathering, processing and reporting (Kaplan & Anderson, 2004). A new strategy is needed to avoid rising costs and overtime associated with frequent costing dataset updates.

Interim Costing

Any cost update during the financial year is an interim costing and fails to represent the actual cost since the general ledger of the current year and clinical service data are still in progress. While there are multiple drawbacks from interim costing some important ones will be described in the next section.

In Victoria, the general ledger lacks blood transfusion and Health Purchasing Victoria expenses. The interim cost update fails to include their actual expenses and is forced to use estimates which may or may not reflect actual resource consumption. Moreover, medical indemnity allocation weights are provided only after the end of each financial year, and estimates are used to allocate medical indemnity costs. As mentioned above, the VCDC business rule and file specifications are received only after the end of the current financial year, usually in September of the next financial year. The arrival of new business rules and file specifications with the actual expenses of blood and Health Purchasing Victoria makes the prior interim costing defective and triggers necessary corrections of interim extracts and allocation rules. Every correction needs rework or replacement of clinical costing processes that waste resources.

Public hospitals usually boost their throughputs to meet performance targets near the end of each financial year. This increased activity affects the mean cost of many patient groups and needs adjustments in the interim allocation rules and weights. For example, thirty-six million Hepatitis C drug expenses appeared in March, which was only three months away from the end of the financial year. This sudden surge of pharmacy costs adversely affected the pharmacy department's mean cost and prior allocation rules. A solution was implemented by creating a specific Hepatitis C cost area with its own service building and mapping, and allocation rules. A post hoc evaluation for the changes was justified to see the reasonableness of the ratio of mean allocated cost to the mean actual charge. Therefore, interim costing and allocation can become irrelevant instead of improving the quality of costing data and its usefulness stated in the standard on costing frequency. The cost update frequency should only be increased if its marginal benefit exceeds its marginal cost according to the cost-benefit principle (Frank & Bernanke, 2009).

Linking Issues

The interim costing poses threats to linking rules. The linking function is a statistical tool matching clinical services to pre-defined encounter types within a specified date range based on the patient unique identifier and service date. Encounter types usually comprises inpatient, outpatient, non-admitted, mental health, radiotherapy, emergency and other based on the scope of activity (Department of Health Victoria, 2016, p. 32). The scope of activity consists of three categories: admitted, non-admitted and emergency patients. The linking rule specifies four algorithms: enable the software to link, create dummy encounters if no link is found, look for the hierarchy of encounter types to link (e.g. emergency followed by admitted patients) within a specified date range (e.g. to look for any inpatient episode one day back and forth from the service date). A problem has arisen when the linking rule fails to find any episode in the loaded encounter file.

For example, intravenous gamma globulin was dispensed from the blood bank on 30th December 2016 to a 51-year old male patient with Common Variable Immunodeficiency for his monthly treatment plan. His next infusion date was 3rd January 2017 and the last infusion was on 29th November 2016 as inpatient episodes in an ambulatory care. The previous infusion date 29th November 2016 was 31 days away from the date of dispensary. The next inpatient episode was in early January 2017, and out of range for the first six month interim costing (July to December 2016). Therefore, the clinical costing software created a 'dummy' encounter for the 30th December gamma globulin in response to the lack of matching inpatient episodes within thirty days. The first priority of linking blood and blood products is inpatient episodes according to the VCDC business rules and AHPCS COST 6.001. The November 2016 linked encounter of the last infusion had a whole range of resource utilisation costs from the gamma globulin infusion and ambulatory care to the respiratory medicine, catering, pathology tests and overheads whereas the dummy encounter only held the gamma globulin cost without any other labour and ancillary service costs. One of the solutions to get a full utilisation cost for the January 2017 infusion would be a full financial year costing from July 2016 to June 2017 (full twelve months), which will build a new encounter database with a complete reloading and relinking of all clinical services. The full year costing also reflects the actual figures and business rules of blood, Health Purchasing Victoria and medical indemnity instead of applying estimates in the interim costing.

The above mentioned linking method is called "soft linked" whereas a "hard link" method is an automated process where the "service-provided" encounters are linked to the corresponding encounters automatically during the service file load process. The purpose is to ensure an alignment of resources to the correct patient. For example, a radiotherapy service provides matching encounter numbers in its service file. The clinical costing software is configured to facilitate the hard link by disabling the soft-linked function and creation of dummy encounters. Therefore, a specific post hoc query could be run to verify this hard link.

New Quality Assurance Checks

New file specifications and quality checks near the submission deadline affect interim costing. The VCDC file specifications are systematic processes of data quality assurance checks to see whether the submission files are meeting specified requirements. The critical errors must be rectified before submission files are accepted. Changes in file specifications and quality checks affect cost data submission processes in terms of time and resources. These specifications are usually received in September, which is only a month away from the submission deadline (October 31st). The changes usually involve a major reconfiguration of data extracts and costing methodologies, and the clinical costing software vendor's support to change or add new functionalities for meeting new reporting requirements. Some health services may not be able to report the newly specified data elements in time. Their interim costing datasets often become obsolete and need rework from the beginning. That is one of the valid reasons for which most hospitals only update their costing datasets after receiving all specification changes at the end of each financial year.

Strategic Tool

Patient-level costing systems are considered more of a strategic tool and have created greater clinical engagement in resource management, for example, disinvesting in unprofitable services (Llewellyn, Chambers, Ellwood, Begkos, & Wood, 2016). Clinical costing, therefore, is a strategic tool for long-term plans, and rarely viewed as an operational instrument, because any operational management tool needs frequent updates such as quarterly or even daily updates. The cost update process usually has a time lag of one or two months between the end of financial year and the updated costing dataset for that financial year.

Clinical costing is based on the principles of activity-based costing. It represents fact-based productive capability (actual activity levels) derived from strategic goals. For example, Weighted Inlier Equivalent Separation (WIES) targets could be set for the upcoming financial year based on the clinical costing information. The clinical costing information is consistent with the relationship between goal achievement and resource intensity.

Every resource decision is a clinical decision and every clinical improvement could be translated as financial performance. Clinical costing shows opportunities to improve such as duplication of tasks and tests. Physicians and nurses could shift their time to patient care activities after removing redundant processes revealed by clinical costing information. Elimination of waste is one of the largest opportunities of reducing costs with equal or enhanced patient outcomes. For example, the endoscopic removals of large colorectal polyps takes 'zero' length of stay in comparison to eight days with surgical approach, and thus, the colonoscopic removals could save $13, 112 per case by removing the resource wastage with the surgical approach ($2, 152 versus $15, 264) (Church & Erkan, 2016). Clinical costing could reveal the proportion of unprofitable clinical services and help eliminate waste such as reducing unnecessary blood, radiograph and test orders.

These are the reasons why clinical costing is used as a strategic tool, especially for its analytic capability in budget preparations, forecasting, goal settings and clinical reviews. Clinical costing is also applied in the area of activity-based management and therefore, nowadays, clinical costing has placed itself at the nucleus of clinical performance management.

The lack of quarterly or monthly cost update is insufficient to suggest any disadvantage in data quality or usefulness, because other factors could influence the result. For example, the lack of operating theatre visit record (usually over ten hours of operation) in the theatre information system could jeopardise the costs of liver transplant cases. The root cause of wrong allocations in these cases is the integrity of the theatre systems rather than frequent costing updates. An active use of costing data could bring improvements in the data quality of clinical costing and other hospital information systems. Liver transplant cases with missing theatre records mentioned above will trigger a theatre information audit to rectify missing theatre records and therefore, the active application of clinical costing information improves the data quality of both clinical costing and theatre information systems.

The current investment in clinical costing and other information management teams in the hospital could also limit their capability to process a regular and frequent cost update, because clinical costing relies on various feeder systems. Victorian clinical costing teams are usually composed of a range between 0.5 and 3.0 full-time equivalents. Their current function is generally limited to compliance reporting to submit annual VCDC to the state department of health. The submission process includes many months of dataset preparation, change implementation, audit, quality checks, feedback, cleaning and resubmissions. An enhanced clinical costing function has recently been expected to assist internal business and put strains on this under-resourced workforce. At the same time, they are involved in multiple research projects, internal process improvement projects, system maintenance, and revenue allocations. A new spectrum of clinical costing is revenue allocations and this new activity involves a steep learning curve to understand public hospital revenue streams and private patient billing. However, having costs and revenue in the system is a clear advantage for both clinical and non-clinical research, because clinical costing will be able to report contribution margins and break-even points. Therefore, the marginal benefit of clinical costing resources spent on these value-added activities seems to exceed their marginal cost.

Summary

Any increase in cost update can result in additional staff time not only from clinical costing teams but also from feeder departments. A semi-annual or annual cost update seems to be sufficient for most strategic needs without incurring opportunity costs of more frequent cost updates. Annually-updated clinical costing information holds valid reference costs for many strategic performance indicators such as cost by diagnosis or surgery, and drives future operational planning, but not the reverse. The cost-benefit principle can inform decisions about the update frequency (the frequency should only be increased if its marginal benefit exceeds its marginal cost). We should not confuse the scalpel with the surgeon, however, the frequent cost update is a tool that fails to substitute many measures that could improve cost data quality and usefulness. More research is needed to verify the effectiveness of frequent cost updates. We must decide how much resource we are willing to spend to improve our data quality.

SOLUTIONS AND RECOMMENDATIONS

Globally-Relevant and Locally-Specific

Users of clinical costing standards require a good understanding of source data issues to make conformity. Flexibility in both interpretation and implementation of standards is necessary, because in the real world, many compliance issues can arise from the availability of data (e.g. direct consumption data) and quality of feeder systems to the resourcefulness of clinical costing teams and strategic directions of the hospitals. A ‘globally-relevant and locally-specific’ strategy would be suitable in this situation without compromising the purpose of disseminating best-practice and carrying out statutory functions with clinical costing data (The Independent Hospital Pricing Authority, 2014, p. 2).

Quarterly cost updates to comply with AHPCS 3.1 COST 4.002 could be implemented without compromising the existing resource level of most clinical costing teams by applying the Pareto principle (Pareto, 1964). This method involves more frequent updates for the twenty per cent of critical cost areas that represent eighty per cent of total costs and usual annual schedules for the remainder (Bragg, 2010).

Overhead allocation statistics from the AHPCS need attentions for flexible interpretation at local levels. The development of new activity-based, consistent, readily available, and locally-reliable statistics is required to address compliance issues. More research is needed to formulate evidence-based preference orders of these allocation statistics. Well-designed studies with control groups could realise the superiority levels of each preference order, and the credibility of standards could then be enhanced.

Empowering the Industry

Clinical costing standards are the reference points where clinical costing communities refer to for their methodologies. These national consensus standards are valuable to generate reliable and consistent datasets that are applied in funding, research and statutory functions. Users are assured that cost variations are from causes other than accounting practice and clinical costing methods. The standards development is a composite net made of national intertwined with local industry elements.

National standards developing organisations and local experts, nowadays, have many opportunities to work cooperatively to fulfil their purpose of disseminating best-practice and maintaining comparable data. While they both have diverse skills to address technical requirements within their specific expertise local business wisdom usually informs national bodies. The approach taken for developing national standards needs to be unique as it is expected to recognise that communities know best when it comes to living with local stakeholders. Sufficient information, explanation and case studies are expected for local users to interpret national standards correctly. The final standards, by taking this collaborative approach, will be comprised of not only locally-reliable but also globally-generalisable guidelines.

Every resource decision is a clinical action, which will, in turn, take care of the basis of cost allocation method. Therefore, clinician participation in clinical costing is the key to success and this increased level of close cooperation between clinicians and clinical costing is urgently required.

Triggers for the requirement of new standards could come not only from clinical costing communities but also from local clinicians, for example, costing of new clinical activities and service delivery models such as online hospitals, robotics, cognitive/artificial intelligence and IoT (Internet of Things)-based biological sensors. These triggers can be prioritised at national and local levels, and then supported by the resourcing and resourcefulness concept to reach the final stage (Joubert & Raeburn, 1998). The concept takes into account of current local workforce capacity and capability in a supportive environment to maximise compliance. Organised efforts of clinicians and national standards developing organisations could then prepare themselves for the innovative means of clinical costing.

FUTURE RESEARCH

Researchers could look at ways to improve better alignment of financial data with activity capture to reduce the need for program fractions (PFRAC). Challenges would be the activity capture of multidisciplinary teams and their case conferences, and mental health and clinical trials. Researchers could also look at ways to capture clinician direct patient care time using smartphones and Bluetooth devices. Future clinical costing standards could formulate the basic partitioning of inpatient, outpatient, emergency, community and operating theatre medical activities and costs in the absence of clinician contact duration. Urgent needs would be uniform ways to partitioning of costs for these clinical settings, because the current practice based on roster and activity levels proves unreliable.

Future research could interrogate the optimal level of investment in clinical costing teams to meet the standards such as the increased frequency of cost updates (COST 4.002), and the optimal level of proportion for resourcing (supportive environment) and resourcefulness (competency). The evaluation of the barriers for compliance and provision of possible solutions need urgent attention.

Future studies are worthwhile to determine the level of flexibility (local relevance) for each finalised standard without compromising the data quality and uniformity. Future studies could look at how to predict the level of future compliance based on the submission data. Researchers need to ask what costing method (e.g. time-driven activity-based costing) would be economic, effective and easily manageable with current resource levels (Kaplan & Anderson, 2004).

Studies that evaluate the governance and operational models of standards developing organisations would be advantageous for setting national and international integration strategies, and building global clinical costing communities to enhance globally relevant clinical costing methodologies.

Knowledge of the degree of accuracy (true cost) from different costing methods will allow appropriate selection of strategies to conform to the standards and ensure that the number of hospitals complying with the standards are maximised within the constraints of the limited and fixed resource available from the current clinical costing teams.

CONCLUSION

Clinical costing standards provide confidence in the data. The application of the standards facilitate statutory functions such as setting National Efficient Price in Australia. Compliance with the standards still represents a challenge for clinical costing communities. The globally-consistent and locally-relevant approaches in the interpretation of standards could maximise compliance. Every standard finalised needs to be evidence-based. Overhead allocation is an important clinical costing function and needs a thorough investigation to allocate correctly, because improper allocations could impact management decisions. The primary data that build the allocation statistics must be consistent, tested and constantly updated on a timely basis. The resourcing and resourcefulness of clinical costing teams and organisational support are critical factors to achieve the goals of standards developing organisations. Local communities could contribute locally relevant standards at national levels such as developing mental health costing standards in Victoria, Australia.

While the immediate goal is focused on best-practice guidelines for costing hospital services the ultimate goal seems to be an adequate financing strategy for achieving equitable and quality healthcare. However, to achieve this end, standards need to be user-friendly, research-based, time-tested, and sensible to clinicians.

REFERENCES

Bragg, S. (Producer). (2010). When should I update standard costs? *Cost Accounting*. Retrieved from http://www.accountingtools.com/questions-and-answers/when-should-i-update-standard-costs.html

Church, J., & Erkan, A. (2016, August 3). Scope or scalpel? A matched study of the treatment of large colorectal polyps. *ANZ Journal of Surgery*.

Council of Australian Governments. (2011). *National health reform agreement*. Canberra, Australia: Council of Australian Governments.

Department of Health Victoria. (2016). *Victorian Cost Data Collection data request specification and business rules for reporting cost data*. Melbourne, Australia: Department of Health Victoria.

Frank, R., & Bernanke, B. (2009). *Principles of microeconomics*. New York, NY: McGraw-Hill/Irwin.

Health Financing & Insurance Department. (2013). *Costing standards version 1.0.2013. State of Qatar*. Supreme Council of Health.

HealthConsult. (2016). *Mental health costing study*. Author.

Jena, A. B., Seabury, S., Lakdawalla, D., & Chandra, A. (2011). Malpractice Risk According to Physician Specialty. [PubMed]. *The New England Journal of Medicine*, *365*(7), 629–636. doi:10.1056/NEJMsa1012370

Joubert, N., & Raeburn, J. (1998, September). Mental Health Promotion: People, Power and Passion. *The International Journal of Mental Health Promotion*, 15-22.

Kaplan, R. S., & Anderson, S. R. (2004, November). Time-driven activity-based costing. *Harvard Business Review*.

Llewellyn, S., Chambers, N., Ellwood, S., Begkos, C., & Wood, C. (2016). *Patient-level information and costing systems (PLICSs): A mixed-methods study of current practice and future potential for the NHS health economy*. Academic Press.

Ma, R. (2015). *From the margins to the mainstream: Clinical costing for clinical improvement*. Melbourne, Australia: IGI Global.

Pareto, V. (1964). *Cours d'économie politique* (Vol. 1). Librairie Droz. doi:10.3917/droz.paret.1964.01

The Clinical Costing Standards Association of Australia. (2013). *Clinical costing standards: version 5.1.17*. Melbourne, Australia: The Clinical Costing Standards Association of Australia.

The Independent Hospital Pricing Authority. (2014). *The Australian Hospital Patient Costing Standards, version 3.1*. Sydney, Australia: The Independent Hospital Pricing Authority.

The Parliament of Victoria. (2014). *Mental Health Act 2014*. Melbourne: The Parliament of Victoria.

The Victorian Government. (2016). *Department of Health and Human Services policy and funding guidelines 2016*. Melbourne, Australia: The Victorian Government.

Webb, P., & Bain, C. (2011). *Essential epidemiology: An introduction for students and health professionals* (2nd ed.). Cambridge, UK: Cambridge University Press.

KEY TERMS AND DEFINITIONS

Clinical Costers: Clinical costing practitioners who process end-to-end data management of the clinical costing system.

Clinical Costing: A discipline which studies the cost of resources used to deliver patient care.

Clinical Data Linkage: It is a statistical tool which allows linking of different datasets kept in different locations that relate to the same individual.

Direct Cost: It is the cost that can be traced back to the direct patient care activity (e.g., nursing costs).

Health Economics: It is a discipline within public health and health systems concerned with efficiency, effectiveness, value, and behavior in the consumption of healthcare.

Indirect Cost: It is the overhead cost that cannot be traced back to the direct patient care activity (e.g., utility and administrative costs).

Patient-Level Costing: It measures and costs resource consumption of each patient care activity. It provides more accurate costs at patient level than the top-down approach. It is also known as micro-costing, bottom-up costing, and activity-based costing.

Public Health: It is the science and art of preventing disease, prolonging life, and promoting health through the organized efforts of society.

Total Cost: It is an addition of direct and indirect costs.

Value-Based Healthcare: It is the healthcare conferring a patient-centered, clinical benefit at lowest unit cost.

Chapter 2
Revenue Allocation

Ronald Ma
Austin Health, Australia

ABSTRACT

Until now, the revenue allocation of a hospital service has not received sufficient attention. Previous research done on this subject overlooked the details of revenue streams in the activity-based funding environment and has not introduced any technical dimension faced by new clinical costers. On the other hand, clinical costers (who manage clinical costing database) have a strong aversion to talking about revenue, because of the exclusion of revenue data collection and submission for most funding authorities. Clinical costing also tries to prevent revenue information from influencing on cost allocation methods. That makes research on this subject extremely difficult. However, the chapter uses a language called "revenue is an integral part of clinical costing" as an alternative way to explore this subject, including fine technical details. The benefits of investing in the revenue allocation process seem to exceed its cost, since the cost, revenue, and clinical outcomes could be analyzed in toto for delivering information on safety and quality of care.

DOI: 10.4018/978-1-5225-5082-2.ch002

INTRODUCTION

Until now, the revenue allocation of a hospital service has not received sufficient attention. Previous research done on this subject overlooked the details of revenue streams in the activity-based funding environment and has not introduced any technical dimension faced by new clinical costers. On the other hand, clinical costers (who manage clinical costing database) have a strong aversion to talking about revenue, because of the exclusion of revenue data collection and submission for most funding authorities. That makes research on this subject extremely difficult. However, the author of this chapter used a language called 'revenue is an integral part of cost analyses' as an alternative way to explore this subject, including fine technical details.

Revenue allocation for a hospital is as important as cost allocation. Understanding revenue streams provides a fairly complete financial picture of a health service, which in turn, enhances the quality of clinical costing and most importantly, financial planning. Having both revenue and cost data opens up a new horizon of analytic possibilities for a clinical service since the revenue data provides a second set of comparison data within and between hospitals. Clinical costers would find it easier to engage clinical services if revenue allocation is incorporated in their analyses. This chapter argues that revenue allocation needs as equal support as cost allocation from finance departments, health departments, clinical services and software vendors. The revenue allocation also needs its own guidelines, business rules and standards as clinical costing.

This chapter will be based on Victorian activity-based funding model of Australia. The contents of the chapter are applicable to other states and countries which have similar activity-based funding models.

THE OBJECTIVES

This paper is aiming to explain why revenue allocation is important in clinical costing and what constitutes revenue allocation in the activity-based funding environment in terms of knowledge, resources, technical expertise and software.

BACKGROUND

Definition

Revenue allocation in clinical costing is the distribution of total income down to the patient level based on appropriate allocation rules in a health service operating under activity-based funding.

In Victoria, it involves a complex process of patient qualifiers (who should get the revenue) and how (allocation statistics or rules) to allocate revenue from the Department of Health Victoria and other funding agencies. The purpose is to maintain the operating structure of the health service. It also requires health services to follow accrual accounting principles that record the cost and revenue of resources when they are consumed in the health service delivery irrespective of the time of the payment (The Independent Hospital Pricing Authority, 2014, p. 32).

History

The revenue allocation in Victorian public hospitals seems to be in its early stages. Uncertainties come from the choice of the allocation methodology, method and software. Revenue standards are not available from any funding and pricing authority. The main purpose of revenue allocation in public hospitals seems to be an internal reporting to investigate profitability and contribution margin linked to patient outcomes. The secondary purpose could be a comparison analysis of own cost and revenue in a timely manner instead of relying on benchmarking organisations.

MAIN FOCUS OF THE CHAPTER

Getting the Data Source

There are two financial data sources for revenue allocations: general ledger (GL) and cash flow (CF). Both sources holds cost or revenue centre/account/amount combinations. Revenue accounts have descriptions on the funded service. For example, cost centre Axxxx/account 5xxxx/amount of 1.5 million for liver transplant. The only difference between these two sources is that CF has detailed information on the separate revenue centre/account/amount combinations rather than an aggregated amount. If the GL is used as the main data source then 'reclassing' or splitting of the aggregated revenue amount would be necessary from the GL revenue centre to the corresponding cost centre to align with costs. Finance Department usually has GL-reconciled cash flow statement for revenue allocations.

Preparation for Revenue Allocation

The CF or GL needs to be formatted with necessary fields and values to suit a chosen methodology and software. There are three main required fields to add to the CF or GL are "Exclude/Include" (the revenue line item to be excluded or included in this revenue exercise), patient qualifiers (who should get it) and allocation rules (how to distribute this revenue).

A typical Victorian hospital under activity-based funding environment has three revenue streams:

- Activity-based funding (ABF) components
- Grants from the Department of Health, and
- Private patient revenue from patient billing systems.

All streams need the same fields to set up in the system such as patient qualifiers and allocation rules. The significant volume of work is needed to configure grant revenue since the knowledge around the type of grants and purpose needs to be built for each grant. This work involves multiple workshops with financial controllers, service managers and management accountants. The aim for holding these workshops is a consensus on what the grant is for and how to allocate it. The credibility and transparency of allocations are gained from these workshops.

Most revenue allocation software could handle ABF components automatically. If the revenue allocation software has a direct link to the private patient billing systems then only qualifiers and allocation rules need to be configured for allocating private revenue.

Activity-based funding (ABF) usually has two types of funding: rate-based and block-based. The most common rate-based revenue is the Weighted Inlier Equivalent Separation (WIES). The Victorian Government uses WIES as its ABF policy for public hospitals (Victorian Department of Health, 2017a). The WIES formula starts with assigning a Diagnosis Related Group (DRG) to each admission with a DRG Grouper software, which reads patient age, gender, diagnoses, procedures and complications. The Government publishes a table of WIES values for each DRG depending on length of stay, the hours of intensive care unit stay and mechanical ventilation, and indigenous status or having certain medical procedures such as stent or Atrial Septal Defect repair. The rate-based grant involves the specified amount (rate) to be distributed to each qualified patient. For example, the WIES revenue is allocated at the rate of AUD4, 248/WIES. This amount will be multiplied by the WIES amount of the recipient patient. The block-based grant, in comparison, specifies the total amount to be shared by the qualifying patients. For example, one of the block-based grants is the Respecting Patient Choice Grant for end-of-life care of terminally ill cancer patients. The amount is distributed to all cancer patients receiving the service (the qualifier) based on the total cost (allocation statistic or rule).

Clinical Service Inputs

Clinical service inputs are required in many areas of revenue allocation except ABF components. The ABF component of revenue is documented in the annual policy and funding guidelines, and therefore, the software vendors are able to programme revenue allocation algorithms without consulting any clinical service on patient qualifiers and allocation statistics whereas the revenue allocation process for specified grants needs the inputs from the clinical services.

Specified grants are provided to a health service to cover the cost which is either incurred beyond the ABF or to carry out agreed services; for example, Victorian Respiratory Support Service provides state-wide ventilator support services in Victoria. Consulting clinical services is necessary to investigate the nature of the grant (one-off or recurring), the recipients of the service and appropriate allocation statistics. The consultation process will uncover their information systems (where the activity is recorded) and the data quality. Therefore, the revenue allocation process provides a complete knowledge of a clinical business, its funded activity unit and counting, and costing and revenue allocation altogether. In the costing world, the revenue allocation is considered to be a complimentary to costing.

For example, the block grant-funded mental health services need multiple revenue allocation workshops to discuss each grant and its allocation methodology. Caveat arises when the total cost is used to allocate revenue in mental health services. Some systems might have pushed all expenses to the discharging financial year for those patients staying across multiple financial years (very long stayers). In this way, the allocated revenue will potentially be ‘boosted’ in the discharging financial year. It is important that the total cost must be partitioned within the financial year before any revenue is allocated for those long stayers.

Finance Inputs

Both GL and CF data sources come from finance departments and are usually reconciled to each other. Finance usually manages patient billing systems which are the backbones of allocating private patient revenue.

Financial controllers could usually provide directions on the nature of the grants (fixed and variable, or recurring and one-off grants), patient qualifiers, allocation rules and service owners. A specific financial knowledge of each grant seems to be the most useful input from finance. The formal documentation for such knowledge seems to be rare in many public hospitals.

Most grants are variable in nature and specific for a cohort of patients receiving a particular service. Defining patient qualifiers involves a complete financial knowledge of cost centres and their service. For example, a specified grant on additional public holidays would cover all patients of the hospital whereas non-cash grant insurance only covers public liability on behalf of the hospital, but is a separate grant from that of medical indemnity.

The main task of clinical costers is transforming the knowledge of patient qualifiers and allocation rules into a software-specific language and system configuration. The next step will involve a search for activity data recording systems on how the activity comes to clinical costing systems. The clinical costing systems need to be configured to balance cost and revenue for the same activity (parallel construction). For example, sundry expenses and revenue are excluded on both cost and revenue allocations to get a balanced profitability statement or 'profit and loss' report.

A linked server or data extract needs to be configured to extract private patient activities and fee amounts for allocating private patient revenue. The finance department could also verify the integrity of the private patient extract information before loading into the costing system. Therefore, engaging finance departments is valuable for the revenue allocation.

System Configurations

Victorian clinical costers mainly have four system configurations to allocate revenue:

- PowerPerformance Manager (PPM) and the revenue dataset approach
- PPM and Idiom Decision Manager combination,
- CostPro Plus, and
- Structured Query Language (SQL) database approaches.

A small hospital could be able to allocate revenue with a simple spreadsheet program.

PPM and Idiom

Idiom Decision Manager is a desktop-based decision engine program producing revenue allocation rule sets for all three revenue streams. Its rule sets come with complete documentation. The rule sets are imported into PPM to allocate revenue down to qualified patients in the costing engine. The revenue outputs are displayed along with costs in standard reports. Therefore, profitability analyses could be done for a specified parameter. For example, reports on profitability are readily available as standard at patient-level by admission type, consultant, DRG, referral source and patient type. The revenue by type is a useful standard report in parallel to costs such as private revenue, grants and activity-based funding revenue.

PPM and the Revenue Dataset Approach

The PPM and revenue dataset approach was introduced in 2016 using the same methodology as the costing engine. The costing system data sources could be used for revenue allocation, for example, the patients, general ledger and revenue account codes. This approach builds on the strength of 'time-tested' costing methodology such as service builders, service mappings and allocation rules. However, the general ledger configuration for the revenue needs to be loaded as a separate financial year. The revenue activity engine relies on the service building of the revenue lines and mapping of these services to the revenue area that holds the dollar amount. Many PPM users welcome this approach because of their familiarity with the system screens and configurations. However, reclassing many new revenue line items for the whole financial year needs an intensive work. This approach may work well for small hospitals.

One of the challenges in New Zealand scenarios is the nature of the general ledger revenue which is the budgeted revenue rather than actuals (Horan, 2018). For example, a capped funding is imposed to provide a thousand first specialist assessments (FSA) and there will be no additional revenue in the general ledger for extra assessments beyond the capped volume. Therefore, there is cost but no revenue for those extra assessments since hospitals have no ability to turn these patients away. The current allocation engine needs to accommodate this logic and write a smarter algorithm. In this regard, Idiom Decision Manager can easily handle this logic and algorithm.

CostPro Plus

CostPro Plus is a web delivered activity based costing and revenue allocation system written within SQL Server. According to S. Rush (personal communication, May 29, 2017), it can also be extended to include nightly activity reporting to provide a powerful patient-level information repository and business intelligence reporting system in one package. It is utilised in seventy percent of New Zealand's hospitals operating within their activity-based funding environment.

CostPro facilitates managing activity, performance and growth strategies as well as understanding the contribution margin for the service lines. The software engine is based around the separation of the bottom up development of product costs for each department and then applying these costs to the patient activity. The system is automated and able to process data nightly on multiple on-line years of data. CostPro is implemented within public and private hospitals within Victoria and Queensland, and available for the Australian health and education sectors. It has a facility to continuously audit the clinical costing activity from within the front end of the user interface. This has been set up within Victoria to incorporate the standard suite of Victorian Cost Data Collection (VCDC) audits, such as missing prostheses, medical, theatre or nursing costs from episodes that would be expected to receive them.

The homepage dashboard includes new cost centre and account mappings at each GL load to alert the users, as well as other costing errors, on an exception basis. It also calculates WIES and other ABF models and incorporates private billing revenue during the overnight load. This information is utilised by the revenue module to allocate revenue as accurately and fully as possible to the patient episodes, based on rules, scope clauses and allocation statistics. This allows the review of full patient costs, detailed patient revenue and the contribution margin by specialty, doctor, DRG or patient on-line, throughout the organisation.

Major international software vendors from other sectors, such as RevPro, IBM, Oracle, Aptitude, Microsoft and SAP, could be of value in revenue allocations of the health sector. These revenue recognition software need further investigation whether they would suit public hospitals' financial planning needs.

SQL Database Approach

Some Victorian hospitals adopt this approach. It involves a creation of Structured Query Language (SQL) database using an open source MySQL or similar in-house software. The major task includes creation of SQL tables in the same costing server to link patient and costing information. There are five main tables to be created:

- The qualified patient cohort or list
- Main allocation statistics
- The revenue bucket or output tables for reporting purposes
- The encounter details table for patients and revenue amount, and
- The revenue line details.

The patient cohort table contains the cohort description (e.g. WIES public patients) and rule (defining the cohort characteristics for selection purposes). The allocation statistics table holds information on the allocation rule set such as total cost or length of stay for distributing revenue amounts to qualified patients. The revenue bucket table is for reporting on the revenue category at the end of allocation, such as WIES public or private practice fees. The fourth table is the encounter details table which contains episode numbers and allocated amounts. The fifth table is the revenue line details imported from the cash flow statement or general ledger. This fifth table is the key table linking revenue dataset by financial year, line items, revenue buckets, patient cohort identifiers, allocation statistic identifiers, revenue amount to be allocated and allocated revenue amount, and revenue include flag and comments.

The advantage of this approach is the speed of the revenue run, which seems to be fast and accurate. One of the reasons of the speed gain is that the calculations are made right inside the SQL database without any intermediary system and application, such as the frontend application and Java platform.

This approach would need a high level of technical expertise and time investment from the clinical costing team. The downside would be the documentation, maintenance and support of this in-house system, especially in the climate of high staff turn-over. In comparison, for example, the PPM and Idiom combination have a comprehensive documentation and support for maintenance.

Vendor Inputs

The revenue section of a costing software vendor is usually limited in comparison to the costing section, because the patient-level revenue is not required to report to the funding authority. However, the revenue consultant could guide the revenue allocation process from the system configuration point of view. The capabilities and weaknesses vary from software to software, but the main functionality is the same such as loading necessary data elements and running different revenue models on patient qualifiers.

There are two different perspectives on working with software vendors. Firstly, it involves a complete configuration of a chosen software and relevant system modifications to process the first revenue dataset. The vendor's revenue consultant usually audits the first revenue outputs to see whether the system setups are correct. The consultant will then hand over the dataset to the local clinical costing team to maintain and improve it (hybrid business model). Secondly, the consultant configures every new financial year (totally outsourced). If the new financial year involves a funding formula or amount change then re-programming is necessary.

The vendor itself sometimes adopts a new system and way of revenue allocation. Therefore, the local clinical costing team needs to decide whether to go with the new approach or stay with the existing one, which may or may not be supported in the future. For example, PPM introduced a new way of revenue allocation called "revenue dataset approach", technically similar to its costing engine in 2016. Its previous software companion Idiom Decision Manager for producing revenue rule sets would become almost unsupported. Client hospitals using PPM could end up re-configuring the whole revenue setups with the new revenue dataset approach. The new process could involve a tremendous amount of time from the already strained local clinical costing teams. However, the revenue allocation clinical business knowledge is transferrable to any new approach in the horizon.

Challenges

Emergency Department Revenue

The emergency department (ED) visits in Victoria, Australia, have two main funding streams: the ED block grant for non-admitted visits regardless of the level of activity and WIES funding for the ED admitted episodes (The Victorian Government, 2016). For example, Patient A is a non-admitted ED episode and gets funding from the ED block grant. Patient B is an admitted ED episode and its journey includes an ED visit and admitted episode. On discharge, Patient B is funded through WIES units that could be translated to actual dollars according to the WIES price (AUD4, 248 in 2014-15 Financial Year) of that particular discharging financial year. The WIES for the Patient B covers both the ED and admitted episodes. The ED block grant revenue allocation excludes admitted ED episodes (revenue = zero) despite these episodes still attract significant costs. The ED revenue model needs to decide on what proportion of WIES revenue belongs to the ED component of these admitted ED episodes, for example, ten percent of WIES revenue. Therefore, the ED revenue model would eventually allocate appropriate amount to both ED and admitted components of the admitted ED episodes along with their costs.

Qualifiers and Allocation Statistics

The main revenue allocation process includes patient qualifiers and allocation statistics. They vary from hospital to hospital but the gap between them is narrowing since revenue allocation standardisation is happening among clinical costing communities, for example, Victorian Clinical Costing User Group (VCCUG) is working on the revenue allocation standards.

Two examples will be provided to demonstrate the formulation of patient qualifiers and allocation statistics. The first example is WIES allocations and the second example a mental health block grant.

The WIES allocation involves thorough understanding of WIES funding model which has been implemented for public hospitals in Victoria for over twenty years. The WIES funding model covers approximately sixty percent of health services' funding in Victoria and additional funding is provided with block funding and specified grants (Victorian Department of Health, 2017a).

Every eligible patient episode is funded at a flat cost weight based on the DRG and paid per cost weight. Therefore, funding starts with the process of clinical coding that is a method of classifying patients into similar conditions and levels of resource use. The coding is followed by counting of eligible patients for WIES funding and recorded in patient management systems. Victorian public hospitals are required to report costs for all state-funded activities and maintain clinical costing systems. The WIES eligible patients are already recorded on these costing systems and the programming for defining patient qualifiers usually follows the definition of the funding policy guidelines.

WIES eligible patients are those in Victorian Admitted Episodes Dataset (VAED) with the care type 4 including qualified newborns (The Victorian Government, 2016). Therefore, patient qualifiers for public WIES revenue could be the care type 4 or Acute Care and the discharge election is "to be treated as a public patient" whereas the qualifier for Department of Veteran Affairs (DVA) WIES could be of the same as the public WIES patients with an additional criterion of the account class of DVA patients (Victorian Department of Health, 2017b).

The qualifiers for the Electroconvulsive therapy (ECT) mental health block grant could be a specified cost area where the ECT activity is delivered and captured, such as Hxxxx acute psychiatry cost area. The ECT activity could be the patients from the community and hospital admissions, and its activity for the community and inpatients is usually recorded in separate systems. It is usually delivered in the procedure room. The allocation statistic would be the total cost of the qualified patients.

In summary, revenue allocation equips clinical costers with a thorough understanding of the hospital-wide clinical business on how it is funded, counted, costed and reported. Therefore, revenue allocation improves clinical costing data quality.

Private Patient Revenue

Clinical costing teams need to have access to the patient billing information systems for adding private patient revenue to the revenue dataset. These information systems usually reside in the finance department and the 'read-only' access would be appropriate. Ways to access and extract this billing information vary from hospital to hospital. There are mainly two ways to extract this information: linked server approach and extract as a separate source system in the clinical costing system.

The linked server approach involves a mapping of the patient billing system server and its tables directly to the clinical costing system. The patient billing system owner typically grants security permission (user name and password) of certain tables to the clinical coster. The clinical coster imports information directly to the clinical costing system as a linked server source system. The patient billing source system of the clinical costing system holds a series of data fields such as patient number, episode number, date of billing, date of admission, revenue type, quantity, dollar amount and invoice number. It is a seamless process and delivers error-free information directly to the clinical costing system.

The second approach is to extract the same information mentioned above as a separate "comma-separated values (CSV)" file for the tabular data, and load into the clinical costing system. It is a manual process and usually goes through an "Extract, Transform, Verify and Load (ETVL)" process. Both approaches need an audit to ensure data integrity.

For example, the patient billing system holds the same date and time for an episode. This same date/time field may cause errors in the clinical costing system even though the same date/time is valid for billing purposes. Clinical costing systems usually prefer a unique date/time which is system-generated.

The patient qualifier and allocation rule for the private practice fees would be an allocation to those billed patients in the billing system based on the total cost of each patient from the relevant cost area. Validation checks on the allocated amount is necessary after each allocation run.

One of the auditing processes could look at episode discrepancy with the clinical costing system. For example, since many hospital information systems feed information to the billing information systems just for billing purposes some episodes may not be in the clinical costing system such as vascular laboratory outpatient tests directly recorded in the billing system without entering in any patient administration system. These episodes need a separate revenue area and services to isolate a matched revenue amount and service. The revenue auditing process may be difficult for clinical costers, because they may not see any complete physical table of the billing system in the clinical costing system via the linked server configuration approach.

Auditing Revenue Dataset

The auditing process could follow the "Rule of Two". The rule of two concept is borrowed from the principle of ordering radiographs in orthopaedics for the triangulation of costing/revenue datasets by comparing two datasets (two views: Antero-posterior and lateral), two sources (two limbs: including the normal side), two groups (study and control) (two joints: above and below the suspected fracture) and two independent 'blinded' researchers whose only involvement is to assess the outcome measure (Webb & Bain, 2011). The principle of research and epidemiology such as comparison by time, place and person, and eligibility and exclusion criteria, and external validity considerations could be the main evaluation technique. Confounding and biases should be taken into account. Statistical principles, such as descriptive and analytic statistics (t-test), and convergence and divergence, could guide every step of the evaluation process. The central tendency, dispersion and confidence intervals of the data are useful techniques for evaluation. Aggregates and averages need to be interpreted with extreme caution. Statistical indices (similar to Consumer Price Index) could be adopted to see any variance in activity or cost/revenue combinations (Lind, Marchal, Wathen, & Magazine, 2006).

Health researchers need to acknowledge that variations in cost and revenue usually come from patients themselves and their associated clinical services, and thus, the only way to eliminate variability in healthcare would involve the elimination of all patients (Morton & Cornwell, 2009; Pandit, Pandit, & Reynard, 2010). Researchers could look at the underlying clinical variability of "time, place, person" principles of epidemiology with risk adjustments, and then move on to the variability of cost and revenue for each cohort if a comparison analysis with peer health services is implemented. It is vital that the auditing and evaluation focus on opportunities to improve based on actionable insights in the cost/revenue data.

Time Constraint

Clinical costers usually allocate their 'submission-free' time (April to June) on revenue processing. The task of revenue allocation involves thorough and lengthy investigations with service managers and clinical directors. The ideal arrangement would be having a dedicated revenue processor staff in addition to the existing clinical coster. This arrangement enables the revenue processor to work on the revenue side while the clinical coster oversees the whole costing and revenue allocation. In this way, the workload is shared among the clinical costing team. The advantage for this arrangement would be a value-added outcome of having a timely revenue dataset on par with the costing dataset. The usual scenario is that in the absence of the dedicated revenue processor, the revenue dataset lags behind the costing dataset's financial year. The workload of maintaining revenue datasets seems to be as equal as the costing.

Organisational Support

The demand for the revenue dataset has been increasing since the clinical costing benchmarking dataset is available for comparison analysis among peer hospitals. The revenue data completes the information needed to run a clinical business. Therefore, senior management support for revenue processing would add business values to the organisation's existing strategic capabilities by knowing what services are not profitable and how to improve efficiency in those services. The cost and revenue combination dataset at patient levels could provide actionable insights where efficiency gain efforts are to be focused on. Investing in clinical costing and revenue processing could expect timely answers for any business question with an aid of exploratory statistical data analysis, data mining and visualisation.

Delirium example

One of the Victorian public hospitals called "Hospital A", for example, investigated the profitability of delirium patients using clinical costing and revenue datasets. Delirium is usually found in 20% of general hospital inpatients and 35% if more than 80 years old (Ryan et al., 2013). A sample of 1, 235 cases was taken based on the delirium International Classification of Diseases (ICD version 10.14) codes of F05.0, F05.1, F05.8 and F05.9 at any position in the clinical coding sequence for 2015-16 financial year. The funding gap for the cohort was AUD13.8 Million at mean length of stay of 14.6 days. The total cost to treat this cohort was AUD42.3 Million (mean cost per episode = AUD34, 257. The 662 males and 573 females had an age ranging from 13 to 101 years (median age = 79).

A research question was asked to see any financial improvement if the delirium cohort was educated, recorded and coded correctly at the position of the secondary diagnosis. An exploratory data analysis was done by running a DRG Grouper with the above ICD codes at the secondary diagnosis on this cohort and populating a new set of WIES revenue. The financial performance improved by AUD2.5 Million at a rate of AUD2, 042 per inpatient episode. The result could be translated as a gain of AUD140 per day of stay. This scenario is similar to the findings of malnutrition coding in Australian and New Zealand hospitals with significant loss of public hospital funding revenue (Agarwal et al., 2015).

However, this coding practice change only failed to make a breakeven point. The Hospital A's financial loss was still at AUD11.3 Million. A marginal cost analysis was further pursued with a multiple regression analysis. It showed that only if in-hospital complications were treated with a principle of "early diagnosis and treatment" then both the human suffering and length of stay would be reduced to a breakeven point. The linear model suggested that improving in clinical outcomes by having any additional reduction in length of stay by a day would save AUD2, 703 ($p < 0.05$), and any additional reduction in complications by one diagnosis would save AUD6, 453.

The cost and revenue dataset successfully demonstrated a series of actionable insights on reducing length of stay and in-hospital complications. Next steps would involve an implementation of locally relevant delirium assessment tools for early diagnosis and treatment. The revenue processing usually serves an addition to the existing business value of clinical costing, and therefore, the marginal benefit of investing in it seems to exceed its marginal cost (the cost-benefit principle).

Reporting

The simple graph has brought more information to the data analyst's mind than any other device - John Tukey

The clinical costing and revenue information system is the 'one and only' system combining all information systems of a hospital in such a way obeying unifying theory of information systems, yet still retaining original characteristics of all data elements (the "Salad Bowl") (Ma, 2015). Therefore, with ever increasing volume of data, it is almost impossible to explore them without appropriate data visualisation.

Standard reports are available in most revenue processing software. Basic reports are those reports showing cost and revenue of a particular measure without any calculation and include 'mean revenue' by DRG, by financial class and by funding. The advanced reports include calculations of descriptive statistics such as mean profitability by DRG, admission type, patient type, funding and referral source, and by consultant clinician. Summary reports are intended for executives to demonstrate the contribution margin in a form of 'S-curve' by showing 'winners' and 'losers' by clinical departments (Turney, 2008).

Clinically-relevant reports would demonstrate areas where clinical improvements could be initiated from the quality of care perspective. The profitability report by any medical complication is an example of clinician-friendly reports, such as Classification of Hospital Acquired Diagnoses (CHADx) by clinical team or department (T. Jackson, Nghiem, Rowell, Jorm, & Wakefield, 2011). These clinically-driven cost/revenue reports for CHADx are aligned with the overarching policy of integrating quality and safety into hospital funding and reduction of avoidable readmission rates in Victoria (Victorian Department of Health, 2017a).

For example, the funding gap with and without CHADx for the delirium was AUD11, 698 versus AUD2, 318 (5 times increase in the loss). The costs of hip replacement with and without CHADx were AUD25, 397 versus AUD21, 930 ($p < 0.05$).

The CHADx was developed by researchers at the Australian Centre for Economic Research on Health at the University of Queensland. The Australian Commission on Safety and Quality in Health Care reviews it regularly, and the latest review was in 2017. The latest version has 17 categories by mapping to ICD-10 Australian Modification Tenth Edition.

The CHADx is the most detailed classification of hospital-acquired conditions based on the "Condition Present on Admission" as a quality tool within hospitals (T. J. Jackson, Michel, Roberts, Jorm, & Wakefield, 2009). The CHADx, therefore, provides an avenue to monitor harm events regularly and highlights specific areas for care quality improvement, such as urinary tract infection and catheter management of spinal cord injuries. One of the Victorian hospitals reports that the prefix "C" or the condition with onset during the episode of admitted patient care is 97.7% agreement between the hospital and auditor (J. Massa, personal communication, January 25, 2016). The CHADx could be used in a similar way to the 3M Potentially Preventable Complications (PPC) Grouping, especially with the implementation of risk adjustments.

Usual CHADx reports include discharges with CHADx by specialty and the mean cost time series with or without CHADx. Clinical reports require some forms of risk adjustment such as age or the Charlson comorbidity index and readmission indicators to be meaningful for clinician scientists (D'Hoore, Bouckaert, & Tilquin, 1996; Huber, Schneeweiss, Signorell, & Reich, 2013; Schneeweiss & Maclure, 2000). Clinical reviews of the CHADx are sometimes required to verify the included hospital-acquired conditions on whether they are natural course of the disease or 'reducible' rather than preventable. Clinical costers need to work with clinical coders and developers of CHADx for expanding its usefulness.

Clinician scientists could aggregate the appropriate measures at the service line level to see whether a diagnostic test or blood transfusion is absolutely necessary according to the established clinical guidelines. For example, in Subacute Combined Degeneration of the Spinal Cord with a haemoglobin level of 6 g/L, we would avoid transfusing packed cells before vitamin B12 replacement as this may irreversibly exacerbate the neurological manifestations, and the blood transfusion in this case could precipitate incipient heart failure and death (Baliga, 2012, p. 285). "Choosing Wisely Australia" runs a series of conversation about unnecessary tests, treatments and procedures, and the cost and revenue dataset could provide cost-effectiveness analyses on these conversations.

Reports on a specific therapeutic modality could also be insightful for choosing a value-based treatment plan (quality care at lowest unit cost), for example, 'zero' length of stay for the endoscopic removal of large colorectal polyps in comparison to 8 days with surgical approach ($2, 152 for colonoscopy versus $15, 264 for surgery) (Church & Erkan, 2016).

In summary, the cost and revenue dataset with clinically-relevant information is one of the best tools for clinician participation in clinical costing to improve patient care, clinically and financially, under the activity-based funding environment. The cost and revenue dataset at clinical service levels is capable of guiding clinicians to choose the maximum quality care, yet cost-effective and efficient, at minimum cost.

SOLUTIONS AND RECOMMENDATIONS

As mentioned before, clinical costers have a strong aversion to talking about revenue, because the clinical costing tries to prevent revenue information from influencing on costing, and the funding authorities usually exclude revenue data collection and submission. However, the demand for the revenue dataset has been growing in the activity-based funding environment to investigate the profitability of clinical services and their contribution margins. According to C. Fan (personal communication, July 11, 2017), it would be difficult to interpret the 'true cost' of care without the revenue component since, in theory, it is the expense and revenue, particularly for private patients, and also provides better clarity over the cost of providing clinical service, because some income is received as a negative expense and others as revenue. If the revenue and costing datasets are interpreted together then service managers and clinicians would get a better picture of their clinical service performance.

The marginal benefit of processing revenue, as mentioned before, seems to exceed the marginal cost of investing in it. Clinical costing teams are expected to provide a series of timely and interactive reports on clinical costing and revenue information at summary and detailed levels. These time series reports could provide internal benchmarking and comparison analyses on key performance indicators.

The CHADx cost and revenue by month could provide a measure of the impact on patient outcomes locally to monitor clinical improvement processes. Clinician participation in revenue and cost allocations would provide a thorough understanding of clinical services and their impact on patient safety and quality of care. Clinical engagement could be a platform for sustainability of clinical costing.

The revenue datasets on private practice fees usually indicate the area of poor financial performance where revenue recovery efforts are to be strengthened when the discrepancy is found between the cost and revenue in patient billing accounts. For example, the Hospital A discovered in 2017 that AUD300, 000 worth of private patient bill was pending after the analysis on the cost and revenue of a 2015 patient with the financial class of Traffic Accident Commission.

The main focus of revenue processing should be providing actionable insights on value-based care which confers quality care at minimum unit cost. Fancy infographics and plots could never replace the role of clinical improvement work on the ground. Only 'real' clinical improvements can confer tangible financial performance.

FUTURE RESEARCH

Researchers could investigate the utilisation rate (the capacity cost rate) (Ma, 2015, p. 192) in relation to clinical outcomes, and the areas of application and practice of cost and revenue datasets in terms of clinical improvements. The barriers (human or material resources) to process cost and revenue datasets need urgent attention for building a comprehensive research data warehouse. The major focus on private patient cost and revenue would be a priority.

Future research could investigate ways to link cost and revenue data with the electronic health record systems and clinical research data warehouses to deliver cost/revenue-conscious health systems (Clinical Data Linkage). Investigations of ways to analyse the clinical value relative to cost and revenue in a complex cost-revenue-outcome relationship need urgent attention to provide 'actionable insights' for improving patient satisfaction.

Future research could focus on "how to improve revenue allocations in healthcare effectively and efficiently" by studying gaps in access to software, cost and quality between healthcare services in different countries based on their budget profiles. For example, researchers need to find answers for why the cost and revenue datasets are always up to date for supporting hospital-wide clinical improvement projects in some hospitals whereas the dataset is always months behind the current operational period in many hospitals. In this way, healthcare researchers would be able to assess the success of innovative healthcare solutions and nurture a supportive environment for these international experiences and innovations to scale locally.

Researchers could also focus on the expansion of 'data science' applications in the area of cost and revenue databases for obtaining best value out of every healthcare dollar (value-based healthcare) and formulating mechanism of action.

The funding of ED admitted episodes needs further investigation on how various ED funding and care delivery models have an impact on their safety, clinical and cost effectiveness.

CONCLUSION

The revenue allocation on the clinical costing dataset completes the life cycle of clinical costing spanning from counting to funding. It improves the quality of costing data, and expands the spectrum of clinically-relevant analyses, which make a valid comparison among cost, revenue and patient outcomes. The revenue allocation is an art, and not a science. It can mislead into wrong performance management decisions if it fails to configure and audit carefully (the Rule of Two). Health services operating under activity-based funding environments require properly configured clinical costing and revenue datasets to drive efficiency. The goal is aimed at achieving sustainable financing of healthcare by utilising the cost and revenue dataset. Local hospital performance could also be measured with this dataset.

Every resource decision is clinical decision that involves cost and revenue. A reporting tool for this dataset is needed to answer fresh business questions for resource decisions linked to patient outcomes, such as contribution margins and profit/loss reports. However, there are obligations to the community by not stopping or reducing the level of service despite of having unprofitable, yet important, clinical services. The revenue dataset with the clinical costing data could close the gap between actionable insights and business goals.

If a health service would like to pursue a proper revenue allocation then it would need to invest a dedicated resource to achieve a favourable revenue dataset. The cost-benefit principle is able to guide the revenue process investment decision on whether the marginal benefit of doing revenue allocation exceeds its marginal cost based on measurable business values. And start, for once, to think about revenue allocations.

REFERENCES

Agarwal, E., Ferguson, M., Banks, M., Bauer, J., Capra, S., & Isenring, E. (2015). Malnutrition coding shortfalls in Australian and New Zealand hospitals. *Nutrition & Dietetics: the Journal of the Dietitians Association of Australia, 72*(1), 69–73. doi:10.1111/1747-0080.12116

Baliga, R. R. (2012). *250 Cases in Clinical Medicine E-Book* (4th ed.). Elsevier Health Sciences.

Church, J., & Erkan, A. (2016, August 3). Scope or scalpel? A matched study of the treatment of large colorectal polyps. *ANZ Journal of Surgery*.

D'Hoore, W., Bouckaert, A., & Tilquin, C. (1996). Practical considerations on the use of the Charlson comorbidity index with administrative data bases. *Journal of Clinical Epidemiology*, *49*(12), 1429–1433. doi:10.1016/S0895-4356(96)00271-5 PMID:8991959

Horan, P. (2018, April 4). [Revenue dataset].

Huber, C. A., Schneeweiss, S., Signorell, A., & Reich, O. (2013). Improved prediction of medical expenditures and health care utilization using an updated chronic disease score and claims data. *Journal of Clinical Epidemiology*, *66*(10), 1118–1127. doi:10.1016/j.jclinepi.2013.04.011 PMID:23845184

Jackson, T., Nghiem, H. S., Rowell, D., Jorm, C., & Wakefield, J. (2011). Marginal costs of hospital-acquired conditions: Information for priority-setting for patient safety programmes and research. *Journal of Health Services Research & Policy*, *16*(3), 141–146. doi:10.1258/jhsrp.2010.010050 PMID:21719478

Jackson, T. J., Michel, J. L., Roberts, R. F., Jorm, C. M., & Wakefield, J. G. (2009). A classification of hospital-acquired diagnoses for use with routine hospital data. *The Medical Journal of Australia*, *191*(10), 544. PMID:19912086

Ma, R. (2015). *From the margins to the mainstream: Clinical costing for clinical improvement*. Melbourne, Australia: IGI Global.

Morton, A., & Cornwell, J. (2009). What's the difference between a hospital and a bottling factory? *BMJ: British Medical Journal (Online), 339*.

Pandit, J., Pandit, M., & Reynard, J. (2010). Understanding waiting lists as the matching of surgical capacity to demand: Are we wasting enough surgical time? *Anaesthesia*, *65*(6), 625–640. doi:10.1111/j.1365-2044.2010.06278.x PMID:20565395

Ryan, D. J., O'Regan, N. A., Caoimh, R. Ó., Clare, J., O'Connor, M., Leonard, M., ... Trzepacz, P. T. (2013). Delirium in an adult acute hospital population: Predictors, prevalence and detection. *BMJ Open*, *3*(1), e001772. doi:10.1136/bmjopen-2012-001772 PMID:23299110

Schneeweiss, S., & Maclure, M. (2000). Use of comorbidity scores for control of confounding in studies using administrative databases. *International Journal of Epidemiology*, *29*(5), 891–898. doi:10.1093/ije/29.5.891 PMID:11034974

The Independent Hospital Pricing Authority. (2014). *The Australian Hospital Patient Costing Standards, version 3.1*. Sydney, Australia: The Independent Hospital Pricing Authority.

The Victorian Government. (2016). *Department of Health and Human Services policy and funding guidelines 2016*. Melbourne, Australia: The Victorian Government.

Turney, P. (2008). *Activity-based costing: An emerging foundation for performance management*. Cary, NC: SAS Institute Inc.

Victorian Department of Health. (2017a). *Department of Health and Human Services policy and funding guidelines 2017*. Melbourne: Department of Health and Human Services.

Victorian Department of Health. (2017b). *Victorian Admitted Episodes Dataset (VAED) manual*. Melbourne: Department of Health and Human Services.

Webb, P., & Bain, C. (2011). *Essential epidemiology: An introduction for students and health professionals* (2nd ed.). Cambridge, UK: Cambridge University Press.

KEY TERMS AND DEFINITIONS

Actionable Insights: Data analytics provide sufficient information into the future for decision makers to act upon.

Allocation Statistic: It is a measure of weighting system for distributing revenue to a specific cohort of patients.

Clinical Coster: Clinical costers are specialists responsible for end-to-end clinical costing data management.

Clinical Costing: A discipline which studies the cost of resources used to deliver patient care.

Clinical Data Linkage: It is a statistical tool which allows linking of different datasets kept in different locations that relate to the same individual.

Cost-Benefit Principle: The level of an activity should only be increased if its marginal benefit exceeds its marginal cost.

Patient Qualifiers: The patient who is entitled to receive a specific revenue stream.

Revenue Allocation: It is an allocation of revenue amount in clinical costing by distributing total revenue streams down to the patient level based on appropriate allocation rules in a health service operating under activity-based funding.

Value-Based Healthcare: It is the healthcare conferring a patient-centered, clinical benefit at lowest unit cost.

Chapter 3
Applying Business Intelligence and Analytics to Clinical Costing Data

Martin Hugo Rennhackkamp
PBT Australia, Australia

Graeme Hart
Austin Health, Australia

ABSTRACT

Most healthcare organizations would like to provide actionable information to the managers of their various service lines. Bringing administrative, clinical, and financial data together is critical to operating the service lines efficiently. It also presents a strategic advantage, as the applications of funding are more closely monitored, and regulatory reporting requirements increase. With a clearer picture of their financial and clinical performance together, organizations are better prepared to put efficient strategies in place to meet their goals and demonstrate value. However, that requires thorough planning and forward-thinking leadership. This chapter discusses approaches to how organizations can empower their stakeholders by providing them with integrated clinical and costing data. It addresses how business intelligence supports the management and reporting of clinical costing data, the utilization of data visualization and advanced analytics, the importance of data governance, and the role of a BI strategy, illustrated throughout with a case study.

DOI: 10.4018/978-1-5225-5082-2.ch003

INTRODUCTION

In the field of information management, the discipline of business intelligence, in its broadest sense, is about transforming the transactional data of an organisation, and providing suitable information to the decision makers and other interested stakeholders in the organisation. Among hospitals and other healthcare providers, clinical costing data forms a key part of the data that requires conversion to useful information for decision makers on various levels of the organisation.

The objectives of this chapter are to illustrate how the following concepts are related to and utilised in the reporting and analysis of clinical costing data:

- Business intelligence.
- Data warehousing.
- Reports and dashboards.
- Data visualization.
- Applied analytics.
- Business-intelligence strategy.
- Data governance.

BACKGROUND

A Data-Oriented View of Clinical Costing

From the point of view of data, clinical costing lies at the intersection of the following subject areas:

- Patients (inpatients or outpatients)
- Services provided
- Providers (e.g., clinicians, nurses, radiologists) of these services
- Resources utilised (e.g., wards, beds, theatres, equipment)
- Consumables used (e.g., medications, bandages, food and beverage)
- Costs associated with:
    - Each aspect
    - Each episode
    - Each ward (or unit)
    - Each hospital

Complicating this further is the fact that each patient receives a unique "bundle" of services for each episode of care, paid for as a collective in some cases—especially when private health insurers pay for it. However, the cost of each separate component must be included and analysed, in order to enable:

- Determining profitability and/or sustainability.
- Classifying diagnoses, episodes of care, and treatment options into identifiable classes.
- Determining efficient pricing.
- Determining and comparing cost weights.
- Informing product and service development of funding models and budget proposals.
- Analysing the cost of healthcare—overall, and by patient or type of diagnosis.
- Benchmarking costs for comparable activity across hospitals.
- Comparing against other healthcare providers providing similar services.
- Informing decision makers of best-practice and quality-improvement initiatives.
- Informing planning of clinical services within a hospital.
- Informing decision makers of resource utilisation.
- Effecting clinical-practice improvement in a hospital.

Clinical costing is also a key building block of activity-based funding (ABF). This discipline entails studying the cost and mix of resources used to deliver patient care. Costing informs the development of classification systems and provides valuable information for pricing purposes. Hospital patient costing is essential for understanding the total cost of treating a patient, including costs for services or products. For example, Victorian public hospitals are required to report costs for all funded operational activity and expected to maintain activity and costing systems as part of good management practice (Victoria Health, 2017).

While many other industries are quite established in using data-driven methodologies to perform and manage cost accounting, healthcare has been lagging far behind. Whether due to high costs, change-management challenges, low priority, or other reasons, hospitals and health systems have put off revising and upgrading the decades-old methodologies they use. In this "old world", data analysts have to manually collect data from different systems – like patient administration and accounting systems, manually collect and integrate it – typically in spread sheets, and then do their clinical costing reporting and analysis on these uncontrolled copies of crucial data. This approach is not only labour-intensive, but it is also error-prone, hard to trace and repeat and it often introduces inconsistencies between various versions of the truth, depending on who's spread sheet gets utilised and when they created it. Executives end up debating for hours which calculations are correct and which indicators to trust and use.

In today's environment of growing amounts of data and clinical electronic medical record (EMR) systems, the old methods and cost-accounting systems do not use the richness and depth of data available to provide an accurate view of costs. The move toward electronic health records, tracking of quality measures, and data collection has come to the forefront, and will only increase. This shift provides a wealth of information that previously was very hard to obtain in an easy-to-understand and analysable format. Between regulatory requirements and a changing reimbursement structure, both hospitals and health systems must adapt in order to compete.

Improving cost accounting within hospitals is no longer a "nice to have" item; it has become a critical component of meeting the increasing pressures of cost containment, changes in reimbursement practices and rates, and greater patient awareness of the cost of services across various providers.

Clinical costing can be calculated bottom-up (e.g., at the patient level) or top-down (e.g., using costing modelling):

- Patient-level costing allocates costs directly to individual patient episodes, using service volumes such as actual tests or minutes in theatre. This achieves more accurate cost allocation at an individual patient level.
- Cost modelling allocates similar costs to all patient episodes, using formulas and assumptions in the absence of detailed patient records.

However, both forms of clinical cost calculation require a number of data items to which the calculation is applied such as patient, episode, ward, procedure, and clinician (or other provider). At the state level, data items such as hospital, facility, region, and state augment these data items. These entities already give an indication of the dimensions for analysing the clinical costing data.

CASE STUDY

Throughout this chapter we present a case study of a public hospital in Australia that used clinical costing data to determine and validate outcomes, and to present the results of predicting 30-day "all-cause" unplanned hospital readmissions (Rennhackkamp & Hart, 2016).

The case study shows how clinical costing data can communicate the impact of correctly predicting unplanned readmissions; and how this clinical data is recorded, incorporated, and reported through data-visualisation capability.

The objectives of the hospital were to:

- Identify the most likely patient groups for 30-day unplanned readmissions;
- Identify the drivers of 30-day unplanned hospital readmission;
- Redesign the admission, treatment, and discharge-planning processes; and
- Predict the impact of avoidable bed-days on costs, throughput, and waiting lists.

The outcome was a validated analytical model that predicts the likelihood of an unplanned hospital readmission occurring within 30 days after a given in-patient episode. An "all-cause" model does not pay attention to any specific disease or diagnosis groups.

The predicted likelihood of unplanned readmission can assist care workers and clinicians in planning treatment and discharge processes. In fact, as the project ran its course, the clinicians involved realized that knowledge of the likelihood of unplanned readmission could also assist in planning admission and triage processes, as well as ward and clinician assignment.

BUSINESS INTELLIGENCE

There is no single definition of the concept of business intelligence (BI). Business leaders, key BI practitioners and specialists, tool suppliers, and academicians have provided various definitions over the years. In this chapter, the definition of business intelligence refers to the concept in its broadest sense.

Business Intelligence (BI) consists of the set of strategies, processes, applications, data, products, technologies, and technical architectures used to support the collection, analysis, presentation, and dissemination of business information (Dedić & Stanier, 2016). Broadly interpreted, BI technologies provide historical, current, and predictive views of the information, which represent the organisation's operations.

Various functions are incorporated under the umbrella of business-intelligence technology, including data warehousing, reporting, online analytical processing, analytics, data mining, process mining, complex-event processing, business performance management, benchmarking, text mining, and predictive and prescriptive analytics. These are typically capable of handling large amounts of structured and sometimes unstructured data, to not only report the current state of the business and some longer-term trends, but also provide information and insights derived from this information that can assist the organisation to identify, develop, and create new strategic business opportunities. Identifying new opportunities and implementing an effective strategy based on such insights can provide businesses with competitive advantage. Tracking current performance against benchmark or target figures can lead to longer-term stability (Rud, 2009). However, the overall goal of BI is to turn data into information, and to allow for easy interpretation of this information, regardless of whether the underlying data is small or big, structured or unstructured, simple or complex.

Business intelligence is typically used to support a wide range of business decisions ranging from operational to strategic. Basic operating decisions include ward or theatre occupation, staff assignment, equipment utilisation, clinician efficiency, and related functions. Strategic business decisions include priorities, goals, and directions at the broadest level, such as theatre or ward re-appropriation, new discharge protocols, new criteria for hospital-in-the-home admissions, and different provider engagement profiles. In all cases, BI is most effective when it combines data derived from the industry in which an organisation operates (external data) with data from systems and sources internal to the organisation, such as clinical, administrative, financial, and operational data (internal data). When combined, external and internal data can provide a more complete picture, effectively creating "intelligence" that no singular set of data could yield (Rud, 2009).

Among their myriad uses, business intelligence tools empower organisations to gain insight into new markets, assess demand and suitability of products and services for different market segments, and gauge the impact of optimisation efforts (Coker, 2014).

In most cases, in order to achieve these objectives, the clinical costing data must be found, obtained, filtered, collected, and transformed into a format that is convenient for various stakeholders. This entails extracting the data, copying it into a work area, often integrating it with other data such as administrative data and quality indicators, and then presenting it in some communicable format, such as in a report, dashboard, or presentation.

However, in organisations that have not yet reached a sufficient state of maturity with respect to their BI and analytics capabilities, finance or costing department staff scrapes together this information, using spreadsheets and other informal means of data collection and reporting. The problem with this approach is that clinical costing staff performing all this work using desktop software translates into a great deal of repetitive and manual effort that is not only prone to error—the staff members involved in these activities spend more time looking for, wrangling, and massaging the data than they spend actually reporting and analysing it.

In a best-practice approach, BI teams using BI tools and solutions should collect, manage, and report much of the clinical, administrative, and costing data, especially since these tools and solutions can automate performing and managing integration across business applications on a more permanent and efficient basis.

BI AND CLINICAL COSTING

At the intersection of clinical costing and business intelligence is a person with a clinical costing background, who is at once a business analyst, a data analyst, and a broad-spectrum BI practitioner. As an example, the following job description recently appeared on the New South Wales Department of Health's website for a "Clinical Costing and Reporting Analyst" for the Sydney Children's Hospital network (NSW Health, 2017):

Purpose of Position

The Clinical Costing and Reporting Analyst has a primarily responsibility for the implementation, refinement and maintenance of clinical costing systems in SCHN. This position is to assist in development of clinical costing methodology including translation of NSW Health Cost Accounting Guidelines into performance based information, development and implementation of an activity based funding; participation in costing data collection and the provision of ad hoc report to meet the organisation's changing priorities. The Clinical Costing and Reporting Analyst is responsible for the completion of the NSW District and Network return (DNR) within the specified deadlines. Prepare and analyse ad hoc and standard costing reports for internal and external stakeholders. This position will report directly to the SCHN Costing & Analysis Manager.

Requirements

1. A degree in Information Management, Finance or Technology or relevant field; or equivalent work experience; or a combination of study and work experience.
2. Demonstrated sound knowledge of clinical costing methodology, standards and principles.
3. Understanding of the concepts of Activity Based Funding, its relationship to costing and knowledge of clinical information data processes including classification systems. Experience with the Health Information Exchange and Power Performance Management (PPM) systems.
4. Highly developed analytical and numerical skills, with the ability to interpret complex information and communicate it to clinical and non-clinical stakeholders. Advanced skills in manipulating and analyse large amounts of data including Microsoft Excel, Access, Business Objects and other reporting tools.
5. Demonstrated experience in assessing information requirements, data analysis techniques and provision of high quality reports that support a performance management framework.
6. Excellent interpersonal skills and a demonstrated ability to communicate with stakeholders at all levels including senior executive and clinicians, and demonstrated capacity to operate as an effective team member.
7. Proven ability to work with minimal supervision and as a team member and in a multi-disciplinary team.
8. Experience in managing data quality and initiating quality improvement practices to ensure data integrity.

Job Functions

- *Clinical Costing:*
    - *Implement programs and procedures to improve costing information capture, flow and analysis of data. Implementation and development of clinical costing systems in line with NSW Health Costing Standards across the Network.*
    - *Responsible for improving costing methodology within the SCHN.*
    - *Collation of SCHN data files for upload into the clinical costing system. This involves the extraction, upload and maintenance of patient data within agreed timeframes.*
    - *Design and analyse performance outcomes in order to support effective management and improvement of services and health outcomes.*

    - *Dissemination and education of staff relating to costing data emanating from the state-wide clinical costing tool.*
    - *Develop and maintain strong effective working relationships and communications with key internal and external stakeholders to facilitate data collection, review, analysis and costing reporting.*
    - *Expand clinical costing to include other feeder systems.*
    - *Lead the provision of advice and expertise to health service executives on costing and case mix issues and be able to consult widely on activity and costing information needs across SCHN.*
- *Analysis and Reporting:*
    - *Provide ad hoc reports including the investigation and analysis of emerging issues to serve the management information requirements of key stakeholders.*
    - *Establish and implement a vision for innovation in the use of analysed information to assist in more effective decision-making and improvements in clinical care.*
    - *Respond to internal and external data requests within requested timeframes.*
    - *Analyse complex data and databases to deliver meaningful information for SCHN. Provision of data to support benchmarking activities, dashboards and business cases using databases and spread sheets.*
    - *Assist in the development of report specifications. Construct technical & user documentation as required.*
    - *Ensure documentation relating to developed reports retains currency and is subject to version control.*
    - *Assist in standard report development to meet the needs of the SCHN.*
    - *Support quality improvement processes for data collections and production to meet current needs and actively manage any risks.*
    - *Assist in the development of Key Performance Indicators to measure performance.*
    - *Other duties as directed by the SCHN Costing & Analysis Unit Manager relevant to/consistent with the award classification.*

This job description illustrates the importance of utilising business intelligence in the reporting and analysis of clinical costing data. The remainder of this chapter addresses how the reporting and analysis of clinical costing data applies and utilises various components and aspects of business intelligence.

DATA WAREHOUSING

Bill Inmon, known as the "father of data warehousing", defined a data warehouse as a subject-oriented, integrated, time-variant, and non-volatile collection of data in support of management's decision-making process (Dyche, 2000). These terms are further explained in context:

- **Subject-Oriented:** A data warehouse can be used to load, store, and analyse the data of one or more specific subject areas. Examples of subject areas in the hospital world are "patients," "episodes," "providers," and "theatres." Each subject area may be defined in terms of a number of entities, reference items, and relationships.
- **Integrated:** A data warehouse integrates data from multiple data sources. For example, administrative data may be obtained from MEDITECH, clinical data from Cerner, financial data from Great Plains, and pharmacy data from Merlin. But in the data warehouse (using a best-practice approach) these various data subject areas are integrated along their corresponding dimensions. "Cost centre" is a data entity that financial data and administrative data have in common, while "Patient" is a common dimension of Patient Administrative System (PAS), quality, and radiology data.
- **Time-Variant:** Historical data is kept in a data warehouse. For example, one can retrieve data from a data warehouse at three months, six months, twelve months, or even older. This contrasts with a transactional system that often keeps only the most recent view of data. A transactional system may hold the most recent address of a patient, whereas the data warehouse holds all the various addresses associated with the patient over time.
- **Non-Volatile:** Data in the data warehouse will not change. So, historical data in a data warehouse should never be altered. The data of most modern data warehouses are stored in a database to achieve this characteristic. Such a database is typically managed by a commercially available database management system (DBMS) such as Oracle, Microsoft SQL Server, IBM DB2, and a few others; or a freely available public database management system such as MySQL.

On a technical level, a data warehouse has many other functional requirements to which it adheres, such as availability, ease of access, security and privacy control, fail-safeness, and backup and recovery. However, this chapter focuses only on the logical storage and processing of the data, and how it is used in the context of clinical costing.

Ralph Kimball provides a more concise definition of a data warehouse—namely, a data warehouse is a copy of transaction data, but specifically structured for query and analysis. However, this simple definition does not convey that Ralph Kimball has been instrumental in specifying, documenting, and training thousands of practitioners on how the data inside the data warehouse should be modelled, structured, stored, and processed. This work includes over 80 concepts and techniques, under the umbrella term "dimensional modelling." Dimensional modelling is a design technique for databases intended to support end-user queries, such as in a data warehouse, oriented around understandability and performance. Dimensional modelling always uses the concepts of facts (e.g., data about measures or KPIs) and dimensions (e.g., data that gives context to the facts). Facts are typically (but not always) numeric values that can be aggregated, while dimensions are groups of hierarchies and descriptors that define the entities to which the facts refer (Kimball & Ross, 2013).

For example, a fact table describing a patient's episode in a dimensional data warehouse will contain measures such as length of stay (LOS) days, direct costs, indirect costs, and other numeric indicators. The dimensions "around" this fact will include data describing entities such as patient, hospital, ward, dates (admission and separation), cost centre, diagnosis, and referring provider. In database terms, the fact table refers to or has referential integrity constraints applicable to the surrounding dimensional tables.

An episode fact table is illustrated in Figure 1.

Note that this is an oversimplification, but it serves to illustrate the relationships between the measurements coupled to an episode (e.g., LOS days, Direct Costs, Indirect Costs), as they relate to the context-providing dimensions (dates, provider, ward, patient, cost centre, and diagnosis). In real life, where many more measurements and descriptive dimensions are associated with an episode, each of the dimension tables will typically have many more descriptive attributes, and quite a number more dimensions will typically be associated with the fact. Actually, the direct and indirect costs may be calculated at a much finer level of detail than by episode, but the two measurements shown may represent a summation of those underlying detailed fact measurements.

An important concept in data warehousing is that of data integration. Although the data may originally be sourced from various transactional systems, in the data warehouse it is structured according to business functional subjects. In essence, each fact table represents a distinct business process, at a particular level of detail, and it may contain data about that business process that has been obtained from a number of transactional systems. The integration is implemented based on the concepts of conformance (Kimball & Ross, 2013).

Figure 1. Example of episode fact table

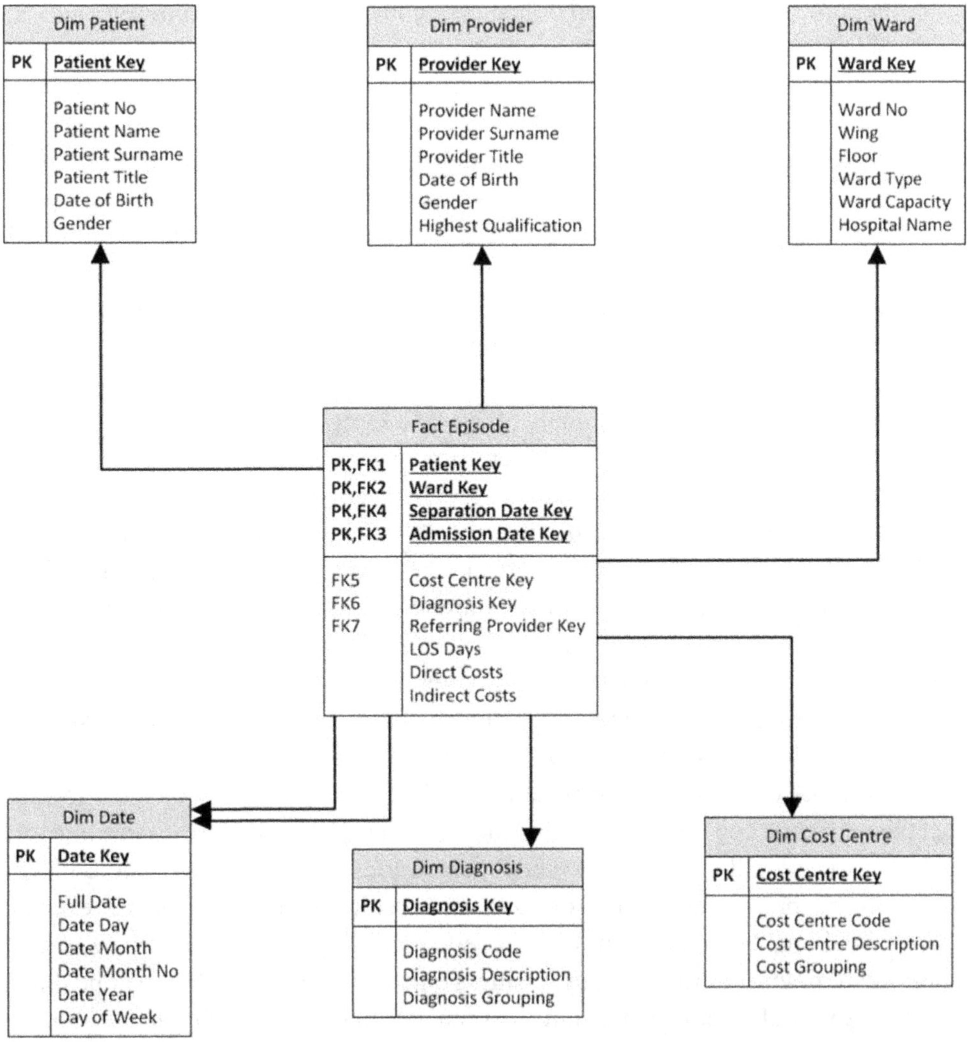

- If the same measurement appears in separate fact tables, care must be taken to make sure the technical definitions of the facts are identical if they are to be compared or computed together. If the separate fact definitions are consistent, the conformed facts should be identically named; but if they are incompatible, they should be differently named to alert the business users and BI applications.

- Dimension tables conform when attributes in separate dimension tables have the same column names and domain contents. Information from separate fact tables can be combined in a single report by using conformed dimension attributes that are associated with each fact table. When a conformed attribute is used as the row header (that is, the grouping column in the SQL query), the results from the separate fact tables can be aligned on the same rows in a drill-across report. This is the essence of integration in an enterprise DW/BI system. Conformed dimensions, defined once in collaboration with the business's data governance representatives, are reused across fact tables; they deliver both analytic consistency and reduce future development costs because the dimension tables are not repeatedly recreated.

As a case in point, in the example above, the Length of Stay days are typically sourced from the PAS, while the direct costs and indirect costs may be sourced from another administrative or financial system. But in the data warehouse, they are integrated in one fact table, because it represents a single business process.

In one form or another, data warehouses have been around for some time. However, the idea of an enterprise data warehouse (EDW) that supports the entire organisation's data needs as a whole is becoming more important in healthcare organisations. An EDW is the physical implementation of a totally integrated data repository along conformed facts and conformed dimensions, for decision-support purposes. A full-fledged mature EDW may contain hundreds of conformed fact tables, and even more conformed dimension tables. There will typically be a conformed fact table for each key business process such as patient admission, ward transfer, and episode of care; and, as illustrated above, operation, separation, consultation; staff appointment, promotion, allocation, transfer; account invoice, payment, reversal; theatre booking, cancellation, refurbishment, cleansing. Likewise, there will be a conformed dimension for each key business entity (e.g., patient, provider, hospital, ward, theatre, staff member, account, cost centre), and one for each standardised list of values, also called lookup codes (e.g., equipment types, provider types, account types, DRG codes, ICD codes, postal codes, state codes). Lookup lists are also considered conformed dimensions.

DATA WAREHOUSING AND CLINICAL COSTING

A hospital's EDW integrates the data from all the various systems, including the clinical cost data. Much more extensive and in-depth analysis—especially to address the data-related objectives of clinical costing listed above—is possible when the clinical costing data is properly integrated with administrative data, human resources and labour data, quality data, and data from allied care such as radiology, pharmacy, pathology, and rehabilitation. Properly implemented in practice, the EDW will become the main source of information for not only the Clinical Costing and Reporting Analyst, but also all other reporting analysts, data analysts, and data modellers working with the organisation's data.

Note, however, that very few healthcare organisations—or any other organisations, for that matter—have fully mature, completely populated, and completely integrated data warehouses. A data warehouse is like a living organism: it must be continuously extended, updated, and changed as the organisation's objectives and operations, and hence its systems and data, change. A data warehouse is always a work in progress; some organisations are just more organised and mature in this progress.

REPORTS AND DASHBOARDS

Business intelligence tools, such as report writers and dashboard-authoring tools, go hand in hand with data warehousing. Once the data is integrated and housed in the (enterprise) data warehouse, these tools are used to productively develop, run, deliver, schedule, and manage reports and dashboards. Note that the report writers and dashboard authoring tools do not require the presence of a data warehouse; they can be configured to report from any data source, including the databases underlying the transactional systems, or even on the data contained in spreadsheets. Most of these tools can also do some form of data integration by combining data from different systems. However, reports are typically better reports, and more consistent and accurate dashboards, when they are run off a structured data source such as an EDW.

A report-writer tool, also called a report generator, is software that allows data from database files to be merged, in the form of graphs or tables, into a document to provide a complete report. It is an application that allows users to create reports by choosing the information to be included, and presenting it in the desired format. Such a program can access a database to obtain data items (data fields) for insertion into charts, graphs, or tabular reports. The report-writer tool usually automates many processes related to developing a report, such as the placement of data items, images, and page headers and footers. Once a report presentation is prepared, subsequent presentations can be automatically generated—for instance, by refreshing the underlying data (Dictionary of Engineering, 2017).

The term dashboard originates from the automobile dashboard that drivers utilise to monitor major functions at a glance, using the instrument cluster located on the vehicle's dashboard. A dashboard provides an at-a-glance view of a collection of related measures, also called key performance indicators (KPIs). Relevant to a particular objective or business process, information is typically in a useful format to conveniently compare the measures to expected or forecasted values (e.g., for episodes, admission, discharge), as described above under fact tables (Alexander & Walkenbach, 2010). The dashboard consolidates and arranges a number of related metrics on a single screen. It may be tailored for a specific role, and display metrics targeted for a single point of view or department. The dashboard-authoring tool provides its user with a specialised set of tools to create custom-designed dashboards.

In effect, "dashboard" is another name for a "progress report" or an "online report." It is often not the content, but the form of display that differentiates a dashboard from a conventional report. To an extent, any dashboard can be printed out as a series of reports. However, the dashboard really starts to provide value when it is presented and utilised as an interactive screen. A user can interact with the dashboard to further investigate the values and ratios, and to perform comparisons to target values. An interactive dashboard often includes more widgets, dials, and graphical elements, some of them active elements with which the user can interact. Often, the dashboard is linked to a database, which allows the report to be constantly updated as the underlying data changes.

For example, a patient dashboard may show the numbers of patients admitted, transferred, or discharged, and these indicators will constantly change as patients move through the systems. Similarly, a human-resources dashboard may show numbers related to staff recruitment, retention, and composition, such as the numbers of permanent staff, temporary staff, unfilled positions, or average days or cost per recruitment initiative (Briggs, 2017).

The business intelligence dashboard is often confused with the performance scorecard. Traditionally, the main difference between the two is that a business-intelligence dashboard is the physical implementation used to display a number of related measures using a dashboard-authoring tool, while a scorecard is the logical grouping of related measures, KPIs, targets, and other related values in a formalised framework. Examples of scorecards are the balanced scorecard (Kaplan & Norton, 1992) and the six-sigma frameworks (Gupta, 2004). Total Quality Management (TQM) is another type of scorecard, often used in quality control (Andersen, Lawrie, & Savic, 2004). A scorecard can be implemented with a BI dashboard tool, using data from an underlying data warehouse. The business users would see it as a particular type of scorecard, implemented using the BI software, while the technical BI developers would see it as a dashboard that contains data relevant to that particular scorecard framework.

Healthcare organisations use business-intelligence tools, such as report writers and dashboard authoring tools, to develop reports, dashboards, and scorecards for reporting various aspects of the organisation, and to track quality indicators across its systems. The value of the information provided, especially at the strategic-management levels in the organisation, increases if the data from various systems are properly integrated in an underlying data warehouse. A data warehouse is not required to develop and implement reports and dashboards, but using one will likely improve the types, value, and quality of information provided.

Financial and clinical costing data form the core contents of many industry-standard scorecard frameworks, such as the balanced scorecard.

An example of a balanced scorecard used in a hospital is shown in Figure 2.

REPORTING AND CLINICAL COSTING

Financial information is an important component of most informational reports produced and used in a hospital. A key part of such financial information is clinical cost data. Reports that relate revenues to costs often include data that comes directly from systems that maintain clinical costing data.

On a hospital's balanced scorecard, a key part of the financial view would include clinical costing data, to illustrate where finances are spent and present the hospital's profitability and financial health, as illustrated in Table 1.

By applying advanced costing methods, a hospital can:

- Directly assign patient-treatment costs as a means to analyse the financial effectiveness of various procedures and service lines;
- Identify physician practice variation:
- Standardise clinical practice patterns; and
- Support more flexible budgeting and payer contracts.

One of the biggest challenges hospitals face, as they seek to improve quality and control costs, is that neither they nor the individual care providers who work with them know how much it really costs to deliver patient care. The reason for this surprising lack of visibility is that costing has historically been based on charges or reimbursement, rather than on the actual cost of providing care. The departmental structure of a hospital does not accurately reflect a patient's journey through the care-delivery system, because a patient being treated for a single condition crosses many departmental and organisational boundaries throughout the continuum. An integrated enterprise data warehouse and enterprise-level reporting system assists in providing information across the entire organisation.

Figure 2. Example hospital balanced scorecard
Source: Chelniciuc, 2013

Clinical/Operations

Metrics	FY2012 Cumulative	FY2011	FY2010	Benchmark	Target
Mortality Index	1.19	0.93	0.92	0.43	<1
Length of Stay	0.89	0.89	0.82	0.97	<0.90
All Readmissions (30 day)	14.01%	15.92%	15.85%	NA	<15%
PCP Communication at Discharge	>80%†	NA	NA	NA	>80%†
Timely Follow Up Appointments	>80%‡	NA	NA	NA	>80%‡
Core Measures Performance: CAP Antibiotic Selection	100%	97%	NA	94%	100%
Hand Hygiene	91%	83%	NA	NA	>85%
Billing and Documentation: H+P Level III	91%	90%	91%	65%	>90%
Patient Satisfaction HCAHPS	77%	NA	NA	80%	>82%*
Direct Cost per Case	$15,565	$15,757	$14,900	NA	NA

Education

Metrics	FY2012 Cumulative	FY2011	FY2010	Benchmark	Target
E-Value Scores-Teaching & Skills	4.66	4.59	4.68	4.66	NA
E-Value Scores-Overall Rating	8.38	8.25	8.3	8.3	NA
E-value Scores-% E-Valuations Completed	81%	NA	NA	NA	100%

Academic

Metrics	CY2012	CY2011	CY2010	CY2009	Benchmark	Target
# of Peer Reviewed Publications (CY)	Pending	66	44	43	44	NA
# of Abstracts Accepted at Meetings (CY)	Pending	33	32	25	32	NA
# of Non-Peer Reviewed Publications (CY)	Pending	19	NA	NA	NA	NA
Total Grant Funding (FY)	$4,494,156	$4,601,119	$4,603,074	NA	$4,601,119	NA

Community & Faculty Development

Metrics	CY2012	CY2011	CY2010	Benchmark	Target
DHM Overall Job Satisfaction Rating	Pending	87%	76%	63%	>80%
Faculty Development Participation	67%	NA	NA	NA	100%

Table 1. Financial perspective of hospital balanced scorecard

BSC Perspectives	Hospital BSC
• Financial Perspective	• Average charges • Length of stay • Daily census • Net operating margin • Positive or negative variance • Net operating margin • No of referrals from outpatient low cost clinic • No of referrals to inpatient

However, this comes with a caveat. A healthcare organisation can have the "best" data warehouse implementation, the "best" data integration across business lines and systems, and enterprise-wide BI and reporting. But if the data is not captured at the right level of detail, then it cannot be allocated to and reported under the appropriate functions, patient journeys, or cost centres.

DATA VISUALISATION

Many disciplines view data visualisation as the modern equivalent of visual communication. It involves the study of the visual representation of data, referring to data that has been abstracted in some graphical or schematic form (Friendly, 2001).

A primary goal of data visualisation is to communicate information clearly and efficiently using statistical graphics, plots, and other relevant information graphics. For example, numerical data may be encoded using dots, lines, or bars, to visually communicate a quantitative message (Few, 2004). An effective visualisation helps business users analyse and debate about the data, using the visual representation as evidence. It makes complex data more accessible, understandable, and usable, reminiscent of the aphorism "a picture is worth a thousand words."

Users may have particular analytical tasks, such as making comparisons or understanding causality. The design principle of the graphic (i.e., showing comparisons or showing causality) enables them to visually perform the task. Users who will look up a specific measurement generally use tables and reports, while charts of various types show patterns or relationships in the data for one or more variables.

Data visualisation is an intersection of the disciplines of art and science (Aparicio & Costa, 2015), viewed by some as a branch of descriptive statistics, but also by others as a grounded theory development tool. Processing, analysing, and communicating information uncovered from a large variety and a large volume of data present a variety of analytical challenges, made easier through applying data visualisation. The field of data visualisation is also considered a subtopic in the field of data science (Press, 2013).

Professor Edward Tufte (1983), a statistician considered one of the "fathers" of data visualisation, explains that users of visual information displays execute particular analytical tasks, such as making comparisons or determining causality, by analysing and comparing visual representations of the data. The design principle of the particular information graphic utilised should support the analytical task, such as showing the comparison or causality.

In his 1983 book, *The Visual Display of Quantitative Information*, Edward Tufte defines graphical displays and discusses the principles required for effective graphical display. He states that an excellent statistical graphic should be able to communicate complex ideas about the data with clarity, precision and efficiency (Tufte, 1983).

Further, according to Tufte, graphical displays should:

- Show the data;
- Induce the viewer to think about the substance (i.e., what the data represents), rather than about methodology, graphic design, the technology of graphic production, or something else;
- Avoid distorting what the data has to say;
- Present many numbers in a small space;
- Make large data sets coherent;
- Encourage the eye to compare different pieces of data;
- Reveal the data at several levels of detail, from a broad overview to the fine structure;
- Serve a reasonably clear purpose: description, exploration, tabulation, or decoration; and
- Be closely integrated with the statistical and verbal descriptions of a data set.

Tufte further states that graphical representations should adequately reveal the data. He postulates that the appropriate graphical representations can be more precise and revealing than conventional statistical computations. The reason is that a statistical measure only represents a single aspect of the data, while an appropriate visual representation may reveal many characteristics of the data at the same time, in a much more understandable format.

In a way, data visualisation technologies are similar to reporting and analysis tools, in that they are used to analyse and report data. The big difference is that using data visualisation tools represents the data in a graphical form.

VISUALISATION AND CLINICAL COSTING

Hospitals use data visualisation technologies to explore clinical and costing data for new insights and trends, and to report these visually. Data visualisations also facilitate storytelling about clinical costing data, and discovering clinical costing patterns.

The example of visualisation shown in Figure 3 illustrates FY2014 data for an Australian hospital. Used as part of an unplanned-readmissions prediction project, it communicates the potential opportunity for "saveable" bed-days and direct (clinical) costs, should interventions on all correctly predicted 30-day unplanned readmissions be successful.

It depicts the top 10 disease categories (by ICD-10 roll-up to three characters) with the most predicted 30-day unplanned readmissions. For this example, all the direct clinical costs related to the correctly predicted unplanned-readmission episodes had to be calculated, and then added per ICD-10 category, and summarised per ICD-10 roll-up.

Figure 3. Predicted potential "saveable" bed-days in 2014
Source: Rennhackkamp & Hart, 2016.

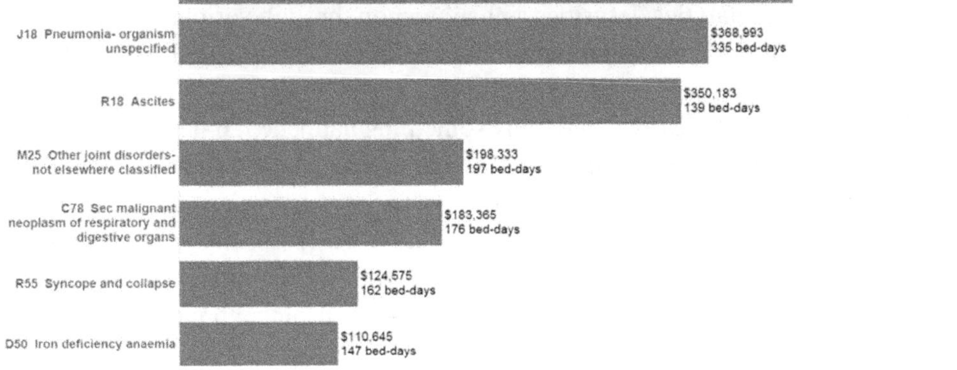

APPLIED ANALYTICS

To analyse is to examine (data) carefully and in detail, to identify causes, key factors, possible results, and trends. The word "analytics" is a very broadly used term, usually defined in practice as any fact-based deliberation that leads to insights and possible implications for planning future action in an organisational context. In general, analytics is the process of analysing data that is done logically, aided by sciences (e.g., statistical, machine learning, artificial intelligence).

Analytics includes any or all of the following:

- Routine tracking and monitoring of business performance;
- "Nice-to-know" validation of facts regarding the business domain;
- Specifically directed diagnosis of "root cause" of business problems; and/or
- Strategic prediction about future business initiatives.

In other words, analytics often incorporates business intelligence.

The commonality across all these processes is that they are driven significantly by facts obtained as a part of data-collection initiatives, where the organisation collects business, marketing, market, publicly available, and other related data, for the purpose of analysis. This makes analytics "rational" by nature.

In the areas of routine monitoring of business performance, there is a large overlap among operational analytics, business performance management, and conventional BI reporting and dashboards.

Applied Analytics, nowadays also popularly called Business Analytics, can be defined as "a set of all the skills, technologies, applications and practices required for continuous iterative exploration and investigation of past business performance to gain insight and drive business planning (Beller & Barnett, 2009).

Depending upon its outcomes, this process can be descriptive, diagnostic, predictive, or prescriptive in nature, as illustrated in Figure 4 (Beller & Barnett, 2009).

- Descriptive analytics describes a phenomenon through various measures that could capture its relevant dimensions. The purpose is to simply unravel what happened, or to alert to what is going to happen.
- Diagnostic analytics evaluates why something happened. It needs exploratory data analysis of the existing data, or additional data if required, using tools such as visualisation techniques to discover the root causes of a problem.
- Predictive analytics seeks options for future business imperatives, predicts potential future outcomes, and explains drivers of the observed phenomena using statistical or data-mining technique—for instance, predicting the sales

of a product for the next month, or the behaviour of a target segment of customers.

- Prescriptive analytics goes beyond describing, explaining, and predicting, to suggest courses of action that may be taken for the future, to optimise business processes in order to achieve business objectives. In other words, it associates decision alternatives with the prediction of outcomes. Prescriptive analytics uses decision analysis that includes tools such as optimisation and simulation.

In a nutshell, business analytics supposedly spans the past, present, and future, to provide more knowledge, better information, and concrete insights. It tends to get more complex and valuable as it moves from descriptive to prescriptive applications.

APPLIED ANALYTICS AND CLINICAL COSTING

Some larger facilities—especially those tied to academic institutions—create clinical data warehouses that clinicians and researchers utilise for advanced and applied analytics projects.

Healthcare organisations apply analytics to a range of functions, from clinical quality reporting to supply chain management. The incorporation of clinical costing data has helped advance this effort, boosting the business case justification and business understanding, especially of the impact of clinical and costing data used for research and analysis. Examples of analytics initiatives are:

Figure 4. Types of analytics
Source: Beller & Barnett, 2009.

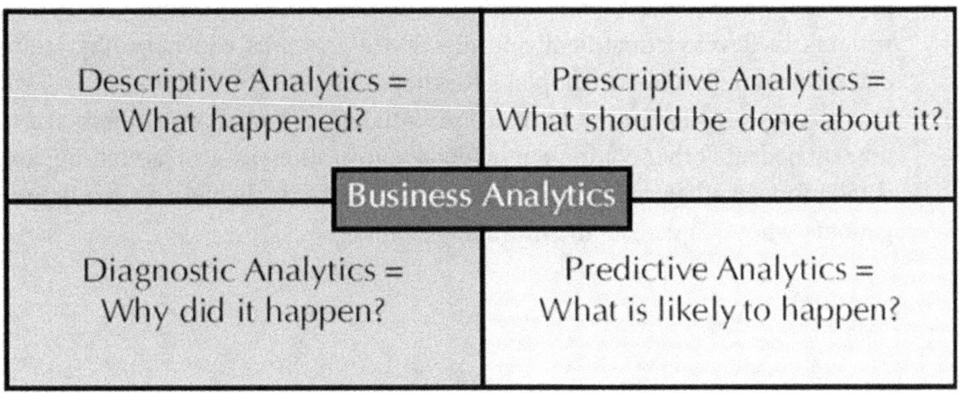

- **Targeting Care to Patient Needs:** By analysing large sets of patient data, caregivers can better understand their needs and predict which patients fall into high-risk categories. Caregivers can also identify gaps in their medical care provision, and adjust their planning and operations accordingly. By incorporating clinical costing data, they can better analyse costs of various treatment options, as well as the business impact of proposed interventions on these cohorts of patients.
- **Reducing Readmissions:** Hospitals may be able to prevent readmitting patients shortly after they have been treated and discharged, or even at the point of primary admission for repeat patients. By incorporating clinical costing data, they can analyse the potential cost and impact of preventative interventions at various points on the patient journey.
- **Streamlining Care for Patients:** From the emergency room to the intensive care unit, prioritising and managing patient needs effectively is essential to keeping costs low and quality high, as well as foreseeing any complications patients could develop once they are admitted. Integrating clinical costing data into the analyses of clinical workflows plays a key role in tracking the business impacts, and in adjusting staff complements, bed availability, and other resources accordingly.
- **Preventing Complications:** The longer patients are in the hospital, the more susceptible they may be to complications such as renal failure, infection, and adverse drug reactions. Though highly preventable, these events are expensive and often result in high rates of morbidity and mortality, leaving providers vulnerable to malpractice suits. Dashboards that incorporate clinical costing data can help managers lower the business impacts of these risks, especially in the ICU.
- **Containing Chronic Conditions**: Chronic health conditions that affect multiple organ systems, such as lupus, rheumatoid arthritis, and other autoimmune disorders, can be challenging and expensive to manage, for both payers and providers. Using health and clinical costing records from these patients to develop treatment optimisation algorithms can help physicians determine efficient treatment plans for these cases.
- **Occupancy and Resource Utilisation:** Analytical models can be utilised to tune up bed and other equipment inventory utilisation, as well as staffing, and it can produce other insights such as how to more quickly and effectively treat patients whose care costs the most.

By using more robust analytics, the organisation can support decision-making in a rapidly changing environment. Applying these principles and using the right information can provide hospitals with valuable data and actionable insights, which they can utilise to get them on the road to long-term financial stability. They will be better able to understand the cost of the full continuum of care, and better apply reimbursement mechanisms such as value-based purchasing, bundled payments, and shared savings

For example, the graph in Figure 5 illustrates the potential saving on bed-days and direct hospital costs by acting timely on patients predicted to have a high probability of an unplanned readmission within 30 days of discharge.

This graph illustrates that six additional targeted interventions per day will potentially affect 1,132 patients and 2,227 episodes per year. If all were effective, these interventions would have reduced unplanned readmissions of all these episodes, which in turn would lead to opportunity for potentially saving 9,287 bed-days, with direct costs of $9,007,799 in FY2014.

To perform meaningful analytics that can be used to transform a healthcare organisation, a strong reporting system is also necessary. With a transparent view and a single source of truth, the efforts of clinicians, operations, and finance can combine to drive informed decision-making. Such a data-driven methodology will enable:

- Improving the assignment of costs based on the actual drivers of expenses.
- Determining a better understanding of the profitability of departments, patients, and other relevant dimensions (e.g., hospital, physician, service line, specialty, disease).

Figure 5. Potential savings on bed-days and direct hospital costs
Source: Rennhackkamp & Hart, 2016.

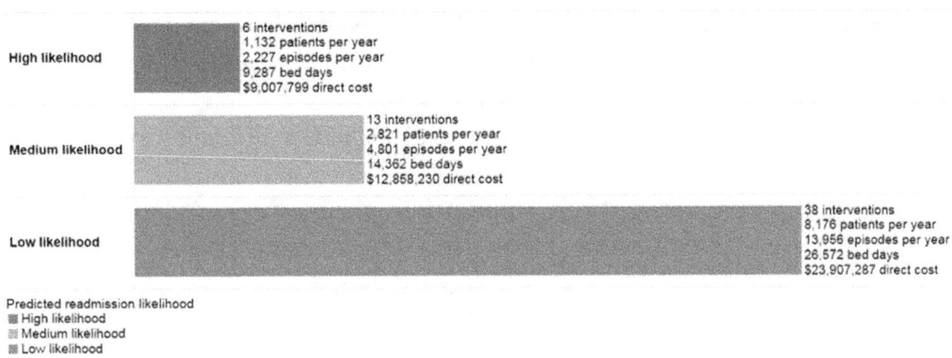

- Generating automated patient and service line profitability data and reports.
- Supporting standardised costing.
- Providing flexible model structure to allow for growth.

OPERATIONALISING ANALYTICS

A key part of implementing analytics in any organisation is to provide the analytical insights in the right format, to the right audience, at the right place:

- **Format:** A score (for example, the likelihood of a patient having an unplanned readmission) can be such a complex figure that it would be meaningless to an untrained individual. However, if that same score is standardised to a percentage, and presented in red, orange, and green to indicate high, medium, and low risk of unplanned readmission, then it makes more sense to most people.
- **Audience:** Providing analytical insights to decision-makers may get a point across, or enable them to make a strategic decision. But enabling day-to-day action on the analytical insights requires providing the analytical outcomes to the line managers, staff, nurses, and clinicians working with the patients on a day-to-day basis. Again, using likelihood for an unplanned readmission as an example, it may assist strategic decision-makers in changing discharge procedures, or post-discharge follow-ups. But it has even more value per individual patient when it is shown to the appropriate staff during admission, triage, and day-to-day treatment of each patient.
- **Locality:** A summary analytical insight has some value on an executive's desk, if he/she is going to use it to make some strategic decision. But a detailed analytical insight has great value if it is displayed right "at the coal face"—at the desk where the patient is admitted, in the ward where the patient is being treated, or even in the theatre where an operation is about to take place.

Technically, analytical outcomes could be displayed in different forms:

- It could be a dashboard-type application when an organisation routinely generates various metrics and uses these data items to monitor a process or various processes across time. All decision support and BI systems fall into this category. This kind of application is used to understand, for example, the financial health of an organisation at a given point of time or to compare it across different points of time. Even in these routine applications, it is important to interpret the numbers and meaningfully connect them, with a good understanding of the underlying processes relevant to decision-making. These are typically "descriptive analytics" applications, used repetitively and routinely in an organisation for its day-to-day monitoring and management of operations.

- The second kind of analytics application is not used routinely, but rather is investigative in nature, and typically used to explore or confirm specific hypotheses. Given a particular business objective, the analysts frame relevant research questions, collect the appropriate data, and analyse it intelligently in order to connect the findings with the business objective. Sometimes during the data collection or analysis, interesting patterns emerge. These applications are useful in understanding the business environment, the customers, or the risks associated with a new product, for making other strategic decisions. As such, this type of analytics is used for forward-looking decision making.

Cost-accounting systems fall short if they cannot provide the required information to enable meaningful analytics on the services provided to a patient, and their fixed and variable costs. With the wealth of data available today, a cost-accounting platform should be able to connect to clinical data sets, such as inpatient/outpatient services provided, physician/nursing time, medications administered, supplies and equipment used, patient room, and ancillary department association (e.g., labs, imaging). It should also link to operational systems and data sets, such as scheduling, patient safety, satisfaction, and quality. But from a clinical costing point of view, the most important data sources are the financial systems and data sets that cover patient accounting, general ledger, payroll system, time and attendance system, and fixed asset system.

BIG DATA ANALYTICS

A special application of analytics is so-called big data analytics, where organisations process many terabytes of data, spread across geographic regions in formats such as texts, photographs, videos, tweets, and blogs. The challenge with big data analytics is to make use of this huge volume and varied sets of data, to derive meaningful insights and drive fact-based decisions for business success. The analytics is largely exploratory and descriptive in nature. Exploratory statistical methods and data mining tools are used to discover meaningful patterns or unknown correlations that could be used for making business decisions.

Newer technologies utilised in healthcare are generating vast amounts of data. This data has to be captured, stored, curated, and analysed continuously, which poses unique challenges for healthcare providers. Large-scale digitisation efforts, the Internet of Things, and each and every new device and new piece of equipment containing a multitude of sensors that generate millions of data points throughout the day compound this problem. Healthcare data is already produced from large variety of sources, such as electronic health records, diagnostics, imaging data, genetic data, clinical records, clinical trials, and adverse-events reporting. Now add sensors, probes, wearable devices, and a massive amount of unstructured text contained in notes, prescriptions, test results, scientific publications, and product schedules. In fact, it is expected that in 2020, worldwide digital healthcare data is expected to reach 25 exabytes (Sowale, 2017). Fortunately, big data technologies can be usefully applied to effectively managing all this data.

Healthcare providers are increasingly utilising big data solutions to transform the way they operate their business, generating new insights from aggregating individual datasets, and analysing these through analytical algorithms harnessing big data. Healthcare providers can also engage big-data prescriptive analytics to simulate high-tech interventions in patient treatment, utilising these simulations to proactively manage and reduce adverse-event occurrences.

For example, if an adverse event occurs, caregivers and analysts together must be able to track the drugs administered, dosage information, subject profile, patient medical history, prior medications, vaccinations, food/nutritional diet provided to the patient, and much more.

Another example of big data analytics is the analysis of medical imaging and radiological data, identifying suitable biomarkers and potentially useful information from treatment purposes through image-pattern identification algorithms.

Big data analytics as such does not affect the utilisation of clinical costing data directly, but the reverse is not the case. An analytics project involving so-called "big data" often uses clinical costing data in conjunction with the "big data," as well as other structured data, to bring the financial view to bear on the analytical insights.

Big data analytics can also enable providers to combine and correlate data from various parts of healthcare spectrum, such as billing, claims, patient history, sentiment data, third-party providers, and pharmaceutical data, to get a 360-degree holistic view of a patient's data. Thus, healthcare providers are increasingly adapting big data analytics to realise improved returns, in terms of better patient care and achieving cost efficiencies (Sowale, 2017).

BUSINESS INTELLIGENCE AND ANALYTICS STRATEGY

Due to the evolving need for more advanced reporting and analysis of healthcare data, especially involving clinical costing data, increasing numbers of healthcare providers now depend on an underlying data warehouse and a good set of reporting and analysis tools.

Developing and implementing a BI platform that empowers clinicians with administrative, costing, and quality data requires an up-front investment. Helping clinicians use costing data to make decisions requires a shared vision and a partnership between finance leaders and physicians. Empowering clinicians with clinical costing data as part of a business intelligence strategy requires collaboration, education, and the right mix of experts.

Getting clinicians to make the most of the costing data requires education and support regarding costing methodologies, and an understanding of what "cost" means. Business intelligence is a new concept for some clinicians, particularly those in not-for-profit health systems, who may get turned off by the "corporate" feel of the term. For this reason, education is vitally important to the success of a BI strategy that places integrated cost and clinical data directly in the hands of physicians.

In addition, the implementation of a BI capability of this size and complexity must be driven through a well-defined and enterprise-wide accepted business intelligence and analytics strategy. Without such a strategy to guide the implementation, a very dysfunctional set of insights may be the undesired end result. The BI and analytics strategy will ensure that:

- The right objectives are achieved.
- The right data is collected, and processed in the correct manner.
- The right data warehouse is implemented correctly.
- The right measures and dimensions are reported.
- The right analytical insights are derived.
- The right information and insights are shared with the right business users, at the right level of detail.

DATA GOVERNANCE

Data governance is defined as a set of processes that ensures that important data assets of the organisation are formally managed throughout the enterprise. Data governance ensures that data can be trusted and that people can be made accountable for any adverse event that happens because of low data quality. Data governance is all about putting people in charge of fixing and preventing issues with data, so that the enterprise can become more efficient (Sarsfield, 2009).

Defining and implementing data governance often entails an evolutionary process for the organisation, changing all stakeholder and staff ways of thinking about data, and setting up the necessary processes to handle data, in a manner that enables the entire organisation to utilise it.

Technology, such as data dictionaries, is utilised when necessary, if it aids the process. When organisations desire, or are required (e.g., by regulation) to gain tighter control of their data, they empower their people, set up processes, and utilise technology to do it (Sarsfield, 2009).

In a way, data governance is a quality-control discipline for assessing, managing, using, improving, monitoring, maintaining, and protecting organisational information. It is a system of decision rights and accountabilities for information-related processes, executed according to agreed-upon models that describe who can take what actions, with what information, and when, under what circumstances, and using what methods (Thomas, 2013).

DATA GOVERNANCE AND CLINICAL COSTING

The financial systems of a hospital can collect many different "buckets" of finance data. The most important areas include labour, direct hospital, and supply costs. Although highly useful to financial managers, these cost components can sometimes overwhelm clinicians if they are not well defined and described. Thus, it is critical to determine exactly which financial information is pulled from the costing system, at what level of detail, and how it is integrated into the BI and analytics solutions for clinicians to access and assess. This action of determining which information is required, and defining it and naming it exactly, falls under the purview of data governance.

Before integrating data from different sources, the BI and finance teams also must determine how they will define certain aggregate data points. For example, strong data governance is required to ensure that everyone is using the same cost data definitions, before the technical experts begin building models and tools.

CONCLUSION

The distinction between clinical data and financial data is becoming blurred, in terms of how data can affect the bottom line. Hospital administrators are increasingly in need of insights on which they can act to improve both business outcomes and clinical outcomes.

Accurate costing has been a missing component of the decision-making process for many healthcare organisations. The future success of healthcare providers and health systems hinges on moving away from traditional cost-accounting methods, using the right systems, and taking advantage of the expanded amount of data now available to make informed decisions. As cost pressures grow, healthcare organisations will need the ability to use BI and analytics to understand which areas of the organisation are profitable, and which are not. Along with the need to cut costs, there is growing expectation of improving quality and managing population health. Without better cost accounting, and improved information and insights about its application, moving to assessment of services and making smart choices about growth strategy is not possible.

REFERENCES

Alexander, M., & Walkenbach, J. (2010). *Excel dashboards and reports*. New York, NY: Wiley. doi:10.1002/9781118257500

Andersen, H. V., Lawrie, G., & Savic, N. (2004). Effective quality management through third-generation balanced scorecard. *International Journal of Productivity and Performance Management*, *53*(7), 634–645. doi:10.1108/17410400410561259

Aparicio, M., & Costa, C. (2015). Data visualization. *Communication Design Quarterly Review*, *3*(1), 7–11. doi:10.1145/2721882.2721883

Beller, M. J., & Barnett, A. (2009). *Next generation business analytics*. Retrieved May 9, 2017 from https://www.slideshare.net/LightshipPartners/next-generation-business-analytics-presentation

Briggs, J. (2017). *Management reports & dashboard best practice*. Retrieved May 8, 2017 from https://www.targetdashboard.com/site/Dashboard-Best-Practice/Management-Report-and-Dashboard-best-practice-index.aspx

Chelniciuc, A. (2013). *Adapting the balanced scorecard for an academic hospitalist group*. Retrieved May 8, 2017 from http://www.performancemagazine.org/adapting-the-balanced-scorecard-for-an-academic-hospitalist-group/

Coker, F. (2014). *Pulse: Understanding the vital signs of your business*. Bellevue, WA: Ambient Light Publishing.

Dedić, N., & Stanier, C. (2016). Measuring the Success of Changes to Existing Business Intelligence Solutions to Improve Business Intelligence Reporting. *Research and Practical Issues of Enterprise Information Systems: 10th IFIP WG 8.9 Working Conference, CONFENIS 2016, Proceedings*, *10*, 225–236.

Dictionary of Engineering. (2017). *Report generator*. Retrieved May 8, 2017 from http://www.dictionaryofengineering.com/definition/report-generator.html

Dyche, J. (2000). *E-data: Turning data into information with data warehousing*. Reading, MA: Addison-Wesley.

Few, S. (2004). *Eenie, meenie, minie, moe: Selecting the right graph for your message*. Retrieved May 8, 2017 from http://www.perceptualedge.com/articles/ie/the_right_graph.pdf

Friendly, M. (2001). *Gallery of Data Visualization*. Retrieved May 8, 2017 from http://www.datavis.ca/gallery/

Gupta, P. (2004). *Six sigma business scorecard: Ensuring performance for profit.* New York, NY: McGraw-Hill Professional.

Health, N. S. W. (2017). *Clinical Costing and Reporting Analyst.* Retrieved May 8, 2017 from https://nswhealth.erecruit.com.au/ViewPosition.aspx?id=228072

Kaplan, R. S., & Norton, D. P. (1992). The balanced scorecard—Measures that drive performance. *Harvard Business Review, 83*(7), 71–79. PMID:10119714

Kimball, R., & Ross, M. (2013). *The data warehouse toolkit: The definitive guide to dimensional modeling* (3rd ed.). New York, NY: Wiley.

Press, G. (2013). *A very short history of data science.* Retrieved May 8, 2017 from https://www.forbes.com/sites/gilpress/2013/05/28/a-very-short-history-of-data-science/#6bea3ea555cf

Rennhackkamp, M. H., & Hart, G. (2016). Predicting unplanned hospital readmissions. *Proceedings of the Scientific Stream at the Health Data Analytics Conference.* Retrieved May 1, 2017 from http://ceur-ws.org/Vol-1683/

Rud, O. (2009). *Business intelligence success factors: Tools for aligning your business in the global economy.* Hoboken, NJ: Wiley & Sons.

Sarsfield, S. (2009). *The data governance imperative.* Ely, UK: IT Governance Publishing.

Sowale, Y. (2017). Effectively using big data in healthcare. *Information Management.* Retrieved May 1, 2017 from https://www.information-management.com/opinion/effectively-using-big-data-in-healthcare

Thomas, G. (2013). *The DGI data governance framework.* Retrieved May 1, 2017 from http://www.datagovernance.com/wp-content/uploads/2014/11/dgi_framework.pdf

Tufte, E. (1983). *The visual display of quantitative information.* Cheshire, CT: Graphics Press.

Victoria Health. (2017). *Clinical costing and activity based funding.* Retrieved May 8, 2017 from https://www2.health.vic.gov.au/hospitals-and-health-services/funding-performance-accountability/activity-based-funding/clinical-costing

KEY TERMS AND DEFINITIONS

Analytics: The process of analyzing data that is done logically aided by sciences.

Business Intelligence: Set of concepts, methods, processes, and systems to gather, integrate, and provide data from multiple sources and present it as information to business users to enable and improve operational, tactical, and strategic business decisions.

Dashboard: Provides an at-a-glance view of a collection of related measures, also called KPIs (key performance indicators), relevant to a particular objective or business process, typically in format that is useful to conveniently compare the measures to expected or forecasted values.

Data Governance: A set of processes that ensure that important data assets of the organization are formally managed throughout the enterprise.

Data Visualization: The study of the visual representation of data.

Data Warehouse: A subject-oriented, integrated, time-variant, and non-volatile collection of data in support of management's decision making.

Report: A document containing information organized in a narrative, graphic, or tabular form.

Chapter 4
Electronic Health Records:
Where They Are Now and Where They Need to Be

Henry R. Glennie
Medilink Australia, Australia

ABSTRACT

The physician often spends far more time gazing at the screen than at the person who has made the appointment. The patient has booked with the expectation their illness or accident will receive undivided attention. Immediately there is a problem, both for the doctor and the patient. Careful medical record-keeping is one of the most important duties of a clinician. How else can a patient's history be documented, the clinical findings recorded, the provisional diagnosis entered, and the chosen treatment pathway defined? But how does the doctor maintain confidence-giving eye contact whilst doing all this? The 19th century physician, as exemplified by the famous painting of "The Doctor" by Luke Fildes in 1891, typifies the devotion to care exhibited by the committed physician. The actuality is that today's physicians display equal amounts of dedication to their work; the difference in 1891 was that there was very little available to treat the great majority of illnesses. EHR, if used to its potential, is the means of pulling all this data together and getting it right every time!

DOI: 10.4018/978-1-5225-5082-2.ch004

INTRODUCTION AND BACKGROUND

Walking through our local hospital corridor recently I passed one of my colleagues, an excellent paediatrician, wheeling a suitcase filled with medical records. I held up my mobile tablet and said, "This is all you need." His reply was predictable and encapsulates the problem medicos have in ditching their traditional paper records, "No, not for me, I'm a hands-on doctor." What does this mean? Surely, we can be hands-on and still be advocates for electronic health records (EHRs).

The computer is often seen by patients to be taking over consultations because the doctor regularly spends more time gazing at the screen than at the person who has made the appointment. The patient has booked with the expectation their illness or accident will receive undivided attention. Immediately there is a problem, both for the doctor and the patient. Careful medical record-keeping is one of the most important duties of a clinician. How else can a patient's history be documented, the clinical findings recorded, the provisional diagnosis entered, the investigation results be displayed and the chosen treatment pathway defined? But how does the doctor maintain confidence-giving eye contact whilst doing all this? The "Sick Woman" (Figure 1) illustrates the 17th Century physician caring for his patient (Steen, c 1663). The difference in the day of Dutch artist Jan Steen (1626-1679) was that there was very little available to treat the great majority of illnesses. Doctors today have the ability to treat their patients effectively so long as they make the right diagnosis. If not sure what they are dealing with they have the ability to access huge amounts of information to make the right call.

EHR, if used to its potential, is the means of pulling all this data together and getting it right every time! Unfortunately, all this knowledge is not being harnessed effectively and the EHR systems in use today have many shortcomings. Evolving technology and increased expectations of health workers and patients is likely to make them obsolete, with all the current problems suitably attended to. To see how this will be achieved it is necessary to look at what healthcare is now and what it will be with optimally functioning EHR systems.

When there is talk of "healthcare" this is largely a misnomer. It is actually "illness care", apart from public health measures which have been around for over a century such as safe water supplies, vaccination, hygienic food handling and alerts at times of disease outbreaks. Worse still, it is illness care of the "snapshot" variety. Hospital admissions, office consultations, home care visits, are all "snapshots" in the ill-health of a person. What is required is effective healthcare. And, because by common usage the word healthcare is almost exclusively illness or accident care, the term will be used throughout the chapter in this context. Perhaps the best way it can be shown to be effective is to provide holistic healthcare, recording health information on every person in a community at times when they are considered to

Figure 1. "The Sick Woman" by Jan Steen

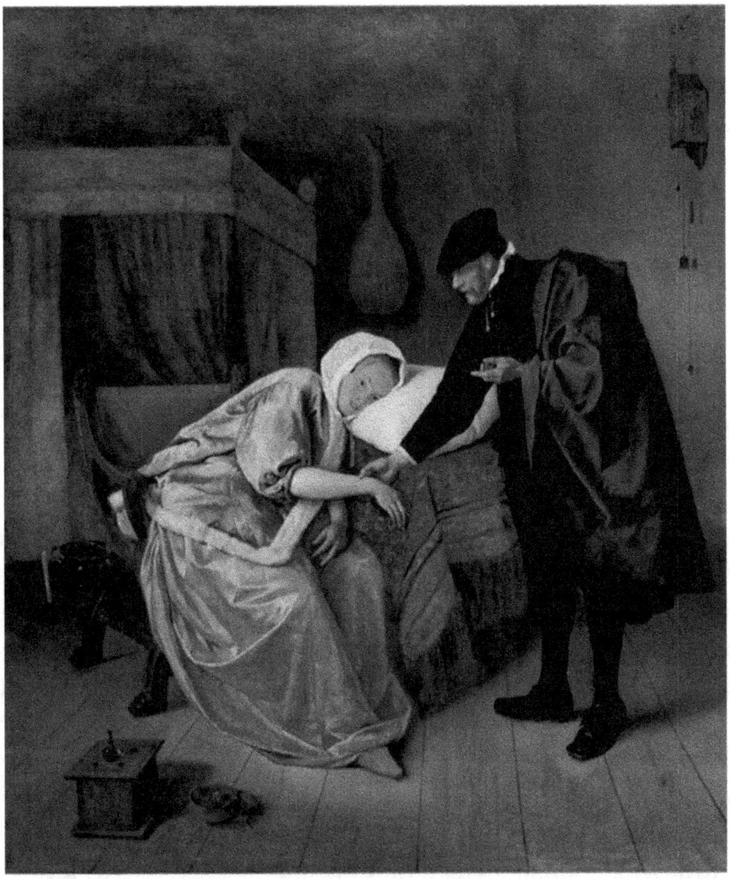

be "healthy" as well as the times they are in poor health, combined with measures to prevent catastrophic physical and mental illness, predicting it and treating it effectively when it does occur.

Everyone, at some time or another, is a "patient". There are the fortunate few who are patients at birth and very infrequently subsequently. But the majority access health care moderately often, if only for active surveillance to prevent serious illness. The benefits are firmly established, as evidenced by protocols for breast and cervical screening, prostate, colon and upper gastrointestinal evaluation and diseases of genetic origin. In this latter regard, it is considered at 25 years of age that 5% of the U.S. population has a disorder with an important genetic component (Snyder, 2016). As genomic knowledge increases it will be discovered that the percentage is far higher, once records of large numbers of patients are scanned with expert system algorithms in conjunction with their genomic data to identify correlations which are currently unknown.

Capturing all episodes of health care in this holistic sense, combined with universal genomic sequencing, may become the means that ill-health is identified before clinical symptoms are manifest. To make this a reality, every person within a population must have a comprehensive EHR, fully secure, with all privacy issues dealt with and, with pre-authorisation from patients, accessible to users when and where it is required, Strict levels of access are integral to this so that information can be retrieved only in areas relevant to the user's particular discipline.

It should also be noted that electronic health record (EHR) and electronic medical record (EMR) are used interchangeably and usually considered to be the same (Hoffman, 2016). However, there is considerable benefit in distinguishing the two. "Medical" comes with the connotation of illness and the term EMR should strictly refer to illness care. The focus for every nation should be "health" and avoidance of illness and hence EHR is the preferable nomenclature. One definition of EMR is that of an electronic medical record created and stored in a single location with EHR as the comprehensive collection of a patient's record created and stored at multiple locations (Health IT.gov, 2016). It is only by aggregation of data from large patient populations, with multiple sites allowing authorised access to the stored information, that electronic records will have any useful role in population health management and cost containment. EMR by that definition will not achieve this. Another definition states that EMR documents the illness and accident history of patients (Garrett & Seidman) whereas an EHR documents the illness and the accident history of every individual in a community as well as the wellness (Garrett & Seidman), recording the measures that people take, or do not take, to lead a healthy lifestyle.

Increasingly, there will be monitoring with mobile devices, externally worn or implanted, to provide continuous recording of vital signs and activity levels, conveying that information on to the person's EHR, with alerts when preset parameters are exceeded. Qualcomm Life, partnering with the EHR company Cerner and health information exchange infrastructure provider, Orion Health (Sukel, 2015), is an example, capturing data from medical devices and sensors within a patient's home, transmitting it to Cerner health care so that providers can remotely monitor chronically ill patients in near real-time to enable proactive engagement to potentially reduce the risk of acute care episodes. Undoubtedly just around the corner, to facilitate remote monitoring, is the availability of electronic health records on mobile phones, with end to end encryption for security and voice commands to display the exact information the clinician requires, providing the appropriate level of authorisation has been authenticated.

Another important facet of EHR development must be full access by patients, or their carers, so patients become custodians of their own health care. Care must be patient-centred, the patient, their carers, their family care doctor, their specialists and their allied health workers all utilising their combined skills to obtain the best possible outcomes. This must include the opportunity for patients to make entries in their record, adding information they consider important and correcting any inaccuracies. But they should not be able to delete any part of the record. This should be retained as entered but added to as considered appropriate by the patient or the caregiver. Gradually this may result in whole populations taking an interest in maintaining their health and it could become the primary means by which early signs of illness are discovered so that optimal treatment pathways can be implemented at an early stage. In cardio-vascular care Medtronic encourages patients to manage their own care through its CareLink product. It is considered to be clinically much more effective and efficient than conventional follow-up (Guedon-Moreau, Mabo, & Kacet, 2013).

For those who consider active surveillance of your health seems unlikely, think again! The financial burden of chronic illness to most nations is unsustainable unless tackled with effective illness prevention strategies. In all OECD nations there is unrelenting upward pressure in health care spending due to population ageing, income growth and technological change, that will continue over coming decades (OECD, 2010). 5% of the population costs almost half of the total expenditure of health care in the U.S. (Stanton, 2006) and figures in other countries are similar (Drouin, Hediger, & Henke, 2008). For example, the cost of health care for the 15.4 million people in England with at least one long-term condition consumes 70% of the NHS's £110bn budget (The Guardian, 2014) as well as £10.9bn of the £15.5bn spent on social care (The Guardian, 2014). 25% of the U.S. population have one or more of five major chronic conditions (mood disorders, diabetes, heart disease, asthma, hypertension) and their care consumes 49% of total healthcare costs (Druss, Marcus, & Olfson, 2001). Concerns are frequently expressed but so far little is being done to rectify the situation. For example, "Costs of this magnitude could make the NHS unsustainable unless these long-term conditions are given better care, with much of it provided by GPs (family physicians) performing enhanced roles rather than hospital doctors (Porter, 2015)."

There are only two ways to reduce chronic illness expenditure. Either reduce the cost of treatment or reduce its incidence. The importance of optimal control of chronic disease processes is well-recognised (Wagner, et al., 2001) and early diagnosis and effective treatment leads to reduced complications (Marshall & Flyvbjerg, 2006). Not only are these associated with pain, suffering and loss of income but, from a national perspective, very considerable additional expense. The benefit of healthy lifestyle is well documented, with increased longevity and better quality of life (Warburton, Nicol, & Bredlin, 2006). National strategies are required to combine medical knowledge with healthy living habits, including regular exercise programs.

A fully functioning EHR system has the capacity to do this and also provides a massive database where algorithms can identify correlations between present health status and the likely development of medical conditions. Early diagnosis can then be combined with optimal treatment pathways. Very considerable work has been carried out in formulating the best treatment pathways for specific conditions (De Blester, et al., 2006). However, patients are individuals and the conditions they have is a complex interplay of their genetic structure and the various environmental influences affecting them (Hernandez & Blazer, 2006). It is only when a sufficiently large population of patients with similar conditions are analysed in appropriate detail, and increasingly this will involve genomic sequencing followed by identification of the various metabolites interacting with the individual's basic genetic structure, that systematic features will become evident which can be used to provide the very best treatment for each individual (Snyder, 2016).

Suitable strategies to prevent illness and accident wherever possible is basic to effective population health, combined with the best treatment pathways when either does occur. Also, and very importantly, a strategy to ensure the ability of a nation to pay for the care its citizens require. The digital revolution, harnessing huge quantities of data and effectively analysing the content, utilising the EHR as the vehicle, will be the means by which the health of nations will be maintained, and where possible improved, within sustainable levels of expenditure.

THE IMPORTANCE OF EHR TECHNOLOGY

From the 1960s the disadvantages of paper records have been tackled utilising computer technology in the health sector. COSTAR became one of the world's first EHR systems (Greenes, Pappalardo, Marble, & Barnett, 1969). The programming language known as MUMPS (Massachusetts General Hospital Utility Multi-Programming System) is the foundation of numerous clinical systems as a Caché database. Users include Veteran's Affairs, Kaiser Permanente and other leading hospitals throughout the U.S. The introduction of computer technology into the health care environment introduced the opportunity to make evidence-based clinical decision-making (Glennie, 1974) but most often clinicians continued to favour intuitive decision-making (Mandell, 1987), just as they had done with their time-honoured paper-based record systems.

However, legislators saw EHR as a priority and by 2004 U.S. President George Bush stated that every American would be obtaining their health care with the support of an electronic health record by 2014 (Bush, 2004). This was reinforced in 2009 during the Obama presidency (Obama's speech on the economy, 2009), with a $30 billion government incentive program to hospitals and office-based physicians who had EHR systems installed (Rowland, 2014). To illustrate, EHRs were installed in only 9.4% of hospitals by 2008 but by 2014 75.5% of hospitals had some form of EHR program (Charles, Gabriel, & Searcy, 2015) and 78% of office-based physicians were using an EHR, from 18% in 2001 (Hsiao & Hing, 2014). Despite the rapid adoption, by 2012, only 42.2% of hospitals met the federal Stage I "meaningful-use" criteria and only 5.1% could meet the Stage 2 criteria (DesRoches, et al., 2013). Obviously, statistics like this caused administrative concern and the Office of the National Coordinator (ONC) for Health Information Technology (HIT) in 2015 published an Interoperability Roadmap "to build longitudinal electronic health records on all Americans and dispense with the disjointed singular episodes epitomising the current health system" (The Office of the National Coordinator for Health Information Technology, 2015). By 2024, the aim is to "push information sharing beyond EHRs to include technologies that empower the American public by putting them at the centre of their own care," with "nationwide interoperability to enable a patient-centred learning health system (Office of the National Coordinator for Health IT, 2016)."

The uptake problems the U.S has experienced have, to some extent, been similar throughout all other nations. Sweden provides an interesting example. By 2012 the whole nation had fully implemented EHRs in hospitals, psychiatry and primary care. However, a single national database for patient records did not exist. Five major software vendors accounted for 96% of the installations but they are not interconnected and even amongst the same software companies there were different configurations. Plans are in place to connect all health care providers, public and private (Falon, 2016). Primary care physicians (GPs) in most OECD nations are the group who have best embraced EHR technology. But, usually the systems are simply used as an alternative to paper records with little or no interoperability between other primary care centres, hospitals, office-based specialists and allied health workers. Initiatives such as the Healthcare Information and Management Systems Society's (HIMSS) Electronic Medical Record Adoption Model (EMRAM) (HIMSS Analytics, 2012) are changing this. EMRAM validation for hospitals and oEMRAM for outpatients is used widely throughout the Western world with eight stages of achievement, from 0 to 7 (HIMSS Analytics, 2017). Many US and European hospitals as well as two

Australian hospitals are in the process of validation. Also, all the New Zealand district health boards are using this model (New Zealand Government, 2017). Universal acceptance of EHR, in ways such as this, is critical if the potential benefits are to materialise.

EHR systems must be universally utilised wherever healthcare is delivered and must be completely interoperable with all other users. The systems must be secure and private, with pre-obtained authorisation for access to healthcare workers involved in the treatment of enrolled patients. They are the logical repository for all this data, providing they are sufficiently user-friendly, instantly available and allowing immediate access to authorised users. They must incorporate comprehensive longitudinal records on their patient population, capturing all outpatient and inpatient "snapshots" through a patient's lifetime as well as wellness profiles detailing all efforts taken to promote and maintain good health. A summarised record must also be included in conjunction with the complete record. The latter could be critical in making a diagnosis and instituting treatment, with pop-down prompts and other devices so that any user can access the information they require without having to plough through masses of information irrelevant to the clinical problem at hand.

But progress towards this utopian health system has been agonisingly slow. The digitally enabled health sector, with interoperable EHR together with real-time mobile recording devices for those with chronic illnesses, is the means to promptly detect any deviation from optimal control of the condition so that appropriate treatment can be instituted.

THE BENEFITS OF ELECTRONIC HEALTH RECORDS (EHRS)

Apart from appointment scheduling and documenting medical histories, drug prescriptions are usually generated electronically; some with direct interoperability with pharmacists. Laboratory and imaging reports are ordered and received electronically and incorporated into the EHR. Drug sensitivities are documented, with alerts when prescribed inappropriately. Online formularies, regularly updated, give additional prescribing information when required.

Additionally, there is huge potential for a host of non-direct care use of personal health information, the so-called secondary EHR uses (Fleischman, Lowry, & Shapiro, 2014). These have been slow to be adopted, despite potential benefit in terms of quality of care provision and cost containment. "Secondary use" is often described as non-direct care use (Safran, et al., 2007); this is misleading. They are clinical activities because they are patient-related and gradually should become mandatory features of all EHRs. However, apart from notable exceptions, such as the health care organisations involved in the SHARP (Health IT.gov, 2013) project and Veterans Health Administration (VHA) in the U.S. (Shulkin, 2016), and some isolated initiatives in other Western countries such as in Finland (EHTEL Connect, 2013) and Estonia (Widen & Haseltine, 2015), most "secondary" uses of EHR are not being widely used despite appreciation of their potential value.

As noted above, many EHR systems in the U.S. are based on the proprietary Cache data model, including Epic systems, with 70% of the nation's HIMSS Stage 7 hospitals as their customers (Gregg, 2014). In February 2014 CVS Caremark's Minute Clinic announced it was switching to Epic and once this transition is complete about 51% of Americans will have an Epic record (Gregg, 2014), despite its "limited interoperability and less-than-ideal usability" (Garber, et al., 2014). What is needed is an integrated and interoperable system suitable for comprehensive population health analytics.

Because of the vast amount of information available to make the best choices for patients, the amount of data collected requires considerable storage capacity combined with analytic capability to the individual patient level. This involves the effective utilisation of re-modelled software platforms and custom-designed algorithms to ensure that particular treatment pathways are the most effective and able to produce the best outcomes at the least possible cost; the greater the granularity of the data that is collected the more useful it is likely to be in optimal clinical decision-making.

It is often not appreciated that doctors, working both in hospitals and community facilities, are the cost drivers in health care. Doctors decide who is admitted to hospital, who is discharged, who has surgery and if so, how much (Glennie, 1992). It has been calculated that physicians direct 80% of healthcare costs (Norbeck, 2012) and improving diagnostic and treatment accuracy directly impacts on the quality of care delivered to patients as well as reducing the overall cost incurred by healthcare systems (Ferruci, Levas, Bagchi, Gondek, & Mueller, 2013). Decisions that are made are completely costless to the prescribing doctor but potentially very expensive to the funder. Also chosen clinical pathways may or may not be in a patient's best interest. Most treatments are instituted without rigorous scientific analysis and patient safety is often compromised when patients requiring urgent healthcare are unaware of the medication they are taking (Kristensson, Modig, Midlov, Hallberg, & Jakobsson, 2010).

In the NHS England 100,000 Genomes Project (Peplow, 2016), one of the largest whole genome sequencing projects in the world, very specific therapy is expected to be delivered to cancer patients and to some with congenital and acquired metabolic conditions. Similarly in the U.S. the Veterans Administration is engaged in a 1 million genome project to promote the future integration of genetic testing in health care delivery, including clinical decision making (Veterans Affairs, 2016), and forecasted to lead to overall savings in expenditure. "The information-poor manner in which medicine is practised today will be replaced with an information-rich system which will be more accurate and more predictive" (Snyder, 2016).

A fully interoperable EHR system is essential in tracking the vast quantities of information which is already collected and which will increase exponentially in coming years, when genomic medicine and continuous monitoring devices become staple components of care. The rate of change in this field of medicine is illustrated in the U.K.'s Wellcome Trust Sanger Institute. The DNA sequencing machines used to create the first map of the human genome have been decommissioned to be replaced by faster Illumina equipment (Mathieson, 2015). By 2025 it has been postulated that genomics will require storage capability of between 2 and 40 exabytes (Elton & O'Riordan, 2016). Obviously if the benefits of genomic sequencing, combined with proteomic analysis, are not realised the lower figure will be operative. If the technology is fully embraced the higher figure may be significantly understated. Clinical decision-making and therapeutic pathways will, very likely, be specific to each individual patient. Analysing the molecular profile of patients, within five years or less, is likely to cost less than $100 and, properly interpreted, the data will provide accurate information about what may be wrong and provide strong clues as to how to correct it (Cullis, 2015).

The time is not too far distant when all newborns in OECD countries will have either had their entire genome mapped during the pregnancy or in the early postpartum period and their proteomes, metabolomes and microbiomes assayed at varying intervals, depending on their likelihood to develop acute or chronic disease processes. The emphasis will change from disease management to prevention; from illness care to wellness management. For those who do develop disease processes targeted therapy will be available to treat the condition promptly and effectively. The result will be increased longevity and overall cost savings when compared with our present "trial and error" system where a treatment pathway is commenced and changed when it is clear that the original therapy was ineffective.

IS EFFECTIVE CHANGE HAPPENING?

Most users are simply using the EHRs currently as a replacement for paper-based records, with electronic prescribing as a convenient adjunct. It is the utilisation of secondary use functions which are going to revolutionise the delivery of healthcare; the right care in the right timeframe in the right clinical setting and at the right cost. And the reluctance of the medical profession to embrace these benefits could be their undoing! Non-physician entrants could take over, providing accurate diagnostic information, together with statistically proven treatment regimes, at very reasonable cost. There will always be a role for physicians treating conditions not cured by the administration of medications but large scale online doctor-patient portals could make a large proportion of the present medical work-force redundant.

Such threats make it vital that doctors ensure the patient-physician interface provides maximum value. Fully functioning EHR systems are an integral part of this, providing all the necessary input to make the right diagnosis and the optimal treatment regime. But this cannot be done by doctors alone. They require software developers to work closely with them to design systems that work very simply, so the doctor can give undivided attention to the consultation, data being entered by a mixture of voice recognition, pen-based technology, typing and scribes where all else fails, to fit every clinical situation, from a routine primary care physician consultation to a life-threatening emergency in a specialised unit. And systems like this must be developed to ensure universal acceptance of EHR technology.

Artificial Intelligence (AI) technologies incorporating advanced machine learning, deep learning, natural language processing and business rules will have an impact on all steps of the software development life-cycle to bring them to their full potential, fully interoperable so that wherever and whenever a patient has been seen in the past, with the utmost privacy and security, authorised users will be able to access that information. Adequate safeguards will be in place to deal effectively with ethical and legal issues; data ownership, fear of lawsuits, security and privacy issues.

In the U.K. a comprehensive EHR system is planned by 2020 (Bunn & Crane, 2016) so that every patient will have all their medical information, including care preferences and lifestyle such as diet and exercise, accessible to all health and social care providers and updated in real time. This will be particularly useful for patients with complex needs and initiatives like this may be followed in many OECD nations.

WHY DO WE NEED ELECTRONIC HEALTH RECORDS?

Healthcare must be respectful of, and responsive to, individual patient preferences, needs and values. These values must guide all clinical decisions (ACSQHC, 2010). This is the very important concept of patient-entered care (Institute of Medicine (US), 2011) (Epstein & Street, 2011) and it cannot proceed optimally without relevant information. Recording patient information in a full and systematic manner is the essence of good medical practice. In an efficient and effective healthcare system, every patient obtains the very best care, with minimal barriers of access, within the shortest possible timeframe. EHR holds the promise to achieve this goal whenever and wherever a suitable system has been installed and when there are sufficient resources to ensure fiscal sustainability. Many EHR promises of quality improvement, cost containment and enhanced access in countries throughout the world have not been realised despite huge investments. This has led to considerable disillusionment, frustration and much wasted expenditure.

Because of this and the inevitable improvements which will occur it is probably best to view current EHR systems as first generation models, providing an alternative to paper-based records but requiring very considerable further development to fulfil the promises made for them.

THE PRESENT REALITY AND THE POTENTIAL OPPORTUNITIES WITH EHR

Introducing electronic health records simply to dispense with paper-based records has too often been seen as an end in itself. Electronic prescriptions and scheduling of on-line appointments is popular as an adjunct but many of the very considerable additional benefits are still to be appreciated by the vast majority of doctors and patients. In this regard there are two main stumbling blocks with regards to the uptake of the EHR throughout the world. Security issues are of great concern and the other has been the failure to appreciate the importance of clinician engagement. Doctors have not been sufficiently involved in the design and implementation of systems. The result has too often been considerable frustration, marked reduction in the number of patients assessed, missing data resulting in clinical errors, less effective communication between patients, their carers and the nurses, doctors and allied health workers responsible for the care. Using the lessons learned from all the nations who have implemented the EHR, the EHRFORUS model is herewith presented, Figure 2.

Ease of Use

Particularly in the assessment and treatment of acutely ill patients many decisions have to be made very quickly. Clinicians often have to view and record salient information very promptly before returning to the patient to make another decision. Any interruption of that process is likely to be negatively received. Medical staff rarely have the luxury of sitting in front of a patient contemplating their next move. A five minute delay in administering an intravenous injection could be fatal.

A computer programmer does not have the same time-frame to work to and there has been insufficient appreciation amongst them of the problems faced by clinicians. An EHR system should:

1. **Maintain Existing Work Patterns as Much as Possible:** It is imperative in the design of any EHR system that clinicians are minimally interrupted in their existing work flow pattern. Too many systems do not allow this, leading to frustration and loss of productivity.
2. **Reliable and Secure Mechanism of Entry to the System:** Perhaps one of the most annoying aspects of EHR is the necessity for a password, entering it, going back to the patient then finding the password has expired!

Iris recognition (Chirchi, Waghmare, & Chirchi, 2011) is one of the most promising of the available mechanisms to allow ease of entry whilst protecting security and privacy, being 1:150,000 secure (1 error in 150,000 users). Radiofrequency identification (RFID) technology is another, with a wristband containing a microchip picking up and sending signals to a reader which allows an authorised user to access the EHR. Both systems are as close as possible to picking up a pen and commencing writing, the way records were kept before the advent of electronic records. Fingerprint recognition is less secure, a typed-in password is only secure if changed frequently.

Figure 2. The EHRFORUS model

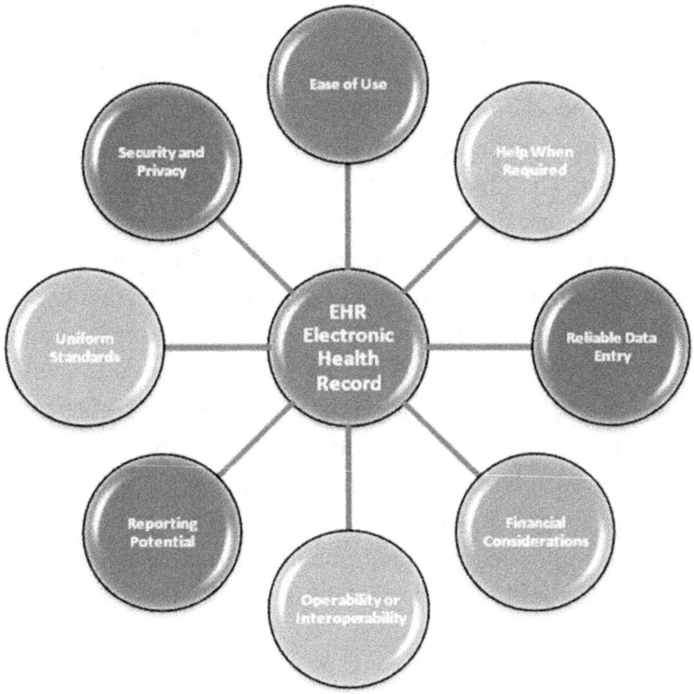

Iris or RFID recognition can be programmed so that activation occurs when the user comes to the screen, with deactivation when he/she leaves it. Also, it can be designed to only allow the appropriate level of access; the physician may be granted complete access, the allied health worker only for the relevant information relating to their area of expertise and no access to persons not specifically authorised by the patient. These appropriate designated levels of access must be incorporated into the EHR design and patients must be able to decide who is able to access their records. Such requests must be adhered to.

3. **Suitable Prompts to. Compartmentalise Records:** Once access to the system has been obtained there must be easy-to-use prompts to obtain relevant clinical information. Summaries are usually rapidly accessible. However, they may not contain critical information. Too often the very considerable information stored within the average record can take an unacceptable period of time to sift through. There are many instances of page after page of electronic data where the same information is repeated again and again.

Different clinicians require different information. An orthopaedic surgeon requires up-to-date information about loss of limb function and the previous orthopaedic treatment the patient has had. Viewing all X-rays and scans is vital and details of previous relevant surgical operations. If a further operation is considered necessary then an overall knowledge of the patient to assess fitness for an elective general anaesthetic is required. The patient's primary care doctor (GP) needs a host of information, sometimes including the detailed specialist reports relating to the orthopaedic problem. The physiotherapist also requires knowledge relating to the orthopaedic condition and the amount of exercise the patient should have.

This means that every person caring for an individual patient requires specific information relating to their discipline and expertise. Time-saving innovations are required within records to allow care to proceed safely, reasonably rapidly and with the highest possible quality. The record has to be structured to achieve this, with suitable prompts to allow each authorised user to obtain the information relevant to their role in caring for the patient, who also must have the right to view any entry in their record. Some will be content with superficial scanning, others will intently comb through their records to identify parts they do not agree with. They should be able to make additional comments, including disagreeing with what has been entered, but nothing should be able to be deleted.

4. **Technology Issues:** Many entries in EHR are less detailed than with paper-based records, particularly when clinicians have limited typing and computer skills. Also, the ability to create useful diagrams in EHR is beyond the technical capacity of most users and, despite electronic prescribing and investigation-ordering capability, many still prefer hand-writing these "because it's quicker."

Less detailed entries often mean that important data is not incorporated into the EHR record and missing data becomes a problem. Suitable drop-down lists and other time-saving aids are required to overcome this, with alerts if particular investigations have recently been carried out and would not normally require repeating within that timeframe.

The opportunity to use voice recognition and pen-based technology should always be available, in conjunction with learning health systems, with the ability to extract relevant clinical information from unstructured data so that meaningful information is shared by converting little-used terminology into standard nomenclature. DeepQA defines a powerful new architecture for structuring and reasoning over unstructured natural language content and provides a foundation for developing decision support systems that can address many of the cognitive challenges clinicians face (Ferruci, Levas, Bagchi, Gondek, & Mueller, 2013).

5. **Alerts:** Considerable acrimony has been created within clinician ranks with patient alerts which have not been urgent enough to disrupt normal workflow and/or leisure activities. Time spent dealing with alerts, often of secondary importance to urgent clinical matters at hand is a common concern (Fihn, et al., 2014). They need to be prioritised in their degree of urgency; those requiring immediate notification and appropriate attention, those requiring decisions within 24 hours and those which can be handled by the practice manager the next working day. Colour coding is a convenient way of achieving this; red, orange and green respectively.
6. Help When Required
    a. **Rapid and Effective IT Support is Essential:** Suitably trained IT personnel must be contactable and available to fix the service problem or replace the faulty server 24 hours a day seven days a week. Medicine has no time barriers and support staff must be available to the same timetable.

b. **The Use of Scribes:** To facilitate data entry, the use of scribes, ideally senior medical students and/or junior doctors, is an innovative solution; the scribe typing in the clinical information as the patient is examined and treated, creating a useful learning environment for themselves and minimal disruption to normal workflow for the senior clinician.

c. **Use of Telehealth:** The use of telehealth to obtain a reliable, high quality picture with synchronous sound, enabled by high speed, reliable broadband technology has many potential benefits in the provision of patient-centred healthcare (Mauney, Furlough, & Barnes, 2015). Information obtained from the telehealth encounter should be incorporated within the record, with appropriate screen-sharing technology so that the two-way conversation with the patient and all relevant investigation results are accessed and recorded simultaneously, with a presumptive diagnosis, the treatment administered and the advice given.

Almost entirely the role of telehealth has been seen to be connecting clinicians with patients separated by considerable distance. Equally valuable is the opportunity to obtain the very best management opinion as soon as possible following a life-threatening accident, physical or mental illness occurs (Glennie, 2012). This includes emergency medicine physicians accessing specialist opinions within minutes of patients arriving at a facility and it should also include paramedics attending motor vehicle accidents and urgent house calls, with head-mounted cameras to allow real-time transmission of high resolution pictures, with synchronous sound, to regional emergency departments. Again, suitable screen-sharing technology is required to allow clinicians to enter all relevant information in real time with high quality voice recognition facilities. All entries should be able to be edited by the clinicians responsible for the care of individual patients once they have completed their assessment and initiated the appropriate treatment, analogous to the way clinicians complete paper-based notes in patient records.

7. **Reliable Data Entry:** Missing data in patient records is currently a very significant problem in reaching valid conclusions and programs should have prompts which advises the user certain relevant questions have not being asked and further operation suspended until the necessary information has been entered. There are three important aspects to this; reliable, unreliable and missing data.

   a. **Separating Reliable Data From Unreliable:** This is a very real problem in EHR usage. A partial solution is a system control which does not allow data entry unless the person's name and designation (e.g. RN, Physiotherapist,

OT, Consultant MD, Resident MD) is inserted. Similarly in the patient portal of the EHR, when the patient, carer or family member has entered information into the record, the name and connection to the patient must be recorded. Unfortunately, the most experienced physician can insert unreliable data, just as a very junior clinician can do. Sometimes this can occur with the time-saving device, the "cut and paste" option. Day after day the same entry may be repeated with minor modifications, sometimes leaving entries from previous days which are no longer applicable to the patient.

b. **Missing Data:** A very significant problem exists when records are being analysed for health status and influence of environmental factors and important information has not been recorded. Data entry may be completely absent or in insufficient detail. This is often the case with environmental irritants such as asbestos and coal dust as well as the onset of chronic diseases such as diabetes, hypertension, etc. Various statistical methods are utilised to obtain valid correlations when missing data is evident.

c. **Misplaced Data:** Occasionally results are placed in the wrong patient's record, the wrong pharmaceutical data is entered and many similar errors occur which lead to erroneous conclusions. Users always have to be cognisant of this, with cross-checking as necessary as well as all other reasonable precautions. End of life directives are particularly sensitive issues in this regard.

8. **Financial:** There are two aspects to this and both must be an integral part of an EHR system:
   a. **Billing Data:** In the U.S. and other nations with fee-for-service systems billing data is a considerable part of the record, vital for revenue generation for hospitals, office-based physicians and all others tendering accounts for services rendered. Current EHR systems are generally well served, with user-friendly input portals.
   b. **Costing Data:** Costing data is relevant whenever and wherever healthcare services are provided, from a solo primary care practitioner to a major hospital. But costing information is rarely incorporated into an EHR system despite it being the logical means to effectively monitor input costs relative to outcomes achieved. A satisfactory program allows the analysis of actual costs incurred relative to expected cost and budgeted revenue projections to ensure the highest possible quality of care within sustainable funding levels.

Effective health care requires the skills of a wide variety of health professionals: doctors, nurses, allied health workers, all working in their respective disciplines. Also administrators, who, if optimally employed, provide the resources required to treat their target population to the highest possible standard in the most cost-effective manner.

The two greatest problems in budgetary control in the health sector are the inefficiency and ineffectiveness of the decisions made by medical personnel in the care of their patients. In this context inefficiency is any decision made when an equally correct one could have been made at lesser cost, such as duplicating a laboratory investigation, prolonging the stay of a patient in hospital unnecessarily, prescribed expensive medication when cheaper medication would have the same or better outcome. Ineffectiveness is when chosen treatment pathways have not resulted in expected improvement to patients.

The following protocol is suggested to overcome these very real deficiencies in patient management. Every intervention ordered on every patient is longitudinally tracked in every EHR record, with mandatory ICD-10 coding whenever a decision is made. There is a precedent in Bosnia and Herzegovina where an ICD-10 presumptive diagnosis is required with every prescription (Mujkic & Marinkovic, 2017). Also, in Canada, detailed annotation is mandatory for every service provided by medical practitioners working both in hospitals and office-based practices (Ontario Medical Association).

In conjunction with this it is suggested that the cost of each intervention, direct and indirect (Power Health Solutions, 2017) is incorporated within each patient's EHR. Each item should appear in the "Cost of Service" record on each patient. When this is accurately calculated to the patient level (Power Health Solutions, 2017), decisions can be made as to whether the service provided has been appropriate and whether it should have been delivered in the home, in an office-based practice or in a hospital setting. Because of the potential savings, as a general rule the former should be chosen whenever the quality and safety of the care is equivalent to care in the other two situations.

This costing information, combined with details of all other interventions, commences when the record is instituted, ideally at birth and continued over the patient's life-time. It incorporates costs associated with presumptive diagnoses, definitive diagnoses, modes of treatment and outcomes over the course of the record. Therefore each patient has a comprehensive longitudinal record of patient care and resource utilisation, monitoring costs and outcomes wherever and whenever healthcare is required. It accurately measures costs, whether they are incurred in hospital, the home or in medical centres.

This data is vitally important in establishing the cost-effectiveness of the care that is delivered. Because it could cause concern to patients it should not be visible to them but only accessible to the staff responsible for the resource utilisation of that patient population. The *raison d'etre* for collecting the information is to obtain the best possible value for every healthcare dollar and analysis must always be with completely de-identified data. The information can be presented to clinicians at regular intervals, adjusted for case complexity and demographics.

The de-identification amongst clinical peer groups must be adequately constructed to ensure that no individual knows the identity of any other. It can be analysed to determine:

1. Outcomes of treatment of similar conditions with similar demographics by other providers regionally and nationally;
2. Cost of treatment of similar conditions with similar demographics by other providers regionally and nationally;
3. Incidence of similar conditions regionally and nationally;
4. The granularity of the data can be increased as appropriate to personalise patient care e.g. the staging and histopathology of tumours, biomarker identification and comparisons of the results of treatment of patients with similar histologic and genetic characteristics regionally, nationally and internationally.

The Canadian and Bosnian experience demonstrates that medical practitioners, both hospital and community-based, will complete the required information on each patient if it is mandated. There is very considerable cost-outcome benefit wherever such legislation is introduced, providing unique population health data, a powerful tool in measuring the quality and cost-effectiveness of the interventions chosen.

Operability (Inter-Operability)

The opportunity for EHR technology to introduce evidence based decision-making was part of the vision of Barnett and his colleagues (Greenes, Pappalardo, Marble, & Barnett, 1969) in the 1960s. But only a small number of conditions, relative to the total number, have been widely accepted in terms of best practice protocols. A far better mechanism exists to obtain consensus but unfortunately it has not been utilised to any extent. EHRs offer this solution by providing clinical insights from observational data collected from large patient populations. Utilising Bayesian algorithms (Heckerman, 1997) improved clinical decision-making can be made in a large range of clinical conditions and presented to users in the form of prompts when the entered clinical data suggests common causality. No longer the roundtable discussions as to best treatment pathways where anecdotal evidence so often prevails.

Clinical decision-making for practically every condition and every manifestation of each condition could be adopted in best practice protocols which would only be superseded when better outcomes were achieved for that condition at the same or lesser cost.

Similarly, many clinical trials could be conducted by evaluating the response to particular pharmaceuticals in large cohorts of patients with similar conditions. Over the course of time these could replace many of the current double-blind trials where conclusions may be drawn from relatively small numbers of patients, particularly for rare conditions. Universal utilisation of interoperable EHR systems in patient populations would mean that all people placed on a particular drug were effectively monitored for clinical benefit and the prevalence of side-effects. Valid conclusions could be obtained within months rather than the years, and at far less cost than with clinical trials.

It should be noted that the benefits of interoperability can only be fully achieved when every individual within a population has a unique identifier and every hospital and community-based provider utilises an EHR system which allows access to all authorised users. The United Kingdom (HM Government, 2014), New Zealand (New Zealand Government, 2017) and Ireland (eHealth Ireland, 2016) are amongst the nations which are introducing systems likely to achieve this.

In the U.S. and in Australia there is legislation preventing a unique identifier linking every citizen throughout the health care system and this is a significant roadblock to effective health information exchange. Changing this would require the repeal of that legislation.

A minority of public and private hospitals in Australia have EHR systems. Primary care physicians (GPs) have a number of software program suppliers and there is limited electronic communication between them. “Firewalls” are in place in many states between public hospitals and GPs and inter-state transmission of health data is almost non-existent except by facsimile.

In the U.S. the Veterans Health Administration (Ibrahim, 2007) is an example of a fully integrated interoperable system but there are only a few such systems in the U.S. To deal with the existing limited operability problem a “final rule” was mandated in October 2015 for “meaningful use” stage 3 criteria (Code of Federal Regulations, 2015). This applies to all eligible U.S. hospitals and health professionals. But even if this rule was adopted universally full interoperability would still not occur because the relevant criterion simply requires users to “facilitate health information exchange”. A stricter criterion is required.

Reporting Potential

This is best considered in terms of advantages and disadvantages:

1. The Advantages of EHR Reporting Capabilities

Advanced analytics allows the development of insights and correlations from large quantities of shared data. Healthcare becomes more precise and quantitative. If a person becomes ill with a particular disease algorithms are coming available to search all other patients with the same disease process, including the identification of cellular mutations when they occur. A complete genetic and molecular characterisation can be made, how they were treated and what the outcome was (Snyder, 2016). A new era of "data-driven medicine" results (Snyder, 2016).

Management of chronic disease and acute neoplastic conditions is greatly facilitated with this approach. The reporting potential is enormous and what better way of storing the data than in a fully functioning EHR system? When nations are currently consuming approximately half of total health expenditure on chronic disease processes (Druss, Marcus, & Olfson, 2001) data-driven medicine not only delivers better care but it is achieved at lesser cost. Clinical decision support systems can be developed for improving diagnostic accuracy and achieving precision medicine (Casteneda, et al., 2015). But most conditions are still being treated according to guideline-directed principles (Cios & Moore, 2002). The Chronic Care Model, which has been implemented by a large number of organisations in the United States, the United Kingdom, Sweden and other OECD nations is an example of this. (Wagner, Davis, Schaefer, Von Korff, & Austin, 1999). Despite the widespread use for nearly 20 years it has been shown that isolated components of CCM are not sufficient to improve clinical outcomes. It is only by combining CCM's six interventions that clinical outcomes are likely to improve (Baptista, et al., 2016). This raises the question of how much expenditure could be saved in chronic disease management if data-driven clinical decisions are made!

It is clear that with full interoperability and analysis of very large databases, which will include real-time data from monitoring devices, improved clinical decision-making will result and with it the potential for very considerable savings by instituting appropriate healthcare in the early stages of disease. In this context wearable health tracking devices (Evenson, Goto, & Furberg, 2015) are destined to be the means that patients, particularly those with chronic conditions, will be continuously monitored to maintain their illnesses in optimal control. Vital signs such as heart rate, exercise, respiratory rate, skin temperature, oxygen carrying capacity (oximetry), stress levels (used for many years in lie detection tests) and sleep monitoring will be continuously measured whilst other transducers will measure blood pressure, cardiac arrhythmias, brain activity, glucose, drug and electrolyte levels in targeted individuals. They will be automatically downloaded to the patient's smartphone and electronically conveyed to central data tracking stations such as local hospitals. 24-hour monitoring of this information, with alerts generated for unusual deviations from normal levels will allow medical personnel to treat chronic illnesses optimally and also to identify illnesses before they become clinically apparent.

Over the course of their life-times individuals will have hundreds of terabytes of data collected, stored, analysed and actioned as appropriate. Reporting of data in this way will not only save lives but also maintain people in their best possible state of health, incorporated into each person's EHR and accessible to that individual, most likely contained within a smartphone or similar appliance, as well as to all medical personnel authorised by that individual. It will be very easy to access and interpret, for instance by using flowcharts in green when results are within the normal range, orange and the upper and lower limits of normal and red when beyond that.

2. The Disadvantages of EHR reporting capabilities

Medical data is collected from many sources and comprises many components; history taking, physical examination, laboratory investigations, radiological imaging, collation of reports from various hospital and office-based specialists, treatment regimes, response to medication, home situation, presumptive diagnoses. All this information needs to be arranged in such a way that the best decisions are made in each clinical situation. All these components may bear upon the diagnosis, prognosis, and treatment of the patient, and cannot be ignored (Campbell, Sittig, Ash, Guappone, & Dykstra, 2006). They must be carefully considered by physicians during consultations; ideally doctors viewing the consultation from the patient perspective.

In this regard it must be borne in mind that patients are intently questioned by their doctors, sometimes with the use of unfamiliar terms. Doctors do what they are trained to do, diagnosing and treating each patient as carefully as possible, usually with significant time constraints. The empathy of the physician, as exemplified in Figure 1, should be the goal of all clinicians because EHRs may cause several unintended consequences, such as increased medical errors, negative emotions, changes in power structure, and overdependence on technology (Menachemi & Collum, 2011). They are often voluminous in their detail, with considerable duplication of information which makes them difficult to negotiate, particularly when clinical details are required quickly. The EHRFORUS model is presented as the means by which these problems will be overcome.

Also, there should always be an alternative to entry and retrieval of data in the event of computer failure. This is a major benefit of the personally controlled electronic health record. If every patient has their record on a suitably encrypted smart device, or cloud based storage is utilised, there is a back-up record which can be accessed as necessary. Where this is not available basic medical care must always be capable of being provided.

Despite these disadvantages, from the foregoing, it is clear that advantages outweigh disadvantages and future EHR developments will make this even more apparent.

Uniform Standards

Oversight (with legislation if appropriate), is needed to ensure the development, implementation, and enforcement of comprehensive national standards for the design, performance, and use of EHR systems to reduce serious EHR-related errors (Bowman, 2013) and EHR system vendors should adopt design and usability standards that optimise system safety and information integrity (Bowman, 2013). Also it is extremely important to include specific minimum data elements within the standards in the design and development of any EHR system (Watzlaf, Zeng, Jarymowycz, & Firouzan, 2005). The American Healthcare Research and Quality (AHRQ) recommended the following policy actions (Armijo, McDonnell, & Werner, 2009):

1. Establishing certification requirements for EHRs that:
    a. Include usability/information design as an essential part of the certification process;
    b. Require/strongly recommend that vendors establish and document their programs for testing the usability of their systems (people and processes), including evaluating potential impacts on quality and safety;
    c. Include EHR design and functionality in standards and guidelines.
2. Developing a national EHR usability laboratory to:
    a. Support public-private collaboration and sharing of best practices in this area;
    b. Develop tools and processes to support evaluation of products and implementations;
    c. Assist health IT vendors in product development and health care.

The Office of the National Coordinator for Health Information Technology's (ONC) Office of Science & Technology (OST) in the U.S. has developed initiatives to standardise *meaning* through the use of standardised healthcare vocabularies, *structure* by leveraging standards in HL7, *transport* using secure email protocols, *security* through National Institute of Standards and Technology (NIST) adopted encryption standards, and *services* through open, and accessible application programming interfaces (APIs) (The Office of the National Coordinator for Health Information Technology, 2015).

ONC enables the health IT community to convene and rapidly prioritise health IT challenges and subsequently develop and harmonise standards, specifications and implementation guidance to solve existing challenges.

ONC is also responsible for curating the set of standards and specifications that support interoperability and ensuring that they can be assembled into solutions for a variety of health information exchange scenarios (The Office of the National Coordinator for Health Information Technology, 2015).

Security and Privacy

The possibility of unauthorised access to computerised health records is considerably greater than breaches of security and privacy with paper records, mainly because the latter are generally either lodged in hospital medical record departments or in office-based physicians' premises, neither being accessible to the public. Breaches of security and privacy are protected by legislation in all OECD countries, with a distinction made between the two terms.

In the EHR context the term "privacy" refers to the collection, storage and use of patients' health information (Hoffman, 2016). "Security" of medical records relates to technical measures and procedures that protect records from being inappropriately accessed or disclosed by hacking or other means (Hoffman, 2016). In the U.S. medical information is protected by the Health Insurance Portability and Accountability Act of 1996 (HIPAA). It defines "individually identifiable health information" transmitted or maintained electronically or in any other form (Code of Federal Regulations, 2015). Risk assessments in order to determine security vulnerabilities with regard to risk management practices are instituted as required.

The Security Rule incorporated within this Act does not apply to the transmission of electronically protected health information in the following circumstances; to another health care provider who is treating the patient, to a group health plan sponsor or to agencies determining eligibility for government programs providing public benefits (Code of Federal Regulations, 2015). The Rule also is designed to ensure that only authorised personnel have access to electronic protected health information (Scholl, et al., 2008). There is no explicit requirement that "covered entities" identify the best current operative security practices (Scholl, et al., 2008).

Other nations have similar security and privacy legislation and all users have an obligation to protect the data entrusted to them by their patients. The number of recent cyber-attacks make it essential that vulnerabilities are actively addressed. End-to-end encryption systems have been designed to ensure absolute privacy between the two parties.

Security of this degree may be necessary in all health information exchanges, with authorised levels of access at each end, creating audit trails in the event that information is inappropriately accessed. Also, EHR systems should have fault-tolerance systems so if one component fails or is experiencing problems the system will switch to a backup component (Harman, Flite, & Bond, 2012).

CONCLUSION

Electronic health records should not be seen simply as a means of dispensing with all the disadvantages of paper-based records. Electronic prescriptions and scheduling of on-line appointments are popular EHR features but many of the very considerable additional benefits are still to be appreciated by the vast majority of doctors and patients.

Privacy and security of records is the main concern of patients, with the thought of unauthorised access preventing many patients from enrolling in digital record systems. From the clinician point of view interruption in normal workflow processes is probably an equally important concern, resulting in considerable frustration, marked reduction in the number of patients assessed, missing data resulting in clinical errors and less effective communication with patients.

This chapter seeks to present a more usable and useful EHR system than has so far been designed, with software developers appreciating the importance of clinician engagement and doctors being more involved in system design.

As stated previously it is best to view current EHR systems as first generation models, providing an alternative to paper-based records but requiring very considerable further development to fulfil the promises made for them. An EHRFORUS model has been presented (Figure 2) and it is the author's expectation that EHR systems will gradually become completely interoperable, extremely secure and of sufficient simplicity that work-flow patterns will not be disrupted.

Also they will be the means by which clinical pathways will be appropriately chosen and accurately costed so that the highest quality of care is delivered at sustainable levels of expenditure. Future EHR development in this manner brings enormous challenges but huge benefits; perhaps most of all by encouraging whole populations to take an informed interest in their health and wellbeing. Better care, better health, lesser cost.

REFERENCES

ACSQHC. (2010). *Patient-centred care: Improving quality and safety by focusing care of patients and consumers*. Discussion Paper. Australian Commission on Safety and Quality in Health Care. Retrieved from https://www.safetyandquality.gov.au/wp-content/uploads/2012/01/PCCC-DiscussPaper.pdf

Armijo, D., McDonnell, C., & Werner, K. (2009). Evaluation and use case framework. *Electronic Health Record Usability, 9*. AHRQ Publication. Retrieved from https://healthit.ahrq.gov/sites/default/files/docs/citation/09-10-0091-1-EF.pdf

Baptista, D. R., Wiens, A., Pontarolo, R., Regis, L., Reis, W. C., & Correr, C. J. (2016). The chronic care model for type 2 diabetes: A systematic review. *Diabetology & Metabolic Syndrome, 8*(7). doi:10.118613098-015-0119-z PMID:26807158

Bowman, S. (2013). *Impact of electronic health record systems on information integrity: Quality and safety implications*. Retrieved from http://perspectives.ahima.org/impact-of-electronic-health-record-systems-on-information-integrity-quality-and-safety-implications/

Bunn, S., & Crane, J. (2016). *Electronic health records*. Parliamentary Office of Science and Technology (519). United Kingdom: Houses of Parliament. Retrieved from http://researchbriefings.parliament.uk/ResearchBriefing/Summary/POST-PN-0519

Bush, G. W. (2004). *Promoting innovation and competitiveness, President Bush's technology agenda*. The White House. Retrieved from https://georgewbush-whitehouse.archives.gov/infocus/technology/

Campbell, E. M., Sittig, D. F., Ash, J. S., Guappone, K. P., & Dykstra, R. H. (2006). Types of unintended consequences related to computerised provider order entry. *Journal of the American Medical Informatics Association, 13*(5), 547–556. doi:10.1197/jamia.M2042 PMID:16799128

Casteneda, C., Nalley, K., Mannion, C., Bhattacharyya, P., Blake, P., Pecora, A., ... Suh, K. S. (2015). Clinical decision support systems for improving diagnostic accuracy and achieving precision medicine. *Journal of Clinical Bioinformatics, 5*(4). doi:10.118613336-015-0019-3 PMID:25834725

Charles, D., Gabriel, M., & Searcy, T. (2015). *Adoption of electronic health record systems among U.S. non-federal acute care hospitals: 2008-2014*. ONC Data Brief. The Office of the National Coordinator for Health Information Technology. Retrieved from http://docplayer.net/4931694-Adoption-of-electronic-health-record-systems-among-u-s-non-federal-acute-care-hospitals-2008-2014.html

Chirchi, V. R., Waghmare, L. M., & Chirchi, E. R. (2011). Iris biometric; Recognition for person identification in security systems. *International Journal of Computers and Applications, 24*(9), 1–6. doi:10.5120/2986-4002

Cios, K. J., & Moore, G. W. (2002). Uniqueness of data mining. *Artificial Intelligence in Medicine, 26*(1-2), 1–24. doi:10.1016/S0933-3657(02)00049-0 PMID:12234714

Code of Federal Regulations. (2015). *Administrative safeguards*. Code of Federal Regulations. Retrieved from https://www.law.cornell.edu/cfr/text/45/164.308

Code of Federal Regulations. (2015). Stage 3 meaningful use objectives and measures for EPs, eligible hospitals: Cornell Law School. Retrieved from https://www.law.cornell.edu/cfr/text/42/495.24

Code of Federal Regulations. (2015). *Technical Safeguards*. Code of Federal Regulations. Retrieved from https://www.law.cornell.edu/cfr/text/45/164.312

Cullis, P. (2015). *The personalized medicine revolution; How diagnosing and treating disease are about to change forever.* Vancouver: Greystone Books. Retrieved from https://vpl.bibliocommons.com/item/show/4176435038_the_personalized_medicine_revolution

De Blester, L., Depreitere, R., De Waele, K., Vanhaecht, K., Vlayed, J., Yen, J., & Sermeus, W. (2006). Defining Pathways. *Journal of Nursing Management, 14*(7), 553–563. doi:10.1111/j.1365-2934.2006.00702.x PMID:17004966

DesRoches, C. M., Charles, D., Furukawa, M. F., Maulik, S. J., Kralovec, P., & Mostashiari, F. (2013). Adoption of electronic health records grows rapidly, but fewer than half of US hospitals had at least a basic system in 2012 [abstract]. *Health Affairs, 32*(8), 1478–1485. doi:10.1377/hlthaff.2013.0308 PMID:23840052

Drouin, J. P., Hediger, V., & Henke, N. (2008). *Health care costs: A market-based view. The McKinsey Quarterly.*

Druss, B. G., Marcus, S. C., & Olfson, M. (2001). *Comparing the national economic burden of five chronic conditions*. Retrieved from https://www.ncbi.nlm.nih.gov/pubmed/11816664

eHealth Ireland. (2016). *eHealth strategy for Ireland*. Department of Health. Retrieved from http://www.ehealthireland.ie/

EHTEL Connect. (2013). *eHealth strategy and action plan of Finland in a European context.* Helsinki: ETHEL Connect. Retrieved from https://www.google.com.au/search?site=&source=hp&q=https%3A%2F%2Fwww.ehtel.eu%2Freferences-files%2Fehtelconnect-support-documentation%2FEHTELconnect-Finland-PeerReview-Public-Report-RAP2013_11.pdf&oq=https%3A%2F%2Fwww.ehtel.eu%2Freferences-files%2Fehtelco

Elton, J., & O'Riordan, A. (2016). *Healthcare disrupted; Next generation business models and strategies.* John Wiley & Sons. Retrieved from http://au.wiley.com/WileyCDA/WileyTitle/productCd-1119171881.html

Epstein, R., & Street, R. I. (2011). The values and value of patient-centered care. *Annals of Family Medicine*, *9*(2), 100–103. doi:10.1370/afm.1239 PMID:21403134

Evenson, K. R., Goto, M. M., & Furberg, R. D. (2015). Systematic review of the validity and reliability of consumer-wearable activity trackers. *The International Journal of Behavioral Nutrition and Physical Activity*, *12*(159). doi:10.118612966-015-0314-1 PMID:26684758

Falon, S. (2016). EHR records in Sweden and what the future brings. *Salus Digital.* Retrieved from http://salusdigital.net/ehr-records-sweden-future-brings/

Ferruci, D., Levas, A., Bagchi, S., Gondek, D., & Mueller, E. T. (2013). Watson: Beyond jeopardy. *Artificial Intelligence*, *199-200*, 93–105. doi:10.1016/j.artint.2012.06.009

Fihn, S. D., Francis, J., Clancy, C., Nielson, C., Nelson, K., Rumsfeld, J., ... Graham, G. (2014). Insights from advanced analytics at the veterans health administration. *Health Affairs*, *33*(7), 1203–1211. doi:10.1377/hlthaff.2014.0054 PMID:25006147

Fleischman, W., Lowry, T., & Shapiro, J. (2014). *The visit-data warehouse: Enabling novel secondary use of health information exchange data.* Academic Press. doi:10.13063/2327-9214.1099

Garber, S., Gates, S. M., Keeler, E. B., Vaiana, M. E., Mulcahy, A. W., Lau, C., & Kellermann, A. L. (2014). *Redirecting spending in U.S. health care: Options to decrease spending and increase value.* Santa Monica, CA: Rand Corporation. Retrieved from https://www.rand.org/pubs/research_reports/RR308.html

Garrett, P., & Seidman, J. (n.d.). EMR vs EHR – What is the difference? *Health IT Buzz.* Retrieved from https://www.healthit.gov/buzz-blog/electronic-health-and-medical-records/emr-vs-ehr-difference/

Glennie, H. R. (1974). Proposals for health reform. *The New Zealand Medical Journal*, (79): 575–578. PMID:4522414

Glennie, H. R. (1992). Downsizing of Hospitals with Effective Community Care. *The New Zealand Medical Journal*, *105*, 202–203. PMID:1625828

Glennie, H. R. (2012). Delivering health care cost-effectively using available technology. In *Proceedings of the Global Telehealth Conference 2012*. Sydney: IOS Press.

Government, H. M. (2014). Using data and technology to transform outcomes for patients and citizens; A framework for action. *Personalised health and care 2020*. NHS. Retrieved from https://www.gov.uk/government/uploads/system/uploads/attachment_data/file/384650/NIB_Report.pdf

Greenes, R. A., Pappalardo, A. N., Marble, C. W., & Barnett, G. O. (1969). Design and implementation of a clinical data management system. *Computers and Biomedical Research, an International Journal*, *2*(5), 469–485. doi:10.1016/0010-4809(69)90012-3 PMID:11697375

Gregg, H. (2014). 10 Things to know about epic. *Becker's Hospital Review*. Retrieved from http://www.beckershospitalreview.com/lists/10-things-to-know-about-epic.html

Guedon-Moreau, L., Mabo, P., & Kacet, S. (2013). Current clinical evidence for remote patient management. *Eurospace*, *15*(1suppl_1), i6–i10. doi:10.1093/europace/eut119 PMID:23737234

Harman, L. B., Flite, C. A., & Bond, K. (2012). Electronic health records: Privacy, confidentiality and security. *AMA Journal of Ethics*, *14*(9), 712–719. Retrieved from http://journalofethics.ama-assn.org/2012/09/stas1-1209.html PMID:23351350

HealthIT.gov. (2013). *Strategic health IT advanced research projects (SHARP); Secondary uses of EHR data*. Retrieved from https://www.healthit.gov/policy-researchers-implementers/secondary-use-ehr-data

HealthIT.gov. (2016). Benefits Of EHR. *What Is an electronic medical record (EMR)? Differences between electronic medical records and electronic health records*. Retrieved from Health IT.gov: https://www.healthit.gov/providers-professionals/electronic-medical-records-emr

Heckerman, D. (1997). Bayesian networks for data mining. *Data Mining and Knowledge Discovery*, *1*(1), 79–119. doi:10.1023/A:1009730122752

Hernandez, L. M., & Blazer, D. G. (2006). *Genes, behavior and the social environment: Moving beyond the nature/nurture debate*. National Academies Press (US). Retrieved from https://www.ncbi.nlm.nih.gov/books/NBK19929/

HIMSS Analytics. (2012). *Electronic Medical Record Adoption Model (EMRAM)*. Retrieved from http://www.himss.org/electonic-medical-record-adoption-model-emram

HIMSS Analytics. (2017). *Healthcare provider models; Adoption and maturity models to move your organization forward through technology*. Retrieved from http://www.himssanalytics.org/healthcare-provider-models/all

Hoffman, S. (2016). Electronic health records and medical big data: Law and policy (Cambridge Bioethics and Law ed., Vol. 32). Cambridge University Press. doi:10.1017/9781316711149

Hsiao, C. J., & Hing, E. (2014). *Use and charactistics of electronic health record systems among office-based physician practices: United States, 2001-2012*. NCHS Data Brief. National Centre for Health Statistics. Retrieved from http://docplayer.net/2252607-Use-and-characteristics-of-electronic-health-record-systems-among-office-based-physician-practices-united-states-2001-2013.html

Ibrahim, S. A. (2007). The Veterans Health Administration: A domestic model for a national health care system? *American Journal of Public Health*, *97*(12), 2124–2126. doi:10.2105/AJPH.2007.125575 PMID:17971535

Institute of Medicine (US). (2011). *Patients charting the course* (L. Olsen, R. A. Saunders, & J. M. McGinnis, Eds.). Washington, DC: National Academies Press (US). Retrieved from https://www.ncbi.nlm.nih.gov/books/NBK91496/

Kristensson, J., Modig, S., Midlov, P., Hallberg, I. R., & Jakobsson, U. (2010). Healthcare utilisation and knowledge concerning perscribed drugs among older people. *European Journal of Clinical Pharmacology*, *66*(10), 1047–1054. doi:10.100700228-010-0837-y PMID:20652233

Mandell, S. F. (1987). *Resistance to computerization. An examination of the relationship between resistance and the cognitive style of the clinician*. Retrieved from https://www.ncbi.nlm.nih.gov/pubmed/3668415

Marshall, S. M., & Flyvbjerg, M. (2006). Prevention and early detection of vascular complications of diabetes. *British Medical Journal*, *333*(7556), 475–480. doi:10.1136/bmj.38922.650521.80 PMID:16946335

Mathieson, S. A. (2015). Genomics big data compels IT to rediscover efficiency techniques. *Computer Weekly*. Retrieved from http://www.computerweekly.com/feature/Genomics-big-data-compels-IT-to-rediscover-efficiency-techniques

Mauney, J., Furlough, C., & Barnes, J. (2015). Developing a better clinical alert system in EHRs. *Proceedings of the International Symposium on Human Factors and Ergonomics in Health Care*, *4*(1), 29-36. doi:10.1177/2327857915041023

Menachemi, N., & Collum, T. (2011). *Benefits and drawbacks of electronic health record systems*. Academic Press. doi:10.2147/RMHP.S12985

Mujkic, S., & Marinkovic, V. (2017). *Critical appraisal of reimbursement list in Bosnia and Herzegovina*. Academic Press. doi:10.3389/fphar.2017.00129

New Zealand Government. (2017). *Digital Hospital. Ministry of Health New Zealand*. Retrieved from https://www.health.govt.nz/our-work/ehealth/digital-health-2020/digital-hospital

Norbeck, T. (2012). *Drivers of health care costs; A physicians foundation white paper.* The Physicians Foundation, Empowering Physicians, Improving Healthcare. Retrieved from http://www.physiciansfoundation.org/uploads/default/Drivers_of_Health_Care_Costs_-_November_2012.pdf

Obama's Speech on the Economy. (2009). Federal News Service. *New York Times*. Retrieved from http://www.nytimes.com/2009/01/08/us/politics/08text-obama.html

OECD. (2010). How much is too much? In *OECD Health Policy Studies - Value for Money in Health Spending* (pp. 21-42). OECD Publisher. Retrieved from http://www.oecd.org/els/health-systems/value-for-money-in-health-spending.htm

Office of the National Coordinator for Health IT. (2016). *2016 interoperability Standards Advisory*. Office of the National Coordinator for Health IT. Retrieved from https://www.healthit.gov/sites/default/files/2016-interoperability-standards-advisory-final-508.pdf

Ontario Medical Association. (n.d.). *Starting a practice; A guide for new physicians*. OMA. Retrieved from https://www.oma.org/wp-content/uploads/1_startingpractice.pdf

Peplow, M. (2016). The 100000 Genomes Project. *BMJ (Clinical Research Ed.)*, *353*. doi:10.1136/bmj.i1757

Porter, M. (2015). An NHS under unsustainable pressure deserves a serious debate. *The Guardian*. Retrieved from https://www.theguardian.com/society/2015/jan/15/nhs-under-unsustainable-pressure-deserves-serious-debate

Power Health Solutions. (2017). *Power budgeting, forecasting and modelling; Business analytics functionality.* Adelaide, Australia: Power Health Solutions. Retrieved from http://www.powerhealthsolutions.com/budgeting

Rowland, C. (2014). Subsidies given for computerizing, but no reporting required when errors cause harm. Hazards tied to medical records rush. *The Boston Globe.* Retrieved from https://www.bostonglobe.com/news/nation/2014/07/19/obama-pushed-electronic-health-records-with-huge-taxpayer-subsidies-but-has-rebuffed-calls-for-hazards-monitoring-despite-evidence-harm/OV4njlT6JgLN67Fp1pZ01I/story.html

Safran, C., Bloomrosen, M., Hammond, W. E., Labkoff, S., Markel-Fox, S., Tang, P., & Detmer, D. E. (2007). Toward a framework for the secondary use of health data: An American medical informatics association white paper. *Journal of the American Medical Informatics Association, 14*(1), 1–9. doi:10.1197/jamia.M2273 PMID:17077452

Scholl, M., Stine, K., Hash, J., Bowen, P., Johnson, A., Smith, C. D., & Steinberg, D. J. (2008). *An introductory resource guide for implementing the health insurance portability and accountability act (HIPAA) security rule.* National Institute of Standards and Technology, US Department of Commerce. Retrieved from http://nvlpubs.nist.gov/nistpubs/Legacy/SP/nistspecialpublication800-66r1.pdf

Shulkin, D. J. (2016). *Beyond the VA crisis: Becoming a high-performance network.* New England Medical Journal.

Snyder, M. (2016). *Genomics and personalized medicine.* Oxford University Press. Retrieved from https://global.oup.com/academic/product/genomics-and-personalized-medicine-9780190234768?cc=us&lang=

Stanton, M. A. (2006). The high concentration of U.S. health care expenditures. *Research in Action,* (19). Retrieved from https://archive.ahrq.gov/research/findings/factsheets/costs/expriach/

Steen, J. (c 1663). The Sick Woman. *Shutterstock.* Retrieved from www.shutterstock.com

Sukel, K. (2015). *Cerner, Qualcomm partner to advance remote home health monitoring.* Retrieved from Healthcare Informatics: https://www.healthcare-informatics.com/news-item/cerner-qualcomm-partner-advance-remote-home-health-monitoring

The Guardian. (2014). The NHS could be 'overwhelmed' by people with long-term medical conditions. *The Guardian*. Retrieved from https://www.theguardian.com/society/2014/jan/03/nhs-overwhelmed-long-term-medical-conditions

The Office of the National Coordinator for Health Information Technology. (2015). *Connecting health and care for the nation; A shared nationwide interoperability roadmap*. The Office of the National Coordinator for Health Information Technology.

Veterans Affairs. (2016). Million veteran program. *Genomics*. US Department of Veterans Affairs. Retrieved from https://www.research.va.gov/topics/genomics.cfm#research2

Wagner, E. H., Austin, B. T., Davis, C., Hindmarsh, M., Schaefer, J., & Bonomi, A. (2001). Improving chronic illness care: Translating evidence into action. *Health Affairs*, *20*(6), 64–78. doi:10.1377/hlthaff.20.6.64 PMID:11816692

Wagner, E. H., Davis, C., Schaefer, J., Von Korff, M., & Austin, B. (1999). A survey of leading chronic disease management programs: Are they consistent with the literature? *Managed Care Quarterly*, *7*(3), 56–66. PMID:10620960

Warburton, D. E., Nicol, C. W., & Bredlin, S. S. (2006). Health benefits of physical activity: The evidence. *Canadian Medical Association Journal*, *174*(6), 801–809. doi:10.1503/cmaj.051351 PMID:16534088

Watzlaf, V. J., Zeng, X., Jarymowycz, C., & Firouzan, P. A. (2005). *Standards for the content of the electronic health record*. Retrieved from http://perspectives.ahima.org/standards-for-the-content-of-the-electronic-health-record/

Widen, S., & Haseltine, W. A. (2015). *The Estonian eHealth and eGovernance system*. ACCESS Health International. Retrieved from http://accessh.org/resource/case-study-the-estonian-ehealth-and-egovernance-system/

Chapter 5
Statistical Inference to Develop Budgets From Activity-Based Funding Costing Data

Harry Chiam
Boston Scientific, Australia

ABSTRACT

Activity-based funding (ABF) is a way of funding hospitals whereby they get paid for the number and mix of patients they treat. In order for governments to fund hospitals using ABF, hospitals use costing to inform the development of classification systems which provide valuable information for pricing purposes. Hospital patient costing is essential for understanding the total costs involved in treating a patient including the services or products used. This chapter outlines a methodology using simple statistics to prepare a budget for an inpatient ward using costing data. This method can be extended to other clinical areas (e.g., residential aged care or non-admitted).

DOI: 10.4018/978-1-5225-5082-2.ch005

INTRODUCTION

Activity Based Funding (ABF) is a way of funding hospitals for the number and mix of patients they treat. In order for governments to fund hospitals using ABF, hospitals use costing to inform the development of classification systems which provide valuable information for pricing purposes. Hospital patient costing is essential for understanding the total costs involved in treating a patient including the services or products used.

This paper outlines a methodology using simple statistics to prepare a budget for an inpatient ward using costing data. This method can be extended to other clinical areas, e.g. residential aged care or non-admitted.

BACKGROUND TO HOSPITAL COSTING

In many jurisdictions across the world where activity-based funding is used to inform healthcare funding, hospital product costing is the process of identifying the inputs used in a hospital and attributing the costs of those inputs to the production of products (patient and non-patient). It should be understated that this process is not simple and requires expertise in identifying inputs and outputs, guidance for allocating the costs, and considerable complex numerical processing, which can only realistically be done using purpose-built product costing software.

Broadly, the process of costing products consists of four steps (IHPA, 2014). "The first step is to manipulate the costs recorded in the general ledger to reflect the products that are being costed (this manipulation is best done inside the costing system, not the general ledger). This process involves identifying those costs incurred in the hospital, as well as those costs generated by the hospital that are necessary for producing the products to be costed. It then requires the alignment of the timing of incurring the costs and producing the products. Once all in-scope costs have been identified, the costs reported in all cost centres are mapped to the standard line items, and the cost centres are partitioned into overhead and final cost centres."

"The second step involves apportioning all costs in overhead cost centres to final costs centres. In performing this function it is important to ensure that the cost centres or parts of cost centres that are associated with non-patient products are allocated their fair share of overheads (if necessary, non-patient product costs centres may then be terminated, and only patient products costed to end-classes, typically individual patient service events)."

"The third step involves partitioning the final cost centres into product categories. Ideally, a final cost centre will fit entirely within a product category. In practice this is often not the case and the costs in some final cost centres need to be apportioned across more than one product category. As the focus is on costing patient products, it is important to clearly identify the costs associated with non-patient products. Ideally these costs should be carried in the costing process all the way through to producing final costs for non-patient products. Great care must be taken in this process, as errors here have significant impact on the final product costs."

"The fourth step involves, within each product category, allocating the costs in final cost centres to end-classes within that category. Ideally for the patient products the end-classes are individual patient services events (i.e. an admitted patient episode, an outpatient service event, or an Emergency Department service event, reflecting patient level costing). The allocation processes are complex, and good allocation requires advanced knowledge of hospital operations."

METHODS

The outputs of clinical costing are usually national hospital costing studies. For example, in Australia, the National Hospital Cost Data Collection (NHCDC) is

Figure 1. Hospital costing process

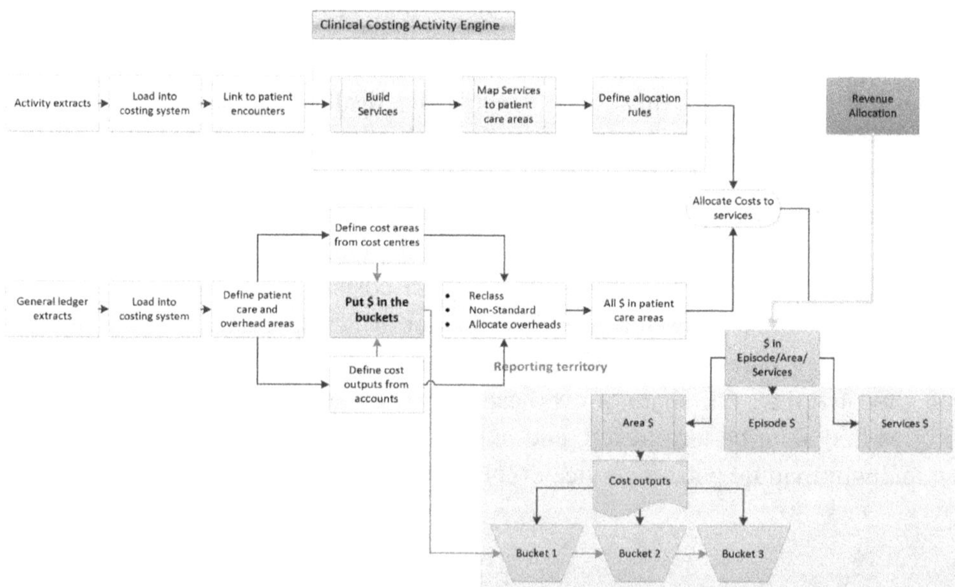

the annual collection of public hospital cost data from a range of public hospital facilities nationally. The objective of the NHCDC is to provide all Australian federal and state/territorial governments and the health care industry with a robust dataset developed using nationally consistent methods of costing hospital activity. The dataset is used for benchmarking, funding and planning hospital services and is the primary data set used to develop the National Efficient Price (NEP) and the National Efficient Cost (NEC).

An extract from the NHCDC is shown in Table 1.

Table 1. Costing data by line item

Admitted acute line item					
	Round 17		Round 18		Change in % contribution Round 17 to 18
Line item	Average $	% of total	Average $	% of total	percentage point
Salary & Wages Nursing	1381	30.0%	1367	29.5%	-0.4%
Salary & Wages Medical (Non VMO)	693	15.0%	713	15.4%	0.4%
Salary & Wages Medical (VMO)	202	4.4%	205	4.4%	0.0%
Salary & Wages Allied Health	214	4.6%	218	4.7%	0.1%
Salary & Wages Other	422	9.2%	426	9.2%	0.0%
On-costs	314	6.8%	321	6.9%	0.1%
Pathology	93	2.0%	96	2.1%	0.1%
Imaging	28	0.6%	26	0.6%	0.0%
Prostheses	146	3.2%	145	3.1%	0.0%
Medical supplies	248	5.4%	249	5.4%	0.0%
Goods and services	399	8.7%	393	8.5%	-0.2%
Pharmaceuticals PBS	28	0.6%	24	0.5%	-0.1%
Pharmaceuticals non-PBS	146	3.2%	140	3.0%	-0.1%
Blood	5	0.1%	5	0.1%	0.0%
Depreciation - building	65	1.4%	74	1.6%	0.2%
Depreciation - equipment	47	1.0%	41	0.9%	-0.1%
Hotel	139	3.0%	148	3.2%	0.2%
Corporate	23	0.5%	25	0.5%	0.0%
Lease	17	0.4%	16	0.3%	0.0%

A hospital may take the results from their own costing study to then drill down into the components of costs.

SUPERVISED LEARNING

Let's start by applying supervised learning to the analysis of hospital costs.

Suppose we have a dataset giving the nursing dollars and patient bed days of 31 patients in a given hospital.

We can plot the data as shown in Figure 2.

Given data like this, how can we learn to predict the nursing costs for this acute DRG, as a function of patient length of stay?

We will discuss a statistical technique called linear regression to analyse this problem. In linear regression, given input variables, e.g. length of stay, we can predict a numerical value, e.g. nursing dollars.

Linear regression captures the relationship between numerical output and input variables. The relationship is modelled as linear. So, in this example, the regression task is given length of stay, predict nursing dollars.

Linear regression consists of finding the best-fitting straight line through the points in the scatter plot above. The best-fitting line is called a regression line. The black diagonal line in Figure 2 is the regression line and consists of the predicted nursing dollars on Y for each possible value of length of stay on X. The vertical lines from the points to the regression line represent the errors of prediction. The red point is very near the regression line; its error of prediction is small. By contrast,

Table 2. Nursing dollars and average length of stay

ALOS	Nursing $
3.42	1599.61
2.21	1283.27
2.92	1292.57
2.26	818.84
2.28	885.8
1.98	856.06
2.03	575.16
2.34	857.57
2.69	856.69
1.32	309.6

Figure 2. Length of stay versus nursing dollars

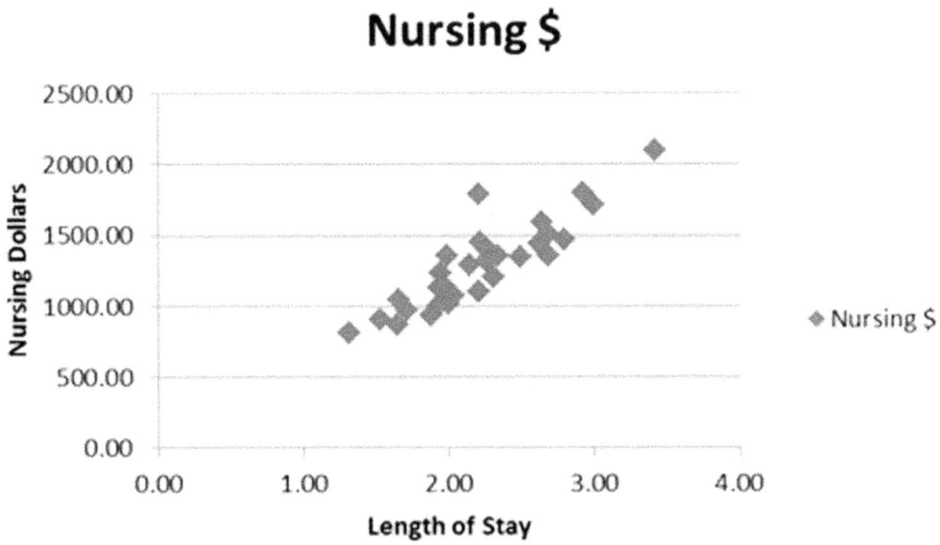

Table 3. Input and target variables

Input variable	Target Variable
ALOS	Nursing $
3.42	1599.61
2.21	1283.27
2.92	1292.57
2.26	818.84
2.28	885.8
1.98	856.06
2.03	575.16
2.34	857.57
2.69	856.69
1.32	309.6

Figure 3. Regression Example

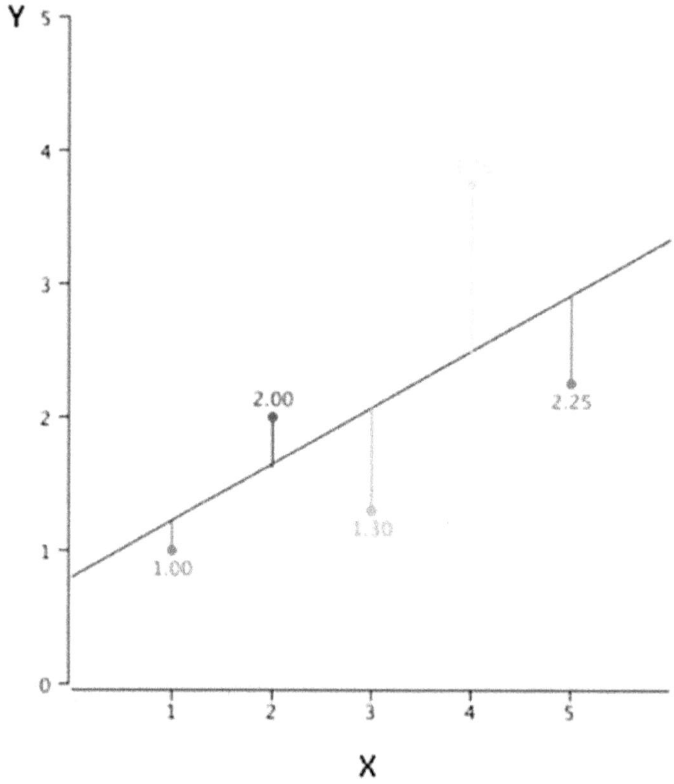

the yellow point is much higher than the regression line and therefore its error of prediction is large.

Numerically, the output of the regression can be written as follows:

$$y_1 = \Theta_0 + \Theta_1 X_1$$

where

- y_1 is predicted nursing costs
- Θ_0 is intercept or base case when bed days = 0
- Θ_1 is the amount that nursing costs changes with a unit increase in bed days
- x_1 is bed days

By far, the most commonly-used criterion for the best-fitting line is the line that minimizes the sum of the squared errors of prediction. In the age of computers, the regression line is typically computed in Microsoft Excel or with statistical software, e.g. R.

The same methodology could be used to predict clinical costs for other departments, e.g. medical, allied health, pharmacy, etc.

CONCLUSION

There is increasingly more data being created with the capture of costing statistics to support activity-based funding. This paper proposes a way of using regression to predict length of stay in a clinical setting and so hopes that it provides a suggested way for clinicians to prepared budgets and bench-mark performance in an activity-based funding environment.

REFERENCES

IHPA. (2014). *Hospital Patient Costing Standards*. IHPA.

Chapter 6
Managing Activity-Based Funding Using Costing Data and Activity-Based Budgets

Stephen A. Cole
Gold Coast University Hospital, Australia

ABSTRACT

This chapter will show how detailed information from an activity-based costing (ABC) system can be used to support activity-based funding (ABF) by providing management with a detailed perspective of the activity and how it can be used to internally model the allocation of target activity to build an activity-based budget (ABB). By building a set of internal cost weights based on ABC data, this chapter will show how activity forecast in a funding agreement can be broken up and applied to the individual cost centers that contributed to the activity in the current year. Building an ABB provides an evidence base for the overarching hospital budget and encourages the adoption of a focus on efficiency by hospital departments.

DOI: 10.4018/978-1-5225-5082-2.ch006

INTRODUCTION

Activity Based Costing (ABC) provides detailed information on the cost of the individual patient encounter and provides the basis for the development of an Activity Based Funding (ABF) model. The challenge for management within the health service is how to best use this detailed patient costing information to allow it to effectively manage the Activity Based Funding.

BACKGROUND

Within the Australian funding methodology, the main source of revenue for most large public hospitals is via Activity Based Funding. This funding is allocated using a standard unit of measure called a WAU or Weighted Activity Unit. A WAU is a measure of the relative resource usage required to generate the output activity. It varies from output group to output group. Australia uses different groupings for different types of activity. For acute inpatients, the output activity is grouped into Diagnosis Related Groupings (DRGs), with a modified version being used in the national model for Mental Health Inpatients. Non-acute patients use the SNAP (Semi- & Non-Acute Patients) grouping, Outpatients use Tier-2 clinic groupings, whilst Emergency Department encounters use URGs (Urgency Related Groupings). All the patients in these different types of activity have their encounters grouped up into the relevant grouping, and each grouping has a relative weight designated in WAU that is indicative of the resources required to produce that activity so, for example, the WAU associated with a kidney transplant is many times more than might be generated by a carpal tunnel release.

Of course, each individual patient encounter has a cost. This cost will vary for every patient, even those within the same grouping. Hence, for example, each individual kidney transplant patient encounter is likely to have a different cost from every other kidney transplant encounter, because they will have a different length of stay, time in theatre, different drugs, diagnostic tests, and all the other items that will vary from encounter to encounter, and consequently change the total cost. From a financial perspective, the key point of interest is the relationship between this cost and the revenue received for the patient. Just as the price weight that determines the revenue is based on an average cost from a statistically large population, then the average cost within the hospital for a particular group of patients should be fairly consistent, as should the manner in which those costs are built up from all the different services the patients receive.

The Independent Hospital Pricing Authority (IHPA) provides a list of price weights each year that represent the average relative resource weights, based on the NHCDC information collected in the previous year. Some states adopt this model with no changes, whilst others implement state-based modifications. For example, Queensland applies a raft of state specific modifications that can, in some cases, significantly modify the revenue generated.

By comparing the cost to the revenue, it is possible to tell if a hospital is making or losing money on a particular patient encounter, and by collectively looking at an ABF group of encounters, identify if there might be an overall profit or loss. Whilst this might seem a little mercenary, it is essential that hospitals understand this and manage it effectively; otherwise, if the hospital ends the year with a net loss, and continues to do this, then the government (and eventually the taxpayer) is obliged to bail them out. There are therefore, a number of performance requirements pertaining to fiscal management that hospital financial managers are obliged to meet.

At the highest level, it is possible to look at the ABF revenue in comparison to the ABF cost of the activity; however, in order to discuss this with the service line managers within the organisation, it is important to be able to produce this at a lower level. Service line managers will want to know if they are efficient. A proxy for efficiency is comparing cost per WAU to the efficient price for the WAU. If your cost per WAU is higher than the efficient price per WAU, then the assumption is that the service line may be inefficient, with the converse being that if the cost per WAU is less than the efficient price, then the service line is efficient. There are, of course, a number of caveats associated with this. It assumes that the costing is accurate, and we know that there are several factors that potentially impact the accuracy of the costing. However, the major factor that causes a problem is that the allocation of activity to a service line is problematic. WAUs are a measure of the activity for the entire patient encounter, so it is generated at the conclusion of the encounter, hence it is an output measure. Therefore, many different areas are likely to have contributed to the care of the patient during their encounter. An admitted patient may have spent time in theatre, possibly ICU, received pathology and imaging tests, received allied health services and potentially been transferred between several different wards. Hence there are multiple different areas that have contributed resources and costs associated with the overall care of the patient. Any measure that only looks at the output cost and revenue is therefore not going to be an accurate measure of the overall efficiency of a service line.

It is also likely that a service line may provide aspects of care for patients not directly associated with the end product. A service line such as infectious diseases is likely to provide consults to patients all over the hospital as well as to patients specifically admitted for an infectious disease. Allowing for the challenges this model of service provides in terms of accurately costing these consults outside of the service line, again, there is a problem if there is only a focus on the output costings and activity.

There is therefore a need to be able to allocate activity to all the services that provide care to the patient so that activity and cost can be aligned and the efficiency of an individual area can be determined. This process can then be further extended to provide allocations of activity to the individual costs centres that combine to make up an area. Aligning activity with the cost centre then provides the basis to build an Activity Based Budget.

Figure 1. Hypothetical encounter timeline

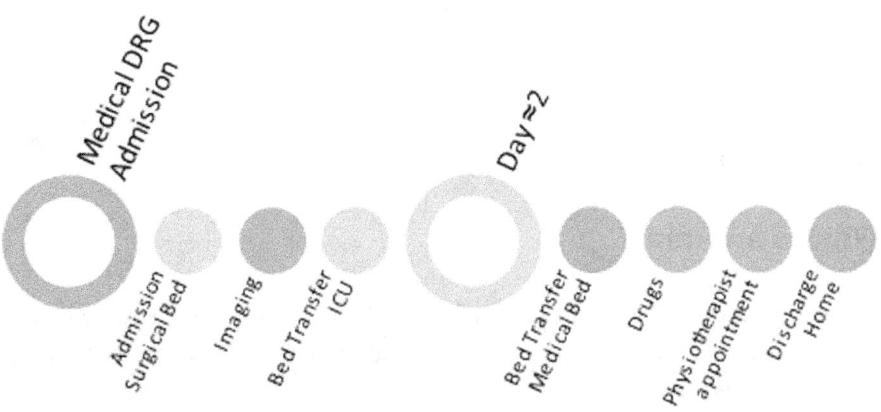

Figure 2. Direct apportionment of activity

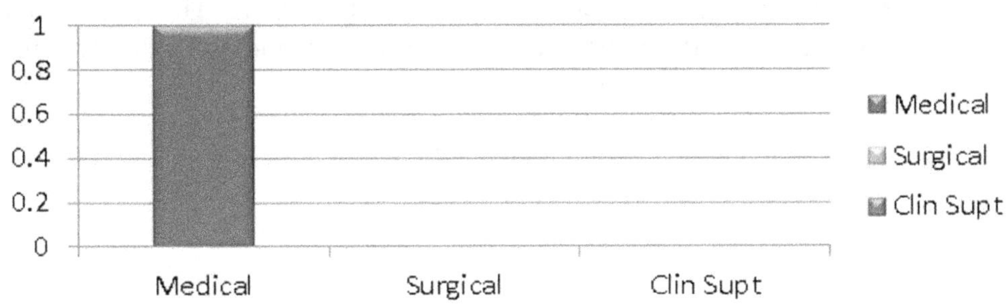

Figure 3. Apportionment to direct clinical areas

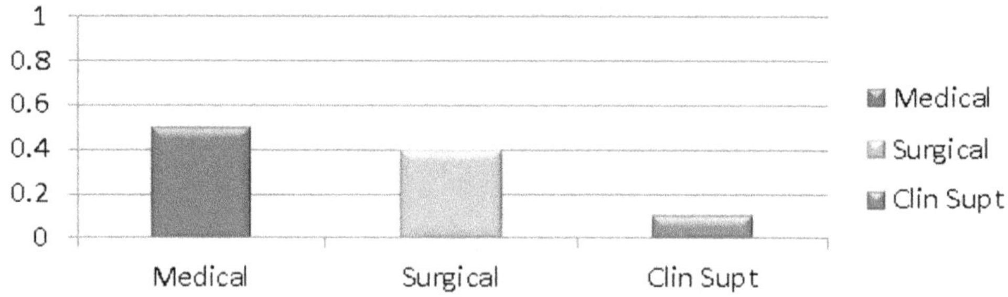

Figure 4. Apportionment including all overhead/indirect areas

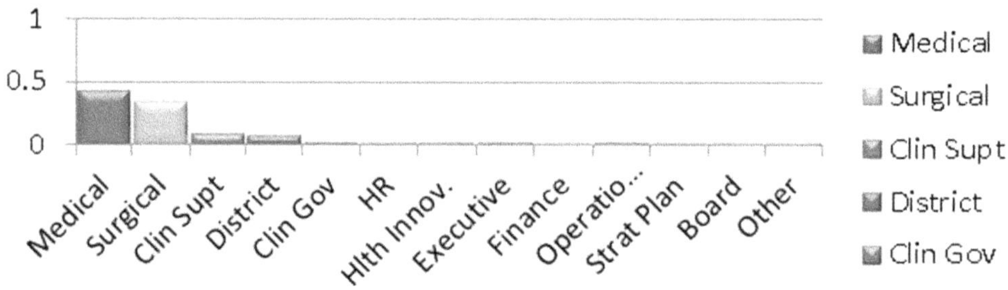

MAIN FOCUS

What Is an Area?

An area is grouping of Cost Centres for which the same costing rules can be applied. This means we do not have to develop allocation rules for every cost centre in the General Ledger.

An Area may be named differently in different costing systems but the general concept is similar.

A grouping of cost centres might consist of all the various radiographer cost centres, or all the cost centres associated with a particular ward. The rationale for grouping cost centres together will be dependent on the situation at an individual site.

Figure 5. Allocation of WAUs to cost centres

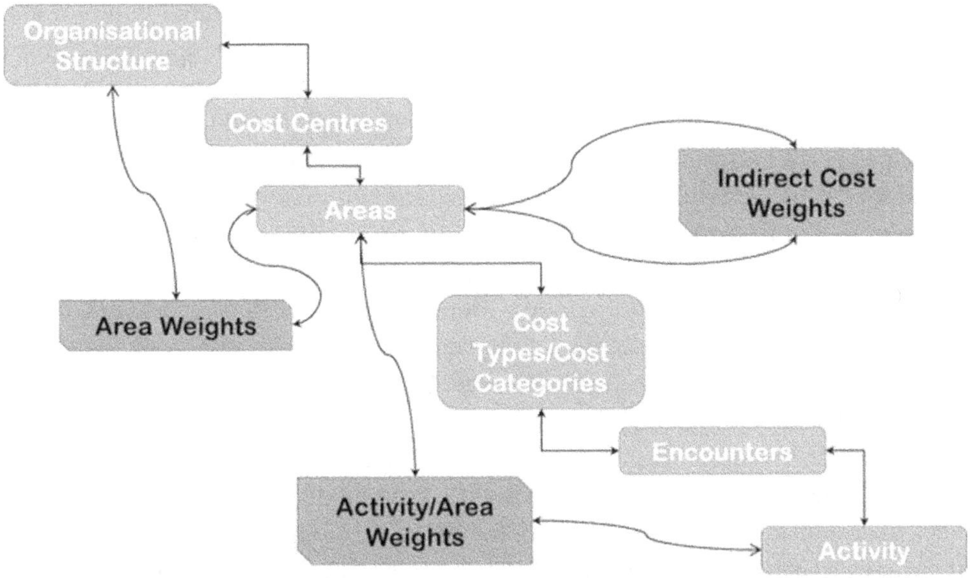

Aligning Activity to an Area

It is essential from a financial perspective to be able to phase this accurately across the year and to be able to apportion this activity to the relevant service lines that are going to generate the activity.

In ABF, activity is generated only by the finished patient encounter, and subsequent to any coding or scoring that might be necessary to determine the ABF group that the encounter belongs to. It is a weight indicative of the relative resource usage that is anticipated to provide the activity. This weight is inclusive of all the different resources and products that would typically provide the activity, but it is a standardised measure based on a state or nationwide average cost for the activity. This means that it is not possible to differentiate all the different types of products and resources that typically contributed to the total patient encounter at an individual hospital. Therefore, when presented with an overarching ABF activity target for the total health service, or even for an individual service within a hospital, it is difficult to determine what that actually means for the individual areas that contribute to the discrete patient encounters that will generate the activity to meet the target.

Financial management within the hospital will often start with the development of the annual budget based on the expected revenue and expenditure for the coming financial year. With large tertiary hospitals often having a budget that may be over 80% ABF, it means that it is important to understand the anticipated activity for the coming year, the expected revenue that activity will provide, and the how that translates into a budget for all the different areas of the hospital. With the expected amount of ABF activity comes an expected amount of revenue, which can then be apportioned based on the budget to all the areas within the hospital and then subsequently to the individual cost centres. Using an Activity Based Budget (ABB) is a method for taking the information within the hospital's Activity Based Costing system to apportion that expected activity and subsequent revenue back to the cost centres. An ABB informs the overall budget build, however it can only reflect the existing internal financial arrangements within the hospital. Planned organisational restructures within the new budget year, changes in clinical practice or the introduction of new services, are just some of the things that can modify resource usage, so these need to be considered independently of the ABB when building a budget. However, there are also activity based tools that allow us to model the possible budget impacts of some of these additional factors.

Most state health departments use a capitation model for ABF expenditure to limit their liability, with some using a purchaser-provider model to purchase a discrete amount of activity from a hospital, usually in discrete patient groupings such as Acute Inpatients, Non-Acute Inpatients, Mental Health, Emergency and Outpatient activity. This means that the hospital is presented with a capped maximum amount of activity that they will receive funding for. Activity in excess of that cap is funded at a severely discounted rate (if at all), whilst failing to meet the activity target (usually with only a very small tolerance) can mean that a financial penalty is applied to the hospital. Hence, one of the first things a hospital must do is understand their own forecast activity independently of any future activity models provided by external analysis.

It may also be important to assign specific activity amounts to discrete purchase groupings, for example if the government launches an initiative to target stroke or cardiac arrest and assigned specific WAU for these initiatives. It would be absolutely essential that the targets are reflective of these initiatives.

Forecasting the Activity

Once the hospital has a forecast of the ABF activity it is expecting, as well as the ABF activity that is forecast, it becomes possible to begin building an Activity

Based Budget. In its simplest form, an ABB reflects the proportional contribution of each cost centre's expenditure to historical activity, by applying those proportional weights to the new activity targets to derive a budgeted expenditure value to meet that new target.

Determining an accurate forecast is often challenging process. Some state Health Departments have set targets at both an overarching level and at certain levels within the model. For example, Queensland Health sets a total ABF target, but also sets targets for Acute Inpatients, Semi- and Non-Acute Inpatients (SNAP), Outpatients, Mental Health as well as Procedures and Interventions, which are typically for procedures that could be done as outpatients or inpatients (e.g. chemotherapy, renal dialysis, endoscopies). There might also be targets forecast at a lower level, such as the SRG (Service Related Grouping) level. There may also be targets for individual initiatives that have been specifically funded. Not all of these lower level targets may need to be followed. The funding agreement with the health service will usually be specific about targets that have to be met, for example Queensland does provide forecast SRG level targets as a means of demonstrating the evidence base behind the purchased acute inpatient target, but does not expect these lower level targets to be rigorously followed.

It is therefore important that hospitals develop their own targets that are reflective of their anticipated activity. There are a number of approaches that can be adopted for calculating targets, based on historical proportions and projected forward. The methods used will often depend on the technical skills of the resources doing the projections. Given the variable nature of activity this is not necessarily an issue, as long as the hospital has processes that will allow it to manage variations in actual activity compared to the projected. The real issue is staying within the capitated total activity purchased.

Activity Above the Cap

Given that there has been a consistent growth in demand for healthcare services, in order to ensure adequate funding, a hospital should be certain that their targeted activity, based on their own growth projections, is consistent with the projections made by their state health department that is purchasing the activity. At the core of any projection should be an understanding of activity that is "unavoidable", that is, activity that cannot be delayed without significantly increasing the risk to the patient. Therefore, unavoidable might include all emergency admissions, emergency triage categories one two and three, as well as consideration of some category four and five encounters, and elective admissions in the two most urgent categories.

With capped activity targets, the ability to manage and control activity to remain within those targets might be essential. If targets are exceeded, then this will usually incur additional cost, but may not necessarily incur additional revenue. If above target activity generates additional revenue but at a reduced rate, if the extra activity is done at marginal cost, then there might be an advantage in doing above cap activity, however, this assumes that costs are being controlled. This would assume that major expenditure items, such as staff levels, are kept at levels that are in line with the budget developed for the capped target. Of course, some types of activity incur costs that may not be able to be contained to a budget level, for example, some types of activity that have a very high drug costs component. It is therefore important to understand not just the type of additional activity, but also the type of costs that this activity is generating.

A Brief Overview of Activity Based Budgets

The core concept in Activity Based Budgets is the proportion that each cost centre contributes to each type of activity. It is up to the individual hospital to determine the level of granularity they wish to use, however using the standard ABF encounter

Figure 6. Concept diagram activity based budgets

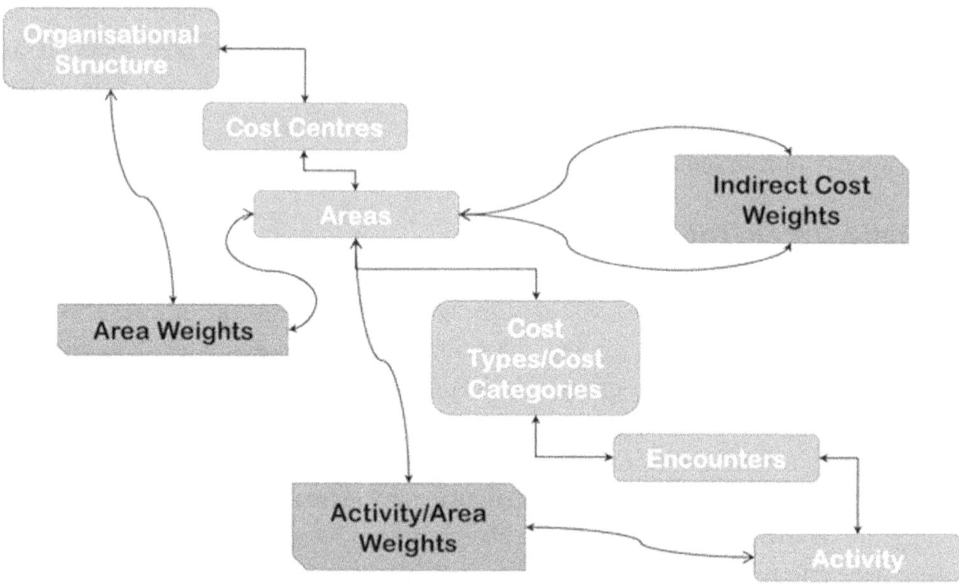

groups such as DRGs, URGs, Tier 2 clinics, SNAP groups may represent the most useful option, as this can allow for the opportunity to use benchmarking components from other sources such a Health Round Table (HRT) and the National Hospital Cost Data Collection (NHCDC) to refine the ABB.

In a simple example, if a particular cost centre provided $10,000 worth of resources for a discrete DRG with 5 encounters during the year for a total cost of $50,000, then the weight for the cost centre would be 0.2 ($10,000/$50,000). Assuming that the hospital expects activity will remain the same in the budget year for the DRG (5 encounters), but due to changes in weights and prices, the amount of revenue expected is $60,000, then the ABB amount for the cost centre derived from the activity for that DRG is 0.2 of $60,000, or $12,000. Of course this is multiplied by over 700 DRGs, and must also be applied for the different classifications for outpatients and emergency, as well as SNAP and Mental Health.

It is also possible to derive the proportional cost centre weights at a more detailed level within each DRG to align with benchmarking standards. This means that the ABB does not need to be built using the historical efficiency of the hospital, but could utilise the bucket components in the NHCDC or HRT costing information to provide an industry standard efficiency level for comparison.

Adjustments must also be made for accounting practices within the hospital. This might mean redistributing pathology and drug costs as well as depreciation. Efficiency adjustments might also be made. The method by which the ABB is to be presented to managers within the hospital will also need to be considered. If the budget process is not properly managed, there is potential for some managers to simply accept the figures and not review them in light of possible changes in practice.

It is also possible to use the costing information to assist with modelling. It is possible to use if for modelling the services, products and resources that can comprise the new activity purchased or targeted in the budget. It can also be used for evaluating the possible impact of changes in clinical services.

The advantage of using costing data to support the budget process is that it provides an evidence base that makes it easier to validate anticipated budget requests. Using modern business informatics tools, it is also possible to develop tools that build on the information in the costing database to support ongoing budget management through the course of the financial year.

The Methodology of Deriving an ABB

The methodology described here will be generic and can be used to calculate an ABB manually, although there are automated systems that offer similar functionality. Different systems may use different methods but the underlying principles are generally similar, in that they will take existing costing information and use it to build a budget for new activity based on anticipated new targets. In essence, there are two processes that must be used. One process that develops a set of weights to apportion the targets associated with activity to the areas, and another process that develops a set of cost weights to apportion the activity from the areas to the direct and indirect cost centres that comprise the areas.

Much of the process is all about assigning proportions, as the total amount of purchased activity might be capped, keeping the total amount of activity absolutely constant through the ABB manual calculations helps ensure that the process is error free. In other words, the total amount of budgeted activity should match the total amount of targeted activity.

ABF Grouping Proportions

Targets are unlikely to be set to the DRG levels, and the mapping of patients to particular target groups may also sometimes be problematic. For example, at the patient level you might have Emergency Department patients with URGs, however the targets are by UDG. There may also be discrepancies between the national funding model and the state as well as subtle distinctions, for example Queensland does not pay for "did-not-wait" patients in ED whilst the national model does, however these patients are different from patients that left after treatment commenced which Queensland classifies as "left at own risk".

Hence, the first step is to align the existing activity which is going to be used to calculated the ABB with the new targets. This might mean mapping each individual encounter to the relevant target. Once activity is mapped to the target, then the proportion of target activity that the historical activity represents can be calculated using the following formula:

$$Encounter\_prop'n\_purchasing\_group = \frac{Individual\_Encounter\_Activity}{\sum Current\_Activity\_for\_purchasing\_group} \times Calculated\_target\_for\_purchasing\_group$$

Once the proportion of purchased activity an individual encounter is linked to is determined, then we have also have a link to the costs associated with the individual encounter and know what amount of purchased activity these costs are a portion of.

Determine the Cost Type Category Proportions

Once the individual encounter is linked to the target, then summaries are built based on the cost type and category for each area for each individual encounter. This sets up the initial values that can then be used for apportioning the activity to the areas and then to the cost centres that comprise those areas. Depending on how you manage budgets as well as the external funding, you might find different summarisation methods advantageous. For example, Queensland funds depreciation separately from their ABF component, so it is important that depreciation can be identified at this point, we differentiate between the direct and overhead costs, we also may need to identify other costs such as drugs.

Summarisation to this level of detail is only necessary to support subsequent differentiation. If this is not required, then there are subsequent savings in terms of database size and processing time. Selecting the level of differentiation is also dependent on what your costing database will support. So, whilst the use of Cost Type and Category is ideal for Queensland purposes, an alternative would be use of the Health Roundtable (HRT) buckets. This would then facilitate using benchmark proportions as an alternative budget allocation method instead of the current allocation proportions. This could prove very useful in determining if budget allocations are significantly at variance with peer facilities.

Figure 7. Individual encounter

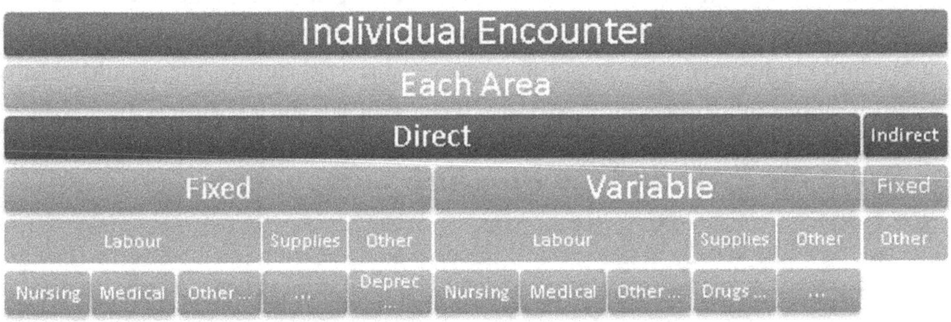

Allocate the Targets to the Areas

Based on the first two steps which map the target activity to the individual encounter and the detail costs within the encounter, it is possible to apportion the targets to the areas. Targets can be apportioned at the very low level of the individual and then summed up for each area. It might seem unusual that we are using existing activity to map new targets, however it is important to remember that the existing activity is only providing a proportional map for the distribution of the new activity. Mapping of the activity will be based on existing efficiencies, so there are also opportunities to evaluate the cost of activity using these calculations.

As an example, in this step, if an area contributed $1,000 of encounter total cost of $4,000, and the total target activity apportioned to the encounter was 1.2 WAU, then the amount of WAUs assigned to the area for this encounter would be ¼ of 1.2 WAU or 0.3 WAU.

By summing the WAUs for each area, then we have the total activity for an area. As we have devolved costs at a high level of detail, it allows for targets to be apportioned to the very detailed level of the cost type and category.

Determine the Proportion That Each Cost Centre Contributes to an Area

Before we can allocate activity back to the cost centre, we must first understand the proportion that each cost centre contributed to the area. Because the costing process handles direct and indirect expenditure differently, it may be more convenient to calculate weights separately for both the direct and indirect cost centres. Given that cost centres within an area are considered very similar as far as costing is concerned, it is possible to allocate the targets to cost centres based on the proportion that each cost centre has contributed to the overall expenditure within the area.

We can then allocate the activity to the individual cost centre. Again, because we are looking to only apportion the targets to the cost centre, we should always end up with the same amount of WAU activity that we started with.

Applying the Price and the Non-ABF Components

Once we have the WAUs at the level of the cost centres, then it is a straight-forward to determine the dollars for each CC by multiplying the WAU by the price. However, this is not necessarily the full picture, as there will always be a number of non-ABF components associated with the budget. The allocation method for these is likely to vary based on the funding supplied for these state by state and might even vary for each site. Therefore, each site will need to develop a methodology that is suitable for their individual requirements.

A suggested method would be to use the historical apportionment of expenditure to the costs centres associated with non-ABF activity, and use the same proportions to allocate the new funding amounts for the different non-ABF activity streams.

Before a full Activity Based Budget can be created, all aspects that contribute to the budget must be considered. This might also include site specific grants, or any anticipated allowances applied part way through the year such as award rate changes. Again, these can vary from state to state, and require specific handling.

Presenting the Activity Based Budget

An ABB helps to inform the development of the full hospital budget; however it should not be the sole input into the budget build. It provides an evidence base which allows informed decisions, however, an ABB reflects the existing activity and expenditure at a site. It is not reflective of new services that might be opening, or revisions of existing service that might change the efficiency or the mix of patients seen by that service.

In addition, hospitals also provide many services that may not be ABF funded, such as community based services. These will have their own budget consideration. There may also be allowances for items such as depreciation which is funded as a separate item in some jurisdictions. Expected salary increases during the year may also have discrete funding allowed. Hence an ABB should not be considered as the only driver of a hospital budget, but it can provide an evidence base for the major portion of a hospital's budget.

These will need to be considered in consultation with the clinical departments. It would be anticipated that any new service or significant change to an existing service would only be initiated with the delivery of a full business case. A business case would include a full analysis of the relative cost benefit based on the activity based costing and funding information, hence this should be possible to integrate into the budget.

It is therefore useful to have a tool which allows the distribution of the budget to the relevant management staff in the hospital in a form which allows them to discuss it with their own staff. To this end, the development of tools in products such as MS Excel can assist, as this can allow the delivery of significant volumes of information, but also allow the workbook to be locked down, allowing updating only of the sections relevant for input into the budget. It can also allow the information supplied to be filtered so that it is relevant to a discrete budget department, or a collection.

The amount of discussion associated with these budgets is not necessarily less than the conventional budget methodology, but it does tend to change the nature of the discussion. The management of the various clinical departments will wish to be assured that the methodologies used do not treat one area significantly better than another, and they will particularly wish to ascertain that none of the budget departments they are responsible for are disadvantaged in any way. Of course, there will be some budget departments which will be disadvantaged, however there should be sufficient evidence in the ABB and the distributed workbook to show why a budget department has been disadvantaged.

The transition from a conventional budget build to an Activity Based Budget, might also require a compromise approach to ensure that budget departments where there is a significant variation between the new and the conventional methodology have an opportunity to adjust. This might mean developing a tailored approach for each department, as some departments might be able to sustain a significant year-on-year change more easily than others. It may also be that the overarching director of a group of budget departments might advise on the advisability of why one of their departments could sustain a significant budget decrement whilst another sees an increment.

Productivity Dividends and Other Adjustments

Just as the Department of Health can apply a productivity dividend to the budget received by the hospitals, so it is possible for the Chief Executive of a hospital to decide to apply an internal productivity dividend or equivalent. The money derived from this dividend can be used for a number of purposes, for instance it might form the basis for a range of quality and innovation incentives.

The methodology used for applying a productivity dividend or any other adjustment should be absolutely clear, so that it is consistent with the evidence based approach of the rest of an ABB. It may also mean that a different approach is required for different departments such as indirect or overhead departments. The methodology used will also be driven by the availability of data within the budget process to support it.

So, for example, a dividend based on efficiency is usually fairly easy to apply within the context of an ABB, as you should have already derived efficiency information for every department in the hospital, i.e. you will have both cost and revenue information for every cost centre allowing the determination of a measure of efficiency. This consequently allows the application of an efficiency dividend that might be more generous for departments that are more efficient and more onerous for those that are less efficient.

If the dividend is anticipated to reward quality, then one methodology might be to apply this based on how well clinical departments manage patients with CHADx (Classification of Hospital Acquired Diagnoses), or HAC (Hospital Acquired Conditions). This might require additional data to be captured, however it can encourage the consideration of quality as a driver of revenue, prior to the application of any penalties for poor quality of care applied to a hospital through a revenue model. In this example, for indirect or overhead departments, a flat percentage might be the easiest way to equitably apply a dividend. Incorporating an incentive into the budget process like this can be applied even without going developing a full ABB.

It is useful that when a dividend is applied like this, that there be suitable reporting tools to allow departments to monitor their performance. This would allow the impact of applying a quality based dividend to be extended through the year by providing feedback information on an ongoing basis.

CONCLUSION

The development and implementation of an Activity Based Budget is a result of having most of the revenue for a hospital being derived from Activity Based Funding and then seeking to internalise the revenue model. It is enabled by having an Activity Based Costing system installed to provide the necessary level of costing information to allow the allocation of funds to the internal cost centres. Conceptually, it is similar to the manner in which the actual ABF revenue model allocates all the funds to the different hospitals – overall funds are allocated based on target activity levels and a series of detail weights derived from the costing information.

An Activity Based Budget can mean that clinicians who would never have paid any attention before, are now interested in costing, as their own annual funding is now being affected by the patient costing information. This forms an effective incentive to improve the quality of data available to build the costing information and on the visibility of the costing information within the hospital.

The ABB however is just one outcome which is possible with improved information that is provided by the implementation of an Activity Based Costing system. There are multiple areas where the dissemination of ABC information within the hospitals may be beneficial. One of these might be associated with quality of care, which allows the cost of care to be linked to complications acquired in the hospital. Another is the opportunity to look at the ongoing costs associated with linked encounters to form a continuum of care. This is also improved as community health is increasingly captured and costed, even though it may not yet be part of an ABF revenue model.

Chapter 7
Health Economic Implications of Complications Associated With Pancreaticoduodenectomy:
A Retrospective Cohort Cost Study

Jason Wang
Austin Health, Australia

Laurence Weinberg
Austin Health, Australia

ABSTRACT

Clinical costing is a powerful tool to bridge the disconnect between financial and clinical information, and is an ideal platform to conduct research aimed at informing value-based clinical decision making. This chapter will provide an example of the utility of activity-based costing to elucidate the costs of complications following pancreaticoduodenectomy, a high acuity procedure with high costs. It will show the significance of clear clinical costing in targeting cost containment in a tertiary hospital environment.

DOI: 10.4018/978-1-5225-5082-2.ch007

INTRODUCTION AND BACKGROUND

As healthcare policy makers increasingly judge quality based on both costs and outcomes, the importance of cost containment has become paramount. Pancreaticoduodenectomy (PD), commonly referred to as a Whipple procedure (Whipple, Parsons, & Mullins, 1935), is a complex, highly invasive and costly surgical procedure performed most commonly in elderly patients and associated with significant perioperative morbidity. It is considered standard treatment for resectable malignant or benign cancers arising in the pancreatic head, ampulla, distal bile duct or duodenum. Despite low perioperative mortality, PD is associated with a morbidity rate of approximately 50% for major complications (Warrillow et al., 2010) due to its invasive nature. Postoperative complications are a greater determinant of mortality than patient and intraoperative risk factors post-major surgery (Khuri et al., 2005), and are associated with both increased length of stay (LOS) and the requirement for further operative intervention (Gupta, Turaga, Miller, Loggie, & Foster, 2011). Furthermore, it has been shown that the development of complications following pancreatic surgery is the most significant factor of increased cost (Enestvedt et al., 2012; Vonlanthen et al., 2011). Complications following PD have significant clinical and economic burden, and therefore represent a target for improvement.

Despite this knowledge, for patients undergoing PD there remains a lack of research investigating the basis of costs and their relationship to the development of complications. Topal et al. (Topal, Peeters, Vandeweyer, Aerts, & Penninckx, 2007) examined hospital cost-categories of PD using an activity-based costing method, and reported that hospitalisation and medical staffing costs were significantly increased in PD patients with complications. Further analyses of this nature are required to determine potential targets for cost containment and sustainable structural changes in the hospital services. Additionally, a dearth of accurate, quality costing data detracts from the ability to make conclusive remarks on the economic burden of complications following major surgery, including major pancreatic surgery (Patel, Bergman, Moore, & Haglund, 2013).

MAIN FOCUS OF THE CHAPTER

Objectives

Our primary objectives were to determine the health economic burden of complications, measured using the Clavien-Dindo classification scheme (Dindo, Demartines, & Clavien, 2004), of PD patients presenting to a high-volume tertiary teaching hospital. In addition, the authors examined the genesis of cost differentials between complicated and uncomplicated stays. Secondary objectives were to identify patient and anaesthetic factors that may influence clinical and economic outcomes.

Our study was conducted to confirm the hypothesis that hospital costs for PD are increased with both severity and number of complications. The authors also conducted exploratory analyses to generate hypotheses related to the relationship between complications and specific cost centres.

METHODS

Study Design

The study was approved by the Austin Health Human Research Ethics Committee. This cohort study considered the index admission and any 30-day readmissions for patients with and without complications following PD.

Setting

The authors considered patients undergoing PD between July 2011 and December 2016 at Austin Hospital, a university hospital with a high-volume hepato-pancreaticobiliary service. Data relating to their preoperative, intraoperative and postoperative details was collected from a prospectively maintained electronic medical database. Collected data included patient demographics, American Society of Anesthesiologists (ASA) class, preoperative blood values, comorbidities, pathological diagnosis, intraoperative and postoperative fluid balance, operation duration, usage of blood products, 30-day readmissions, and the presence and grade of any complications.

Participants

Patients undergoing classic PD (Whipple) or pylorus-preserving PD (PPPD) for any indication were identified from the Austin Health Information Services database using the ICD-10 code "30584-00: Pancreaticoduodenectomy with formation of stoma" for the desired date range. The operation type was further validated by examining the operation report in electronic medical records. Patients undergoing total, distal or completion pancreatectomy were excluded.

Ten consultant surgeons performed at least one PD during the study period. All patients underwent a standardised Enhanced Recovery After Surgery (ERAS) protocol introduced in our institution in August 2009 with the program fully established in 2010. As part of our institutions ERAS protocol, all patients underwent preoperative multidisciplinary assessment and where necessary were optimised prior to surgery. Preoperative haemoglobin optimisation was based on the National Blood Authority of Australia's patient blood management initiative(Authority, 2012). General anaesthesia was managed using a hospital ERAS protocol designed to standardise care with regards to perioperative fasting, analgesia, fluid intervention, antiemesis, antibiotic and chemo-thromboprophylaxis use. Regular dietitian input was routine in all patients to determine graduation from nasogastric feeding. Postoperative analgesia was optimised by a dedicated acute pain service and all patients received daily physiotherapy. Postoperative surgical care was standardised for nasogastric tube, surgical drain and urinary catheter removal. Discharge criterion included unassisted mobilisation, full dietary intake, satisfactory pain control, and absence of medical or surgical complication.

Variables

The presence of complications was coded from electronic medical records and then manually cross-checked with the patients' medical records by two independent investigators, before being further stratified according to the Clavien-Dindo system. The Clavien-Dindo system is a validated schema classifying complications based on the level of treatment required: Grade I, a deviation from the normal postoperative course without requiring intervention, excluding antiemetics, antipyretics, analgesia, diuretics, electrolyte and physiotherapy; Grade II, requiring pharmacological treatment, blood transfusion or total parenteral nutrition; Grade III: requiring radiological, surgical or endoscopic intervention; Grade IV: life-threatening complication; Grade V: death(Dindo et al., 2004). The presence of postoperative pancreatic fistula (POPF) was adjudged using the International Study Group on Pancreatic Fistula (ISGPF) definition (Bassi et al., 2005); delayed gastric emptying was defined as per the International Study Group of Pancreatic Surgery (ISGPS) definition(Wente et al., 2007).

The principal diagnosis was ascertained from ICD-10-CM codes. Preoperative demographic and disease-related data was collected. This included American Society of Anesthesiologists (ASA) score, preoperative bloods, and comorbidities. Cost analysis included the index admission for PD, and did not consider the preoperative course or readmissions. Costs were calculated using an activity-based costing methodology, which allocates costs according to service volume. A general ledger for the relevant costing period was loaded into specialised software, and relevant clinical cost buckets were created. These cost buckets were then matched with patient care activities to allocate costs. Twelve cost categories were then created to combine costs in a simplistic form – "anaesthesia" (anaesthetic drugs), "operative theatre", "intensive care unit", "ward" (cost of hospital bed, nursing, catering, etc.), "consults" (surgical, anaesthetic, medical and ICU consults), "allied health" (e.g. dietitian, diabetic educator, physiotherapy), "pathology" (e.g. blood tests, microbiology), "blood products" (e.g. red blood cells, albumin), "pharmacy" (drug dispensing), "radiology" (e.g. x-rays, CT, radiological procedures), "MET call" (medical emergency team call) and "hospital in the home". The present study combines both direct and indirect costs to compute a total cost for each patient. Only in-hospital costs were considered. No cost discounting took place due to the limited time horizon. Costs were inflated by average Australian Consumer Price Index (CPI) between 2011-2017 and then converted to 2017 USD ($) using the market rate on 25th May 2017.

Data Sources/Measurement

Clavien-Dindo grading allocation was assessed independently by two authors (JW and LW) and a consensus reached for each patient. Where exact volumes of blood products were not recorded, one unit of fresh frozen plasma and packed red blood cells were assumed to be 250mLs and 310mLs respectively.

Bias

Potential selection bias was reduced by including all consecutive patients within the study dates.

Study Size

The availability of economic data only from the 2011-2012 financial year, as well as the number of cases performed at our institution, determined the sample size.

Quantitative Variables

The authors grouped the number of complications into five groups: zero, one, two, three and four or above complications. The authors chose this grouping because they were interested in the economic burden of complication clustering, and the predictability of not only the grade of complication but the number of complications on cost.

Statistical Methods

Discrete and continuous variables were described as medians and interquartile ranges, whilst hospital costs were described as means and standard deviations. Categorical variables were described as totals and frequencies (%). Univariate analyses were conducted using Fisher's exact test, Pearson's χ-square test, unpaired *t*-test or Mann-Whitney test as appropriate. Differences in cost between patients grouped by complication number or severity were determined with the one-way analysis of variance test. A p-value of ≤ 0.05 was considered statistically significant. GraphPad Prism 7, version 7.0c, was used for all analyses.

RESULTS

Participants

One hundred consecutive patients underwent PD during the study period. Preoperative, intraoperative and postoperative characteristics are summarised in Table 1.

Main Results

100 consecutive patients undergoing PD at our institution between July 2011 and December 2016 were included. The median age was 67 years (IQR 58-74) with 52 males and 48 females. Median BMI was 26.1 kg/m^2 (IQR 23.5-28.7). 78 classic PD and 22 pylorus-preserving PD (PPPD) were performed, with malignant lesions the most common indication for surgery (n = 84). Median duration of surgery was 445 minutes (IQR 390-516) with a median blood loss of 300 mLs (IQR 200-450).

Table 1. Descriptive statistics of patients with and without complications. Data presented as median [interquartile range], number (proportion), or mean ± standard deviation

Characteristic	No Complications (n=19)	Complications (n=81)	p value
Age	66 [54:76]	67 [59:74]	0.7953
Male	10 (53%)	42 (51.9%)	>0.9999
Body mass index (kg/m^2)	25 [24:26]	26 [23:30]	0.2016
ASA			0.3721
II	6 (32%)	18 (22%)	
III	13 (68%)	57 (70%)	
IV	0	6 (7.4%)	
Diabetes	4 (21%)	27 (33%)	0.4113
COPD	3 (16%)	12 (14.8%)	>0.9999
Preoperative bloods			
Haemoglobin (g/dL)	132 [117:142]	131 [119:144]	0.9461
White cell count (×10^9/L)	6 [5.2:7.8]	7.7 [6.1:9.8]	0.0112
Platelets (×10^9/L)	260 [203:303]	268 [197:342]	0.5693
Albumin (g/L)	36 [32:41]	36 [31:39]	0.5421
Bilirubin (μmol/L)	15 [9:50]	18 [8:42]	0.3787
Urea (mmol/L)	5.2 [3.8:7.2]	5.5 [4.1:7.1]	0.9844
Creatinine (mmol/L)	72 [55:85]	68 [58:83]	0.9392
eGFR (mL/min/1.73m^2)	88 [69:90]	89 [74:90]	0.5477
Intraoperative fluid balance (mLs)	3300 [2040:4120]	3235 [2420:4283]	0.4893
Surgical technique			0.065
Classic Whipple	18 (95%)	60 (74%)	
Pylorus-Preserving	1 (5%)	21 (26%)	
Principal diagnosis			
Benign	2 (11%)	9 (11%)	>0.9999
Malignant	17 (89%)	67 (83%)	>0.9999
Other	0 (0%)	5 (6.2%)	0.5799
Surgery duration (min)	425 [385:540]	445 [390:514]	0.8977
Intraoperative blood transfusion	1 (5%)	7 (8.6%)	>0.9999
Blood loss (mLs)	300 [300:450]	300 [125:450]	0.4175
Day 1 fluid balance (mLs)	675 [82:2077]	1197 [672:1927]	0.252
Day 2 fluid balance (mLs)	-210 [-778:540]	191 [-736:806]	0.3236

continued on following page

Table 1. Continued

Characteristic	No Complications (n=19)	Complications (n=81)	p value
Number of complications			
1		13 (16%)	
2		19 (23.5%)	
3		19 (23.5%)	
4+		30 (37%)	
Clavien-Dindo grade			
I		17 (21%)	
II		50 (62%)	
III		10 (12%)	
IV		3 (4%)	
V		1 (1%)	
Postoperative median length of stay (days)	8 [7:9]	13 [9:20]	<0.0001
30-day readmission	2 (11%)	14 (17%)	0.7297
ICU time (hours)	18 [14:23]	20 [15:48]	0.2747
Total cost (2017 $USD)	$28,330 ± 11,964	$57,150 ± 52,161	0.019

Overall morbidity rate was 81%, and in-hospital mortality was 1%. Among complicated patients, 17 (21%) were Grade I, 50 (62%) Grade II, 10 (12%) Grade III, 3 (4%) were Grade IV, and 1 (1%) was Grade V. When stratified into number of complications: 19 experienced zero complications; 13 experienced one complication; 19 experienced two complications; 19 experienced three complications; and 30 experienced four or more complications. The uncomplicated and complicated cohorts were largely similar pre- and intraoperatively, except for preoperative white cell count (p=0.012). Median length of stay was significantly higher in complicated patients (8 days vs. 13 days, p<0.0001), and increased across severity grades, except for grade V (Table 2) (p<0.0001). Length of stay strongly correlated with total hospital costs (p<0.0001). There was no difference in 30-day readmission rates, ICU stay or mortality between patients with and without complications.

Mean hospital cost per patient was $51,674 (IQR $25,824 - $57,408). The mean total hospital costs in complicated patients more than doubled those of uncomplicated patients ($28,330 vs. $57,150, p<0.0001). Total hospital costs significantly increased with both severity and number of complications (Table 3). This cost increase was influenced by medical consult, pathology, pharmacy, radiology, ward, intensive care, and allied health costs, but not operating theatre or anaesthesia costs (Figure

1). The hospital costs of operating theatre (29%), ward (22%), intensive care unit (15%), anaesthesia (10%) and medical consults (9%) constituted the majority of total costs in all patients. Comparisons of actual and proportional costs for individual cost centres are shown in Table 4 and Figure 2. Postoperative pancreatic fistula (n=12), postoperative haemorrhage (n=9), delayed gastric emptying (n=21) and infection (n=34) were associated with significant increases in cost ($p<0.05$) and length of stay ($p<0.0001$) over uncomplicated patients ($93,768, 21 days; $102,409, 19 days; $63,950, 21 days; and $74,646, 18.5 days respectively).

Table 2. Hospital costs (2017 US dollars) defined by specific cost centres, and complications graded by the Clavien-Dindo (C-D) classification

	C-D Grade 0	C-D Grade I	C-D Grade II	C-D Grade III	C-D Grade IV	C-D Grade V	p value
Allied health	738	1,039	1,402	1,790	2,619	325	0.0238
Anaesthesia	3,990	5,062	5,212	6,192	1,707	6,871	0.4493
Blood products	5	421	1,117	2,561	134	124	0.5058
Hospital in the home	48	879	820	4,255	1,058	0	0.0198
Intensive care unit	3,558	3,316	8,796	13,298	31,274	7,126	0.0177
Medical consults	2,206	4,358	3,985	13,726	11,585	302	0.0005
Medical emergency team call	0	0	45	0	166	0	0.0593
Operating theatre	9,849	15,854	16,609	15,674	12,010	29,905	0.1484
Pathology	1,390	1,616	1,899	3,154	3,446	1,795	0.0147
Pharmacy	582	586	1,243	1,849	3,524	0	0.0019
Radiology	374	574	1,316	3,905	4,756	864	<0.0001
Ward	5,590	10,036	10,832	23,013	20,864	747	0.0002
Grand total (2017 $USD)	28,330	43,740	53,277	89,419	93,145	48,060	0.0089
Median length of stay (days)	8	9	12.5	20.5	37	2	<0.0001

Table 3. Hospital costs (2017 US dollars) defined by specific cost centres, and number of complications

	0 complications	1 complication	2 complications	3 complications	≥4 complications	p value
Allied health	738	1,086	1,105	1,020	1,979	0.0018
Anaesthesia	3,990	5,957	4,345	4,261	5,986	0.3639
Blood products	5	1,350	61	381	2,106	0.255
Hospital in the home	48	693	429	813	2,302	0.1352
Intensive care unit	3,558	5,876	4,038	4,543	16,356	0.0187
Medical consults	2,206	3,313	3,095	3,766	9,076	0.0077
Medical emergency team call	0	51	0	34	48	0.3898
Operating theatre	9,849	15,260	15,096	16,511	17,458	0.1248
Pathology	1,390	1,677	1,872	1,491	2,680	0.0212
Pharmacy	582	773	606	868	2,104	0.0002
Radiology	374	836	693	1,055	2,855	<0.0001
Ward	5,590	8,336	8,805	9,016	18,625	<0.0001
Grand total (2017 $USD)	28,330	45,209	40,144	43,759	81,575	0.0009
Median length of stay (days)	8	9	10	12	20.5	<0.0001

DISCUSSION

Key Results

The authors performed a detailed cost analyses of patients undergoing PD in a high-volume university hospital for pancreatic surgery. The authors found that severity of complication and number of complications were significantly related to increased total hospital costs and length of stay. The presence of a complication more than doubled total hospital cost in our cohort. The authors also evaluated the cost centres associated with the patients' hospital journeys and found that the

Figure 1. Costs (2017 US dollars) defined by specific cost centres and complications graded by Clavien-Dindo (C-D) classification

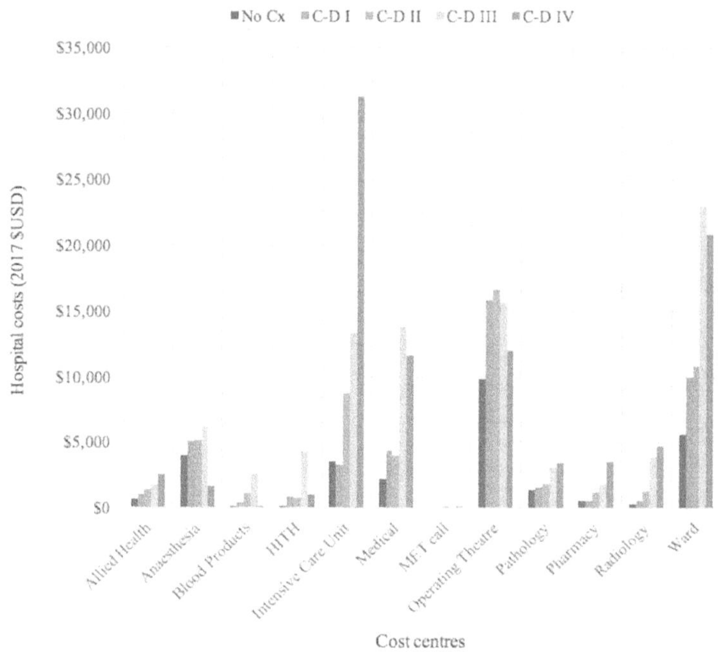

Table 4. Cost in US dollars (proportion of total costs by each cost centre) defined by specific cost centres in patients with and without complications

	All Patients	No Complications	Complications
Allied health	1,278 (2%)	738 (3%)	1,405 (2%)
Anaesthesia	4,963 (10%)	3,990 (14%)	5,192 (9%)
Blood products	892 (2%)	5 (0%)	1,100 (2%)
Hospital in the home	1,026 (2%)	48 (0%)	1,255 (2%)
Intensive care unit	7,977 (15%)	3,558 (12%)	9,014 (16%)
Medical consults	4,876 (9%)	2,206 (8%)	5,502 (10%)
Medical emergency team call	28 (0%)	0 (0%)	34 (0%)
Operating theatre	15,098 (29%)	9,849 (35%)	16,329 (28%)
Pathology	1,925 (4%)	1,390 (5%)	2,051 (4%)
Pharmacy	1,122 (2%)	582 (2%)	1,249 (2%)
Radiology	1,369 (3%)	374 (1%)	1,602 (3%)
Ward	11,119 (22%)	5,590 (20%)	12,416 (22%)

Figure 2. Comparison of costs between patients with and without complications (HITH: hospital in the home, MET: medical emergency team)

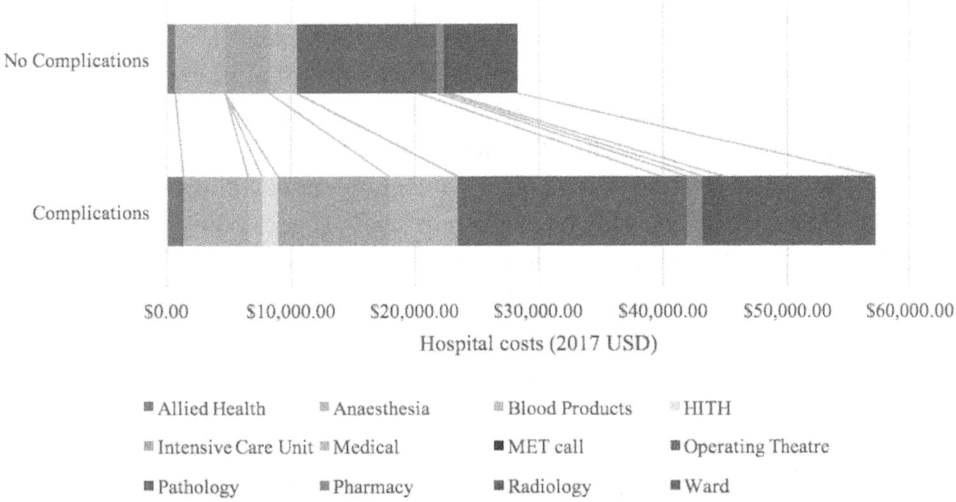

major contributors of costs in all patients, in order of decreasing proportion, were operating theatre, ward, intensive care, anaesthesia and medical consult costs. The occurrence of postoperative pancreatic fistula, postoperative haemorrhage, delayed gastric emptying, and infection, were associated with significant increases in cost.

The authors used actual costs, inflated and converted to 2017 USD, derived from a bottom-up activity-based costing methodology. This methodology allows a more specific cost allocation to each patient's individual journey, capturing local variation in costs (Chapko et al., 2009). The overall morbidity in our cohort was surprisingly high at 81%, given previously published literature from both our institution and others (Brown, Yang, Canter, & Bold, 2014; Knechtle et al., 2015; Topal et al., 2007; Warrillow et al., 2010). However, our major morbidity (Clavien-Dindo Grade III or above) and mortality rate were more akin to contemporary literature at 14% and 1% respectively. The high complication rate may be explained by our stringent adherence to the Clavien-Dindo classification, as well as our thorough perusal of electronic medical records for complications despite a lack of hospital complication coding. For complete accuracy, the authors also included minor complications that were unlikely to affect patients' outcomes, such as minor electrolyte imbalances.

It is unsurprising that postoperative complications following PD have a significant health economic burden, given their impact on requirement for therapeutic intervention and on increased hospital stay. The link between PD complications and an increased hospital cost has been previously established internationally. Enestvedt et al. (Enestvedt et al., 2012) found that major complications in PD patients almost doubled costs;

however, this study utilised median rather than mean costs. A systematic review performed by Patel et al. (Patel et al., 2013) similarly found that complications following pancreatic surgery led to considerable economic burden; however, this review did not delineate between different pancreas surgeries.

The authors used the Clavien-Dindo classification system (Dindo et al., 2004) and once again reinforced its utility for stratifying morbidity for both clinical and economic outcomes in PD patients. The authors also stratified patients by the number of complications, and found that a higher number of complications was associated with higher hospital costs. This has been previously suggested by Knechtle et al. (Knechtle et al., 2015), who reported exponential cost increases with the number of complications in a cohort of 260 patients. This paper, however, did not consider the severity of complications.

Our study identified the increases in cost centres across both complication severity grades and number of complications. Although the costs of the operating theatre and anaesthesia were substantial proportions of the total cost, they did not significantly increase across either severity or number of complications. This may be due to relatively few patients developing complications requiring surgical, endoscopic or radiological management; furthermore, radiological procedures are classified under 'radiology' rather than 'operating theatre'. Instead, the cost increases were of hospitalisation, intensive care, pathology, radiology, pharmacy, allied health consults, and medical consults. Many of these cost centres can be interpreted as necessary costs during a longer length of stay due to complications. In fact, the authors found that length of stay was significantly correlated with total hospital costs ($p<0.0001$). The low overall requirement of medical emergency calls and blood products in our cohort may have led to the non-significance of cost differences between complication grades and number.

Topal et al. (Topal et al., 2007) also investigated cost centres using an activity-based costing methodology in PD patients, and found that hospitalisation, operation room, medical staffing and pharmacy costs were the largest contributors to total cost. Similar to our findings, costs of hospitalisation, laboratory work, medical staffing and pharmacy work were significantly different between patients without complications, with complications other than POPF, and with POPF. POPF is traditionally regarded as the most common major complication following PD, with morbidity between 30-50%(Bassi et al., 2005). It is characterised by leakage of pancreatic juices due to disruption in pancreatic ducts, potentially leading to serious sequelae such as abdominal abscess and haemorrhage (Machado, 2012). The incidence of POPF in our cohort was only 12%, yet led to significant burden when it occurred. POPF increased costs more than threefold and hospitalisation length more than twofold over uncomplicated patients, agreeing with several cost studies of POPF (Santema et al., 2015; Topal et al., 2007).

Post pancreatectomy haemorrhage (PPH) is an uncommon complication with high rates of mortality, which is often only recognised after severe bleeding has occurred (Rajarathinam et al., 2008). PPH was the costliest individual complication in our cohort, with an incidence of 9%. Our results correspond with Santema et al.'s (Santema et al., 2015) study, which found that PPH was costlier than POPF and DGE, with an incidence of 12%. ISGPS-defined delayed gastric emptying (DGE) occurred in 21% of our patients, and had an average cost and length of stay more than double that of uncomplicated patients. This coincides with the results of Eisenberg et al.'s (Eisenberg, Rosato, Lavu, Yeo, & Winter, 2015) study focussing on the costs of primary and secondary DGE; they defined primary DGE as one that was believed not to have occurred secondary to another complication, such as POPF. Indeed, the usefulness of evaluating DGE is compromised by its common occurrence as a secondary complication (Welsch et al., 2010). Additionally, the increased cost from DGE may be due to the requirement to stay in hospital alone, rather than any costly therapeutic measures (Brown et al., 2014).

Infections following PD, both local and systemic, are common and can range from a minor wound infection to life-threatening sepsis. Infection occurred in 34% of our patients and led to costs increasing more than two-fold over uncomplicated patients. In a study investigating infections in elective pancreatic resections, Kent et al. (Kent, Sachs, Callery, & Vollmer, 2013) found an infection incidence of 31%. They also found that costs increased across Clavien-Dindo grades for cases with infection, with 38% of the cost differential incurred by infection. This study included 356 PDs out of 550 major pancreatic resections (Kent et al., 2013).

Our study adds to the substantial body of evidence linking postoperative complications associated with PD with a significant economic and clinical burden. The authors investigated the genesis of the increased costs by breaking down costs into cost centres, and found that similar cost centres were more burdensome across both the number and severity of complications. By identifying these specific cost centres, the authors have established potential targets for cost containment and future research efforts.

Preoperative physiology (Pratt, Callery, & Vollmer, 2008; Vollmer, Pratt, Vanounou, Maithel, & Callery, 2007) has been shown to be economically significant in pancreatic surgery. Pratt's group measured baseline physiology using POSSUM, a scoring system of 12 preoperative variables (Copeland, Jones, & Walters, 1991; Pratt, Callery, et al., 2008), and found that baseline physiology accurately predicted morbidity and mean hospital costs for PD (Pratt, Joseph, Callery, & Vollmer, 2008). In another study, however, Pratt et al. found that improved surgical performance tempered the risk of poorer baseline physiology (Pratt, Callery, et al., 2008). Vollmer et al. also used POSSUM to estimate morbidity for their pancreatic resection population, and compared this estimate with observed morbidity to establish an observed/estimated (O/E) morbidity ratio (Vollmer et al., 2007). They found that a 0.10 decrease in O/E morbidity ratio was associated with cost savings, median blood loss, thromboembolic prophylaxis and early oral intake (Vollmer et al., 2007). These studies give evidence to the potential impact of preoperative optimisation, and likely targets to improve clinical and economic outcomes.

Many approaches have been applied to reduce complications in PD patients. Preoperative optimisation with oxygen (Davies & Wilson, 2004) and inotropes (Lobo et al., 2006) before high-risk surgeries, to compensate for the large inflammatory response and oxygen requirement during major surgery, has been shown to reduce complications. Inotropic optimisation has also been shown to be cost-effectiveness in major elective surgeries, including resection for upper gastrointestinal malignancy (Fenwick, Wilson, Sculpher, & Claxton, 2002). The utility of preoperative optimisation in PD specifically, however, is yet to be determined.

Goal-directed therapy (GDT), a strategy to aggressively monitor and haemodynamically optimise patients with fluids and inotropes to achieve a set haemodynamic endpoint, has previously been shown to have significant clinical (Dalfino, Giglio, Puntillo, Marucci, & Brienza, 2011; Giglio, Marucci, Testini, & Brienza, 2009; Hamilton, Cecconi, & Rhodes, 2011) and economic (Bartha et al., 2012) benefits in high-risk surgical procedures. A meta-analysis of GDT in a variety of major surgeries, including of the abdomen, found reduced complication rates in all studies and a mortality benefit in high-risk patients (Cecconi et al., 2013). Recent studies have shown the morbidity benefits of either fluid restriction or goal-directed fluid therapy perioperatively to avoid excessive intravascular volumes post major surgery (Corcoran, Rhodes, Clarke, Myles, & Ho, 2012; Rahbari et al., 2009). Indeed, high intraoperative (Weinberg et al., 2014) and postoperative (Wright, Koehler, Davis, & Chung, 2014) fluid balance during PD has been shown to be associated with a higher complication rate and length of stay. However, Melis et al. did not find an association between intraoperative fluid volume and morbidity (Melis et al., 2012). Similarly, our current study did not show any differences in intraoperative or postoperative fluid balance at day one or two between complicated and uncomplicated patients; further investigation is warranted.

The implementation of enhanced recovery after surgery (ERAS) pathways has proven efficacious in pancreatic surgery, including PD, in reducing length of stay whilst maintaining morbidity and mortality rates (Coolsen et al., 2013; Pecorelli et al., 2016). This has also been shown in our institution (Nikfarjam et al., 2013). Stowers et al. reviewed the health economics of ERAS programs in a variety of abdominal surgeries, including two pancreatic surgery papers, and found that they appear to be cost effective (Stowers, Lemanu, & Hill, 2015).

A meta-analysis by Koti et al. (Koti, Gurusamy, Fusai, & Davidson, 2010) showed that somatostatin analogues reduce the rate of complications, including POPF, but not mortality in pancreatic surgery patients. Economic evaluations of somatostatin analogues to reduce POPF in PD patients have demonstrated cost-saving (Goyert et al., 2017; Vanounou, Pratt, Callery, & Vollmer, 2007). The studies differed, however, on whether to administer the analogues in all patients (Goyert et al., 2017) or only those with 'high-risk' glands (Vanounou et al., 2007).

Increased hospital volume has consistently shown improved outcomes following PD, including reduced morbidity, mortality and cost (Enomoto, Gusani, Dillon, & Hollenbeak, 2014; Gouma et al., 2000; Schmidt et al., 2010; Yoshioka et al., 2014). Surgeon volume has shown similar outcomes in some studies (Enomoto et al., 2014; Schmidt et al., 2010), although its effect on mortality is more controversial. The present study was conducted in a quaternary hospital with an experienced hepato-pancreato-biliary unit and a volume averaging between 10 and 25 PDs per year.

Strengths and Limitations

Our study has several strengths and limitations. The authors reported cost data on a relatively large sample size and provided a detailed description of the health economic burden of complications, measured using the Clavien-Dindo classification in PD patients presenting to a high-volume tertiary teaching hospital. Our study was performed at single centre, which limits the external validity of our findings, however our hospital has all the typical characteristics of many tertiary institutions and surgical and anaesthesia protocols are similar to those of other tertiary centres. Second, the recording, collection and entering of the data could have been subject to human error both in terms of interpretation and transcription. However, the authors consider it unlikely that this had an impact on the outcomes of this study, due to the electronic medical recording systems in place in our institution, comprehensive cross checks required for data entry and detailed information provided by the hospital's Business Intelligence Unit, which independently collects and reports all adverse outcomes. In addition, complications were manually cross-checked with the patients' medical records by two independent investigators, before being graded into the Clavien-Dindo classification. This allowed for an objective and accurate description and classification of costs associated with complications following PD. The authors only considered the occurrence of a 30-day readmission, and did not consider long-term follow up for both clinical and economic outcomes. Readmissions after major pancreas surgery has been shown to be largely due to procedure-specific complications and lead to significant costs (Kent, Sachs, Callery, & Vollmer, 2011). Finally, the authors did not classify POPF and DGE into grades of severity, although this was not our study's aim.

CONCLUSION

In conclusion, complications following PD are common, and are associated with increased costs and length of stay. The Clavien-Dindo classification applied to our cohort of patients, and increases in severity grade were directly associated with increased cost. Any measures to reduce complications can be expected to lead to cost containment and improved patient care. The present study has provided an in-depth cost analysis by stratifying total costs by cost centres, and therefore has identified individual target areas.

FUNDING

The authors declare no funding or conflicts of interest.

ACKNOWLEDGMENT

The authors would like to acknowledge the contribution of Dr. Ronald Ma, Dr. Paul Eleftheriou, Prof. Leonid Churilov, Mr. David Debono, Mr. Ray Robbins, A/Prof. Mehrdad Nikfarjam and Prof. Christopher Christophi in the preparation and critical review of this manuscript.

REFERENCES

Authority, N. B. (2012). *Patient Blood Management Guidelines: Module 2 Perioperative*. Retrieved from https://www.blood.gov.au/system/files/documents/pbm-module-2.pdf

Bartha, E., Davidson, T., Hommel, A., Thorngren, K. G., Carlsson, P., & Kalman, S. (2012). Cost-effectiveness analysis of goal-directed hemodynamic treatment of elderly hip fracture patients: Before clinical research starts. *Anesthesiology*, *117*(3), 519–530. doi:10.1097/ALN.0b013e3182655eb2 PMID:22814385

Bassi, C., Dervenis, C., Butturini, G., Fingerhut, A., Yeo, C., Izbicki, J., ... Buchler, M. (2005). Postoperative pancreatic fistula: An international study group (ISGPF) definition. *Surgery*, *138*(1), 8–13. doi:10.1016/j.surg.2005.05.001 PMID:16003309

Brown, E. G., Yang, A., Canter, R. J., & Bold, R. J. (2014). Outcomes of pancreaticoduodenectomy: Where should we focus our efforts on improving outcomes? *JAMA Surgery*, *149*(7), 694–699. doi:10.1001/jamasurg.2014.151 PMID:24849180

Cecconi, M., Corredor, C., Arulkumaran, N., Abuella, G., Ball, J., Grounds, R. M., ... Rhodes, A. (2013). Clinical review: Goal-directed therapy-what is the evidence in surgical patients? The effect on different risk groups. *Critical Care (London, England)*, *17*(2), 209. doi:10.1186/cc11823 PMID:23672779

Chapko, M. K., Liu, C. F., Perkins, M., Li, Y. F., Fortney, J. C., & Maciejewski, M. L. (2009). Equivalence of two healthcare costing methods: Bottom-up and top-down. *Health Economics*, *18*(10), 1188–1201. doi:10.1002/hec.1422 PMID:19097041

Coolsen, M. M., van Dam, R. M., van der Wilt, A. A., Slim, K., Lassen, K., & Dejong, C. H. (2013). Systematic review and meta-analysis of enhanced recovery after pancreatic surgery with particular emphasis on pancreaticoduodenectomies. *World Journal of Surgery*, *37*(8), 1909–1918. doi:10.100700268-013-2044-3 PMID:23568250

Copeland, G. P., Jones, D., & Walters, M. (1991). POSSUM: A scoring system for surgical audit. *British Journal of Surgery*, *78*(3), 355–360. doi:10.1002/bjs.1800780327 PMID:2021856

Corcoran, T., Rhodes, J. E., Clarke, S., Myles, P. S., & Ho, K. M. (2012). Perioperative fluid management strategies in major surgery: A stratified meta-analysis. *Anesthesia and Analgesia*, *114*(3), 640–651. doi:10.1213/ANE.0b013e318240d6eb PMID:22253274

Dalfino, L., Giglio, M. T., Puntillo, F., Marucci, M., & Brienza, N. (2011). Haemodynamic goal-directed therapy and postoperative infections: Earlier is better. A systematic review and meta-analysis. *Critical Care (London, England), 15*(3), R154. doi:10.1186/cc10284 PMID:21702945

Davies, S. J., & Wilson, R. J. (2004). Preoperative optimization of the high-risk surgical patient. *British Journal of Anaesthesia, 93*(1), 121–128. doi:10.1093/bja/aeh164 PMID:15121729

Dindo, D., Demartines, N., & Clavien, P. A. (2004). Classification of surgical complications: A new proposal with evaluation in a cohort of 6336 patients and results of a survey. *Annals of Surgery, 240*(2), 205–213. doi:10.1097/01.sla.0000133083.54934.ae PMID:15273542

Eisenberg, J. D., Rosato, E. L., Lavu, H., Yeo, C. J., & Winter, J. M. (2015). Delayed Gastric Emptying After Pancreaticoduodenectomy: An Analysis of Risk Factors and Cost. *Journal of Gastrointestinal Surgery, 19*(9), 1572–1580. doi:10.100711605-015-2865-5 PMID:26170145

Enestvedt, C. K., Diggs, B. S., Cassera, M. A., Hammill, C., Hansen, P. D., & Wolf, R. F. (2012). Complications nearly double the cost of care after pancreaticoduodenectomy. *American Journal of Surgery, 204*(3), 332–338. doi:10.1016/j.amjsurg.2011.10.019 PMID:22464011

Enomoto, L. M., Gusani, N. J., Dillon, P. W., & Hollenbeak, C. S. (2014). Impact of surgeon and hospital volume on mortality, length of stay, and cost of pancreaticoduodenectomy. *Journal of Gastrointestinal Surgery, 18*(4), 690–700. doi:10.100711605-013-2422-z PMID:24297652

Fenwick, E., Wilson, J., Sculpher, M., & Claxton, K. (2002). Pre-operative optimisation employing dopexamine or adrenaline for patients undergoing major elective surgery: A cost-effectiveness analysis. *Intensive Care Medicine, 28*(5), 599–608. doi:10.100700134-002-1257-y PMID:12029409

Giglio, M. T., Marucci, M., Testini, M., & Brienza, N. (2009). Goal-directed haemodynamic therapy and gastrointestinal complications in major surgery: A meta-analysis of randomized controlled trials. *British Journal of Anaesthesia, 103*(5), 637–646. doi:10.1093/bja/aep279 PMID:19837807

Gouma, D. J., van Geenen, R. C., van Gulik, T. M., de Haan, R. J., de Wit, L. T., Busch, O. R., & Obertop, H. (2000). Rates of complications and death after pancreaticoduodenectomy: Risk factors and the impact of hospital volume. *Annals of Surgery, 232*(6), 786–795. doi:10.1097/00000658-200012000-00007 PMID:11088073

Goyert, N., Eeson, G., Kagedan, D. J., Behman, R., Lemke, M., Hallet, J., ... Coburn, N. G. (2017). Pasireotide for the prevention of pancreatic fistula following pancreaticoduodenectomy: A cost-effectiveness analysis. *Annals of Surgery*, *265*(1), 2–10. doi:10.1097/SLA.0000000000001889 PMID:27537539

Gupta, P. K., Turaga, K. K., Miller, W. J., Loggie, B. W., & Foster, J. M. (2011). Determinants of outcomes in pancreatic surgery and use of hospital resources. *Journal of Surgical Oncology*, *104*(6), 634–640. doi:10.1002/jso.21923 PMID:21520092

Hamilton, M. A., Cecconi, M., & Rhodes, A. (2011). A systematic review and meta-analysis on the use of preemptive hemodynamic intervention to improve postoperative outcomes in moderate and high-risk surgical patients. *Anesthesia and Analgesia*, *112*(6), 1392–1402. doi:10.1213/ANE.0b013e3181eeaae5 PMID:20966436

Kent, T. S., Sachs, T. E., Callery, M. P., & Vollmer, C. M. Jr. (2011). Readmission after major pancreatic resection: A necessary evil? *Journal of the American College of Surgeons*, *213*(4), 515–523. doi:10.1016/j.jamcollsurg.2011.07.009 PMID:21840738

Kent, T. S., Sachs, T. E., Callery, M. P., & Vollmer, C. M. Jr. (2013). The burden of infection for elective pancreatic resections. *Surgery*, *153*(1), 86–94. doi:10.1016/j.surg.2012.03.026 PMID:22698935

Khuri, S. F., Henderson, W. G., DePalma, R. G., Mosca, C., Healey, N. A., Kumbhani, D. J., & Participants in the V. A. N. S. Q. I. P. (2005). Determinants of long-term survival after major surgery and the adverse effect of postoperative complications. *Ann Surg, 242*(3), 326-341.

Knechtle, W. S., Perez, S. D., Medbery, R. L., Gartland, B. D., Sullivan, P. S., Knechtle, S. J., ... Sweeney, J. F. (2015). The Association Between Hospital Finances and Complications After Complex Abdominal Surgery: Deficiencies in the Current Health Care Reimbursement System and Implications for the Future. *Annals of Surgery*, *262*(2), 273–279. doi:10.1097/SLA.0000000000001042 PMID:25405558

Koti, R. S., Gurusamy, K. S., Fusai, G., & Davidson, B. R. (2010). Meta-analysis of randomized controlled trials on the effectiveness of somatostatin analogues for pancreatic surgery: A Cochrane review. *HPB*, *12*(3), 155–165. doi:10.1111/j.1477-2574.2010.00157.x PMID:20590882

Lobo, S. M., Lobo, F. R., Polachini, C. A., Patini, D. S., Yamamoto, A. E., de Oliveira, N. E., ... Cunrath, G. S. (2006). Prospective, randomized trial comparing fluids and dobutamine optimization of oxygen delivery in high-risk surgical patients [ISRCTN42445141]. *Critical Care (London, England)*, *10*(3), R72. doi:10.1186/cc4913 PMID:16696864

Machado, N. O. (2012). Pancreatic fistula after pancreatectomy: Definitions, risk factors, preventive measures, and management-review. *International Journal of Surgical Oncology*, *602478*. doi:10.1155/2012/602478 PMID:22611494

Melis, M., Marcon, F., Masi, A., Sarpel, U., Miller, G., Moore, H., ... Newman, E. (2012). Effect of intra-operative fluid volume on peri-operative outcomes after pancreaticoduodenectomy for pancreatic adenocarcinoma. *Journal of Surgical Oncology*, *105*(1), 81–84. doi:10.1002/jso.22048 PMID:21792977

Nikfarjam, M., Weinberg, L., Low, N., Fink, M. A., Muralidharan, V., Houli, N., ... Christophi, C. (2013). A fast track recovery program significantly reduces hospital length of stay following uncomplicated pancreaticoduodenectomy. *JOP*, *14*(1), 63–70. doi:10.6092/1590-8577/1223 PMID:23306337

Patel, A. S., Bergman, A., Moore, B. W., & Haglund, U. (2013). The economic burden of complications occurring in major surgical procedures: A systematic review. *Applied Health Economics and Health Policy*, *11*(6), 577–592. doi:10.100740258-013-0060-y PMID:24166193

Pecorelli, N., Nobile, S., Partelli, S., Cardinali, L., Crippa, S., Balzano, G., ... Falconi, M. (2016). Enhanced recovery pathways in pancreatic surgery: State of the art. *World Journal of Gastroenterology*, *22*(28), 6456–6468. doi:10.3748/wjg.v22.i28.6456 PMID:27605881

Pratt, W., Callery, M. P., & Vollmer, C. M. Jr. (2008). Optimal surgical performance attenuates physiologic risk in high-acuity operations. *Journal of the American College of Surgeons*, *207*(5), 717–730. doi:10.1016/j.jamcollsurg.2008.06.319 PMID:18954785

Pratt, W., Joseph, S., Callery, M. P., & Vollmer, C. M. Jr. (2008). POSSUM accurately predicts morbidity for pancreatic resection. *Surgery*, *143*(1), 8–19. doi:10.1016/j.surg.2007.07.035 PMID:18154928

Rahbari, N. N., Zimmermann, J. B., Schmidt, T., Koch, M., Weigand, M. A., & Weitz, J. (2009). Meta-analysis of standard, restrictive and supplemental fluid administration in colorectal surgery. *British Journal of Surgery*, *96*(4), 331–341. doi:10.1002/bjs.6552 PMID:19283742

Rajarathinam, G., Kannan, D. G., Vimalraj, V., Amudhan, A., Rajendran, S., Jyotibasu, D., ... Surendran, R. (2008). Post pancreaticoduodenectomy haemorrhage: Outcome prediction based on new ISGPS Clinical severity grading. *HPB*, *10*(5), 363–370. doi:10.1080/13651820802247086 PMID:18982153

Santema, T. B., Visser, A., Busch, O. R., Dijkgraaf, M. G., Goslings, J. C., Gouma, D. J., & Ubbink, D. T. (2015). Hospital costs of complications after a pancreatoduodenectomy. *HPB*, *17*(8), 723–731. doi:10.1111/hpb.12440 PMID:26082095

Schmidt, C. M., Turrini, O., Parikh, P., House, M. G., Zyromski, N. J., Nakeeb, A., ... Lillemoe, K. D. (2010). Effect of hospital volume, surgeon experience, and surgeon volume on patient outcomes after pancreaticoduodenectomy: A single-institution experience. *Archives of Surgery (Chicago, Ill.)*, *145*(7), 634–640. doi:10.1001/archsurg.2010.118 PMID:20644125

Stowers, M. D., Lemanu, D. P., & Hill, A. G. (2015). Health economics in Enhanced Recovery After Surgery programs. *Canadian Journal of Anaesthesia*, *62*(2), 219–230. doi:10.100712630-014-0272-0 PMID:25391739

Topal, B., Peeters, G., Vandeweyer, H., Aerts, R., & Penninckx, F. (2007). Hospital cost-categories of pancreaticoduodenectomy. *Acta Chirurgica Belgica*, *107*(4), 373–377. doi:10.1080/00015458.2007.11680078 PMID:17966528

Vanounou, T., Pratt, W. B., Callery, M. P., & Vollmer, C. M. Jr. (2007). Selective administration of prophylactic octreotide during pancreaticoduodenectomy: A clinical and cost-benefit analysis in low- and high-risk glands. *Journal of the American College of Surgeons*, *205*(4), 546–557. doi:10.1016/j.jamcollsurg.2007.05.011 PMID:17903728

Vollmer, C. M. Jr, Pratt, W., Vanounou, T., Maithel, S. K., & Callery, M. P. (2007). Quality assessment in high-acuity surgery: Volume and mortality are not enough. *Archives of Surgery (Chicago, Ill.)*, *142*(4), 371–380. doi:10.1001/archsurg.142.4.371 PMID:17438173

Vonlanthen, R., Slankamenac, K., Breitenstein, S., Puhan, M. A., Muller, M. K., Hahnloser, D., ... Clavien, P. A. (2011). The impact of complications on costs of major surgical procedures: A cost analysis of 1200 patients. *Annals of Surgery*, *254*(6), 907–913. doi:10.1097/SLA.0b013e31821d4a43 PMID:21562405

Warrillow, S. J., Weinberg, L., Parker, F., Calzavacca, P., Licari, E., Aly, A., ... Bellomo, R. (2010). Perioperative fluid prescription, complications and outcomes in major elective open gastrointestinal surgery. *Anaesthesia and Intensive Care*, *38*(2), 259–265. PMID:20369757

Weinberg, L., Wong, D., Karalapillai, D., Pearce, B., Tan, C. O., Tay, S., ... Nikfarjam, M. (2014). The impact of fluid intervention on complications and length of hospital stay after pancreaticoduodenectomy (Whipple's procedure). *BMC Anesthesiology*, *14*(1), 35. doi:10.1186/1471-2253-14-35 PMID:24839398

Welsch, T., Borm, M., Degrate, L., Hinz, U., Buchler, M. W., & Wente, M. N. (2010). Evaluation of the International Study Group of Pancreatic Surgery definition of delayed gastric emptying after pancreatoduodenectomy in a high-volume centre. *British Journal of Surgery*, *97*(7), 1043–1050. doi:10.1002/bjs.7071 PMID:20632270

Wente, M. N., Bassi, C., Dervenis, C., Fingerhut, A., Gouma, D. J., Izbicki, J. R., ... Buchler, M. W. (2007). Delayed gastric emptying (DGE) after pancreatic surgery: A suggested definition by the International Study Group of Pancreatic Surgery (ISGPS). *Surgery*, *142*(5), 761–768. doi:10.1016/j.surg.2007.05.005 PMID:17981197

Whipple, A. O., Parsons, W. B., & Mullins, C. R. (1935). Treatment of Carcinoma of the Ampulla of Vater. *Annals of Surgery*, *102*(4), 763–779. doi:10.1097/00000658-193510000-00023 PMID:17856666

Wright, G. P., Koehler, T. J., Davis, A. T., & Chung, M. H. (2014). The drowning whipple: Perioperative fluid balance and outcomes following pancreaticoduodenectomy. *Journal of Surgical Oncology*, *110*(4), 407–411. doi:10.1002/jso.23662 PMID:24861716

Yoshioka, R., Yasunaga, H., Hasegawa, K., Horiguchi, H., Fushimi, K., Aoki, T., ... Kokudo, N. (2014). Impact of hospital volume on hospital mortality, length of stay and total costs after pancreaticoduodenectomy. *British Journal of Surgery*, *101*(5), 523–529. doi:10.1002/bjs.9420 PMID:24615349

KEY TERMS AND DEFINITIONS

ASA: American Society of Anesthesiologists.

C-D: Clavien-Dindo.

CPI: Consumer price index.

DGE: Delayed gastric emptying.

ERAS: Enhanced recovery after surgery.

GDT: Goal-directed therapy.

HITH: Hospital in the home.

ICD: International Statistical Classification of Diseases and Related Health Problems.

ICU: Intensive care unit.

ISGPF: International Study Group on Pancreatic Fistula Definition.

ISGPS: International Study Group of Pancreatic Surgery.

LOS: Length of stay.

MET: Medical emergency team.

O/E: Observed/estimated.

PD: Pancreaticoduodenectomy.

POPF: Postoperative pancreatic fistula.

POSSUM: Physiological and Operative Severity Score for the enUmeration of Mortality and Morbidity.

PPH: Post pancreatectomy hemorrhage.

PPPD: Pylorus-preserving pancreaticoduodenectomy.

USD: United States Dollar.

Chapter 8
The Integration of an Extra-Corporal Life Support (ECLS) Service at Austin Health

Yvonne Ballueer
Austin Health, Australia

ABSTRACT

Extra-corporal membrane oxygenation (ECMO), also known as extracorporeal life support (ECLS), is a globally established treatment option in modern intensive care medicine for patients suffering from severe but reversible respiratory and/or cardiac failure. If refractory to other advanced treatment options, early instatement of ECLS therapy is closely associated with reduced mortality and improved long-term patient outcome. ECLS, in many ways, has replaced other, less effective treatments and future modelling predicts increased demand. ECLS has routinely and successfully been applied to neonates and pediatrics for many years. This field study however will exhibit focus only on the viability of the introduction of ECLS therapy in the Victorian adult population at Austin Health.

DOI: 10.4018/978-1-5225-5082-2.ch008

INTRODUCTION

Austin Health is ready for the introduction of a fully integrated Extra Corporal Life Support (ECLS) service, adding value to our patients, strengthening the Austin Brand and keeping us in vogue with global and local industry standards.

ECLS is a highly invasive life support mechanism for critically ill patients suffering from severe but reversible cardiac and/or respiratory failure. ECLS maximises gas exchange (CO2 & O2) and supports cardiac function, allowing time for organ (heart or lung) recovery.

Globally, ECLS therapy itself is survived by 54% of the effected adult population (66% in neonates / paediatrics), resulting in an average alive discharge or transfer rate of 43% (51% respectively).

Extra Corporal Membrane Oxygenation (ECMO) devices are operated by an advanced clinical skilled workforce of clinical perfusionists & medical and nursing teams within tertiary critical care settings.

Since 2009, 47 patients have received ECLS treatment at Austin Health. Each of these patients was overseen by the critical care medical teams and cared for by critical trained nursing staff in the Intensive Care Unit. The ECMO device for its duration however, was operated by the clinical perfusionist team, impacting adversely on operational flow within the cardiac operating theatres.

Some of the 47 episodes Austin Health incurred unnecessary marginal costs due to the requirements for locum clinical perfusionist services and overtime paid to medical consultants. In some instances, cardiac cancellations due to the lack of clinical perfusionist services led to loss of opportunity costs. Notably, particularly over the past 24 months, each ECLS episode induced high stress levels for all treating teams involved.

The following proposal investigates and reports on the financial viability and value-add of a fully integrated ECLS service at Austin Health, where each episode is initiated and supervised by the treating medical teams and the ECMO device is operated by fully trained and accredited critical care nursing staff, gradually increasing the degree of independence from the clinical perfusionist services.

The fully integrated ECLS service will:

- Positively impact on patient outcome and patient experience
- Promote Austin's Brand and re-strengthening its competitive advantage
- Create marginal benefits (small revenue)
- Meet demand for future growth
- Support specific related research activities
- Fulfil Austin's Strategic Priority of being a: Global Leader in Specialised Care and Research

- Underpin Austin's Vision of: Outstanding Patient Care, Research and Education
- Add value to a variety of key-stake holders within Austin Health
- Attract and retain high performing clinical specialist staff, nursing & medical

To make the launch of the fully integrated ECLS service at Austin Health a reality, I am requesting funding of $300,000 for the first year.

The funding will be utilised to cover

- Capital Investment
- Workforce Training (Nursing/Medical)
- Nursing Roster Backfill
- ECLS Coordinator
- Annual Simulation Fees

Taking in to account the predicted growth demand for ECLS episodes, it is anticipated that the service will create a small profit margin in the second year and further, will create an accumulated revenue of $500,000 over a timeframe of five years.

I will call your Personal Assistant to schedule an appointment to discuss this proposal with you.

Sincerely,

Nurse Unit Manager, Intensive Care Unit

EXECUTIVE SUMMARY

Extra Corporal Membrane Oxygenation (ECMO), also known as Extracorporeal Life Support (ECLS), is a globally established treatment option in modern intensive care medicine for patients suffering from severe but reversible respiratory and/or cardiac failure. If refractory to other advanced treatment options, early instatement of ECLS therapy is closely associated with reduced mortality and improved long-term patient outcome. ECLS, in many ways, has replaced other, less effective treatments and future modelling predicts increased demand.

ECLS has routinely and successfully been applied to neonates and paediatrics for many years, this field study however will exhibit focus only on the viability of the introduction of ECLS therapy in the Victorian adult population at Austin Health. The study will discuss:

The Business Opportunity

The business venture aims to introduce a model to provide ECLS which is of highest quality, cost effective and sustainable. ECLS will be medically initiated and supported, nurse-led and mainly clinical perfusionist-independent.

The Industry

ECLS commenced in 1971 and today modern tertiary centres offer ECLS as an advanced treatment form for critically ill patients with reversible cardio/respiratory failure refractory to conventional intensive therapy. ECLS therapy is well established globally and nationally and over 70,000 patients have been treated with ECLS to date. Within Victoria, The Alfred Hospital is the industry leader, by providing an average of 1.9 ECLS episodes on any given day. The Alfred model is cost effective by being nurse-led and Clinical Perfusionist independent. Most centres, globally and nationally, rely heavily on costly clinical perfusionist service.

The Competitive Analysis

Austin has several competitors. Main direct competitors are The Alfred and St Vincent, with the latter also being insipient to Austin. According to unconfirmed reports from the DHHS, it is predicted that one of the hospitals (Austin or St Vincent) will have government funding withdrawn for their cardiac service. Austin's cardiac activity

Figure 1. ICU team with perfusionist support

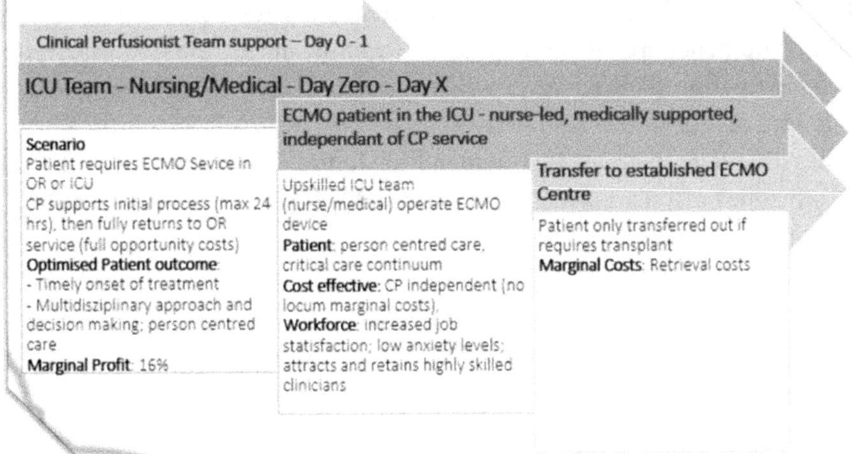

and ECLS episodes are higher than those at St Vincent's. By introducing a fully integrated ECLS service, Austin's competitive advantage will increase significantly. Austin also competes advantageously by geographical location, covering the Northern Corridor of Melbourne, domineering the Northern Hospital. St Vincent geographical location is in close vicinity to the two largest metropolitan health care services, The Alfred and The Royal Melbourne Hospital (RMH). Both have fully established large cardiac services. However, RMH does not offer ECLS and refers patients to The Alfred instead.

The Marketing Plan

All internal key stake holders will be included when the new model rolls out. Externally, Austin ICU will register with ELSO (Extracorporeal Life Support Organisation) and with the Department of Health Victoria. A partnership of collegial nature will be entered with The Alfred.

The Operating Plan

Physical location, facilities, inventory and most equipment, with the exemption of the ECMO devices, is in place and covered by sunk costs. Additional equipment costs are included in the financial feasibility section. The critically trained workforce requires acquisition of additional skill sets. The supplier, Maquet, is already under contract with different equipment, such as mechanical ventilators.

The Financial Feasibility

The Service is financially feasible. On average, activity funding covers costs by 116%, creating a profit margin after the first year. Sunk costs are excluded. Marginal costs are equipment purchase and workforce training during the first year, requiring $300,000 in funding. This however will be partly offset by the activity based WIES funding. Exit and or Growth Strategy

Forecasting demonstrates that demand for future ECLS episodes will increase annually by one episode. Formal training (refresher) requirements will reduce with greater exposure to ECLS therapy.

With research also advancing, new, game changing therapies, such as liver or brain ECLS, might be introduced in the future.

An exit strategy is not required as the service is activity based funded. If demand decreases, costs will also decrease. Training costs can be absorbed into the overall budget for some time.

Day in the Life: The Patient and the Family

Ria, 36, has been feeling lethargic, exhausted and extremely unwell with flu-like symptoms, shortness of breath and coughing. When she develops a fever, her partner decides to take her to the nearest public emergency department (ED) at Austin Health. Whilst undergoing several diagnostic tests in the ED, her condition deteriorates and the medical team decides to place her on a breathing machine to optimise the oxygen levels in her blood. Shortly after, Ria is admitted to the Intensive Care Unit (ICU) with suspected pneumonia. Despite being attached to a ventilator, Ria's breathing condition continues to worsen over the next 12 hours as her sick lungs are no longer able to perform efficient gas exchange, and the oxygen supply to Ria's vital organs is becoming severely compromised.

Ria is commenced on an advanced mode of mechanical ventilation and Nitric Oxide treatment to improve gas exchange. To no avail. Crucial time passes with Ria deteriorating further. Ria's parents, partner and her two small children are called to the hospital as her oxygen levels are now dangerously low, placing her at risk of irreversible hypoxic brain injury. The nurses appear nervous and stressed. The medical team is talking about instating something called 'ECMO' and potentially transporting Ria to a different hospital across town. This is distressing as Ria is attached to all these tubes, lines and beeping machines. The family is anxious about the delayed instatement of the lifesaving ECLS treatment. In what seems like a terrible eternity, 'ECLS' is commenced on the second day. Ria does not look like herself any longer and the family is frightened. Her oxygenation levels however, improve with the treatment.

With the ECMO in place, there is another staff, a 'perfusionist' at the bedside, operating the device. The perfusionist appears very tired and the family is anxious about her staying overnight with the ECMO. The next day, there is another perfusionist. Oddly, the following night, one of the medical ICU doctors mans the ECMO. He too, looks very tired. The family had seen him around in the morning. At some point during day 3 of Ria's admission, the ECMO machine is not manned for 5 hours at all. The bedside nurse appears very stressed and concerned about this and clearly, the nursing shift supervisor is also unhappy. There are a lot of conversations out of earshot. On day 4, there is yet another perfusionist. They all seem to be external employees, reassuringly, they all seem to know what they are doing. On day 5, the medical team makes it known that Ria will be transferred to ICU at The Alfred Hospital across town as a bed has finally become available.

Apparently, The Alfred operates ECMOs routinely. Ria is transferred. On day 14 at The Alfred, Ria is not waking up as planned and is consequently diagnosed with irreversible hypoxic brain injury due to the low oxygen levels during her stay at The Austin. The decision is made by her family to withdraw treatment and Ria passes away on day 15, leaving behind two young children, a partner and parents.

Ria is one of nine patients annually requiring ECLS in the ICU. Some estimated 5 other patients who would also benefit from ECLS treatment, potentially undergo less effective conventional treatment as there is such high threshold to instate ECLS. See Appendix 17 for the continuing of 'A day in the Life … for:

- The Clinical Perfusionist Team
- The Nursing Team
- The Medical Team
- The Cardiac Patient on the surgical waitlist
- The Head of Cardiac Surgery
- The ICU Nurse Unit Manager

The Pitch

The introduction of a fully integrated ECLS service, medically supervised, nurse-led and clinical perfusionist-independent, will close the gap in seamless care provision at the most critical and advanced level. The service will align with global and local best practice optimising patient outcome, positively impact on patient and family experience, attract and retain highly performing clinical teams, meet demand for future growth in critical care, and promote Austin's Brand whilst creating revenue.

INTRODUCTION

The history of Extracorporeal Membrane Oxygenation (ECMO) dates back to 1975 when it was successfully instated for respiratory failure in neonates. Since then, many tertiary centres globally have fully integrated an ECLS service, offering treatment to those neonatal, paediatric and adult patients in severe but reversible respiratory and/or cardiac failure who do not responded to conventional critical care therapies. Depending on indication (Appendix 13 – Indications for ECLS Therapy, ECLS therapy is applied in va or vv mode, for cardiac failure and respiratory failure respectively. 73,596 patients worldwide have been registered for treatment with ECLS therapy to January 2016. Global adult survival rates lie at 43%. Annually, >6000 patients receive ECLS world-wide.

At Austin Health, 47 patients with acute cardio and/or respiratory failure have received ECLS therapy since 2009, nine in 2015/16. Austin Health's current model of care to effectively meet ECLS demand is financially non-economical and potentially compromises best patient outcomes.

This report investigates the feasibility and value adding potential of a fully integrated ECLS service at Austin Health and arrives at a conclusion by conducting detailed analyses of:

In Scope

- The Business Opportunity
- The Business Concept
- The Industry
- The Competitive Analysis
- The Market Analysis
- The Business Model Overview
- The Marketing Plan
- The Management Feasibility
- The Operating Plan
- The Financial Feasibility
- The Exit and or Growth Strategy

Out of Scope

- Project implementation plan (Next Stage: Appendix 15 - Setting up an ECMO Service)
- Micro Economy: quality-adjusted life-years (QALYs) for surviving ECLS patients
- Annual Variations in government funding DRG – WIES

THE BUSINESS CONCEPT

Overview

- This business venture aims to introduce an ECLS service at Austin Health which is financially viable, adds value to our communities and strengthens the Austin Brand.

- The new business model encompasses medical supervision, nurse-led device operation with declining dependency on Clinical Perfusionists Services, allowing those to operate at full capacity in the cardiac operating suites.
- Anticipated benefits are non-disrupted operational flow of cardiac surgery, optimised ECLS patient outcome and positive patient experience, marginally positive cost-benefit, improved workforce satisfaction and an increase in Austin Health's reputation.

Methodology

Methodologies used in this report are:

- Best practice analysis (Literature research)
- Benchmarking
- Cost-Benefit Analysis
- Domain Experts Opinions
- Internal Business reports
- Strategic Canvas (factors of competition)
- Strength-Stature Grid
- Surveys and Interviews with Domain Experts Opinions

Purpose

The purpose of the report is to demonstrate the economic viability of a fully integrated ECLS service and its value adding characteristics. The report is asking for executive commitment and upfront funding of $300, 000 for the first year, with a view of creating a small marginal profit of $170, 000 in its second year.

The Industry

Benchmarking

ECLS (offered on national and global level) is an established treatment form for critically ill patients with reversible cardio/respiratory failure refractory to conventional intensive therapy.

Centres registered with ELSO reported over 70,000 patients who have been treated with ECLS to date (Figure 2).

Figure 2. Extra corporal life support organisation, 2016 – international summary

ECLS Registry Report
International Summary
January, 2016

Extracorporeal Life Support Organization
2800 Plymouth Road
Building 300, Room 303
Ann Arbor, MI 48109

Overall Outcomes

	Total Patients	Survived ECLS		Survived to DC or Transfer	
Neonatal					
Respiratory	28,723	24,155	84%	21,274	74%
Cardiac	6,269	3,885	62%	2,599	41%
ECPR	1,254	806	64%	514	41%
Pediatric					
Respiratory	7,210	4,787	66%	4,155	58%
Cardiac	8,021	5,341	67%	4,067	51%
ECPR	2,788	1,532	55%	1,144	41%
Adult					
Respiratory	9,102	5,989	66%	5,254	58%
Cardiac	7,850	4,394	56%	3,233	41%
ECPR	2,379	948	40%	707	30%
Total	73,596	51,837	70%	42,947	58%

During 2015, >6000 people world-wide received ECLS therapy (Figure 3).

In 2012 in the United States alone, 3000 patients were hospitalised and therapized with ECLS (Figure 4).

Major industry players within Victoria are The Alfred, Barwon Health (Geelong), St. Vincent's Hospital public, Monash Health and Epworth Health Private.

Public healthcare providers compete against each other in terms of government funding, tangibles, such as mortality, most optimal clinical outcomes and best patient experience, but also intangibles, such as reputation and international recognition underpinned by research and advanced clinical practice.

The Alfred Hospital is the largest industry player for adult ECLS nationally and domineers both the public and private healthcare market within Australia and New Zealand.

The Alfred has been providing Adult ECLS since 1990 and eliminated their dependence on the Clinical Perfusionist Services in 2003 to improve 'ECMO delivery and beside care'. Since, the ECLS service has grown and on average 1.9 patients/day (Exhibit 4) receive ECLS therapy in the Alfred ICU. This number should be seen in the context of The Alfred providing Victoria's State Service for Heart &

Figure 3. Extra corporal life support organisation, 2016 - total numbers and centres by year

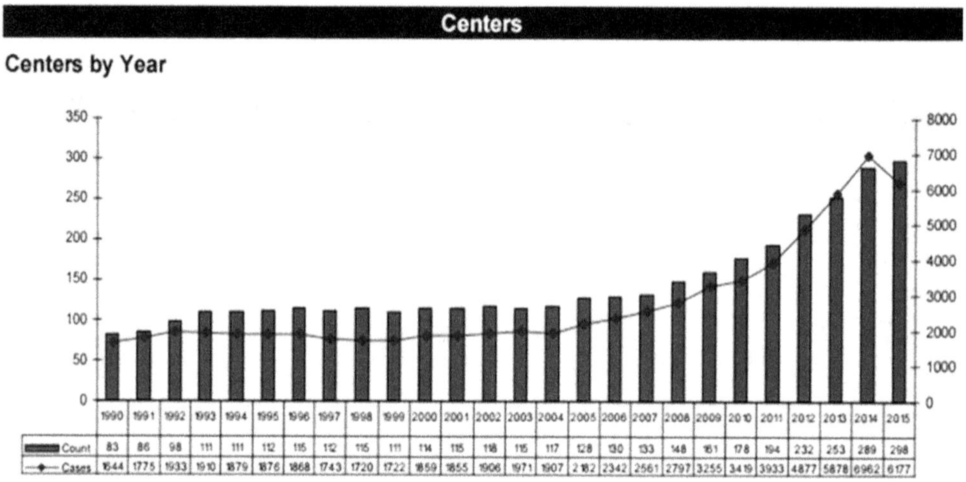

Figure 4. US ECLS cases and mortality, 2002 – 2012

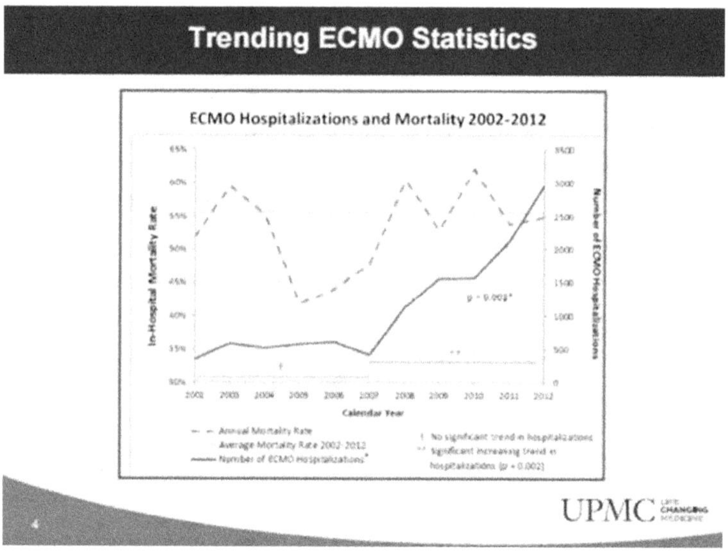

Lung Transplant and ECLS is applied as bridging time to transplant. Further, The Alfred, in cooperation with ARV (Adult Retrieval Victoria), has grown to be the State Service provider for ECMO retrievals; is listed and recognised as a 'Centre of Excellence' on the ELSO website; offers internal and world renowned external education courses; runs a bi-annually International ECMO / VAD (Ventricular Assist Device) symposiums; and conducts extensive research.

A recent visit to The Alfred was a promising start to a collaborative approach to the Austin model.

In 2013, Barwon Health (Geelong Hospital) ICU, entered a partnership with The Alfred, adapting the Alfred Model establishing the first regional ECLS service nation-wide. The model of care enables a nurse-led extracorporeal membrane oxygenation (ECMO) service. Total ECLS numbers are not publically available.

Monash Health covers Melbourne's South-East Corridor. Its current new development of the Victorian Heart Hospital will encompass advanced cardiac surgery and it can safely be assumed that an ECLS service will be included. Specific data on ECLS at Monash could not be obtained for this report.

St. Vincent's Hospital (public) currently undertakes a development of a nurse-led model (Alfred based). This model is in its infancies. Specific data on ECLS episodes is not publically available.

Figure 5. Alfred Hospital, ECLS – weaning success 1990 – 2015

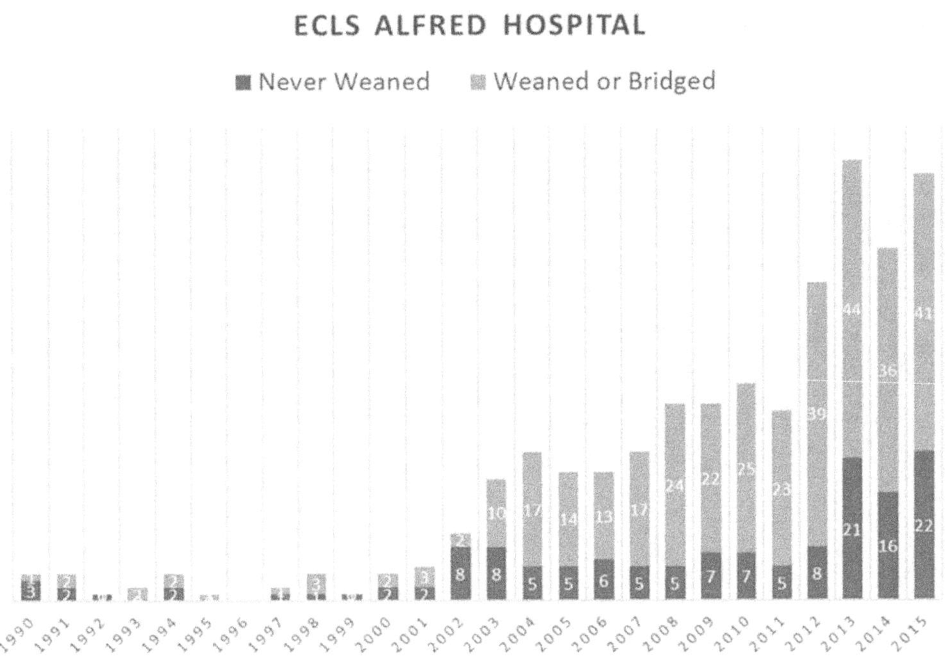

Appendix 16 - PATIENT STORIES describes the patient experience of an ECLS recipient at St Vincent's Hospital (Brett Purcell's Story - St. Vincent's Hospital Melbourne).

Epworth Health Richmond (Private) operates an ECLS service which is perfusionist-led and spans 3 - 5 days. After that time, patients are being transferred to The Alfred. Annually, Epworth Richmond operates less than 5 ECLSs.

Austin Health's current ECLS model is clinical perfusionist-led. There were 47 ECLS episodes since 2009 (Exhibit 5). A patient experience story can be read here: Appendix 16.

With the exemption of 2009, when Australia was severely affected by the world wide swine flu (H1N1) epidemic, Austin ECMO cases have been relatively stable over past 5 years – averaging between 6 to 8 cases annually.

ICU medical consultant A/Prof Andrew Hilton and Cardiology Service Director Omar Farouk estimate that approximately 5 to 10 Catheterisation Laboratory episodes annually might benefit from having an ECMO service available.

Therefore, an estimated 10 to 20 combined cases per year appears a reasonable projection (Exhibit 6) at this stage. According to ELSO guidelines, this is considered an efficient number with which to teach and maintain competencies, and build a safe, efficient, and viable ECLS service for Austin Health.

Figure 6. ECLS episodes at Austin Health

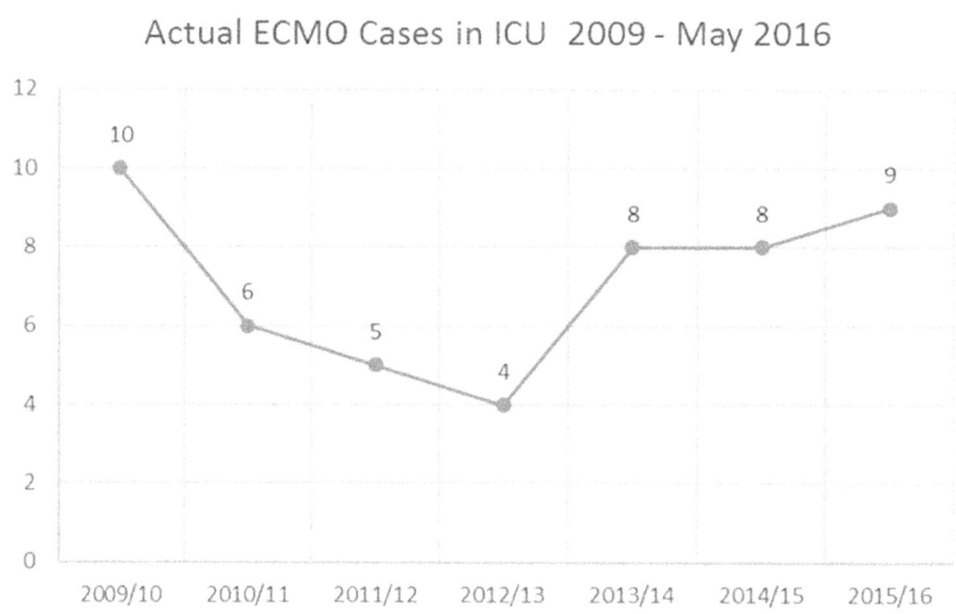

Patients, who currently would benefit from ECLS are often referred to the next ECMO Centre (The Alfred Hospital). Treatment might be delayed, possibly compromising clinical outcome, affecting morbidity and mortality. The retrieval service is costly and the transport itself poses a significant clinical risk to the patient.

It should be noted that the benchmarking component for this report is not yet complete and visits of two European Intensive Care Units, are planned for July 2016.

COMPETITIVE ANALYSIS

Direct and Indirect Competitors: Determining the Potential of the Competitors

Cost leader (C) or differentiator (D)

Appendix 18 - Breakdown of the analysis of competitor potential and degree of competition.

Traditionally, market leaders for ECSL services are large public health care providers only. Increasing access demand to ECLS services state wide due to a growing population in combination with advanced technologies, greater business efficiency and improved marketing brokers, allow for competitors previously considered to be potential competitors to migrate into positions of indirect or direct competitors.

Figure 7. Future modelling for Austin ECLS episodes

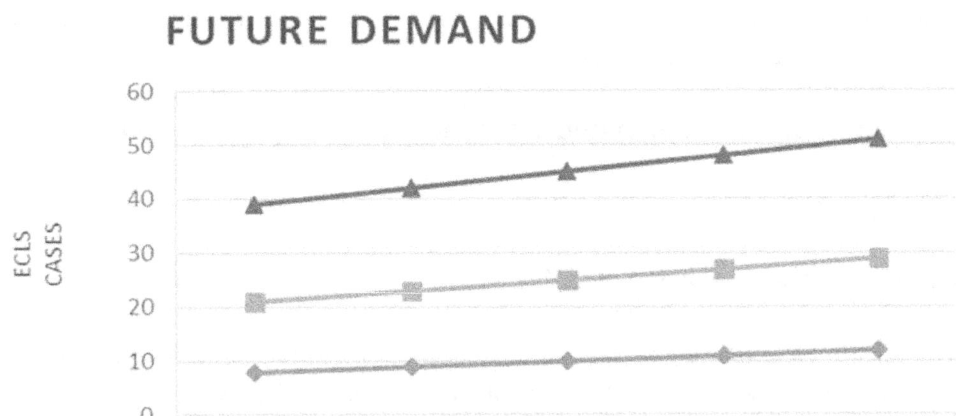

	2016/17	2017/18	2018/19	2019/20	2020/21
max	18	19	20	21	22
average	13	14	15	16	17
min	8	9	10	11	12

Table 1. Summary potential of the competitors and degree of competition

All Competitors – Summary		**What is offered**		
What is considered	(D)(C) (D) (D)	**Direct Competitor** The Alfred Monash St Vincent	**Potential Competitor** Barwon	(D)
	(D) (C)	Indirect Competitor Epworth	Incipient Competitor St. Vincent	(D)

Austin itself competes by favourable geographic location covering the northern corridor of Melbourne and dominating the closest public healthcare service, the Northern Hospital. The Northern Hospital is not considered a competitor. Austin further competes by its specialist services and its world renowned research activities.

Austin Health and The Alfred pursue strategies of differentiation (patient experience, place, promotion), whereas private providers usually differentiate by cost and by differentiation. The private, not-for-profit Epworth Hospital is higher priced (private healthcare cover for customers) but occupies a smaller (yet expanding) market share, differentiating by products (i.e. special surgery), by providing great patient experiences and by being located in an attractive easily accessible location. There is potential for The Epworth Hospital to expand their critical care services, anticipating tomorrow's needs. Other, somewhat smaller public healthcare providers such as St. Vincent's require close monitoring about their strategic directions. Potentially St Vincent's can differentiate by location (place), product and/or promotion. However, required infrastructure and workforce expansion (i.e. additional ICU beds, additional operating theatres and employment of a skilled workforce) is timely and costly and can be viewed as a barrier to entry.

Strategy Canvas: Austin and Competitors

See Figure 8.

ERRC Analysi: Austin Health

The Austin Health strategic profile depicts the correlation between the 'level of offerings' from low to high and 'factors of competition'. It displays the Austin Health 'as-is' (blue) & 'to-be' (orange) curve (Appendix 19).

It was identified from this exercise that Austin Health needs to:

- RAISE its Presence/Visibility of its critical care services

Figure 8. Competitor strategic profile comparison

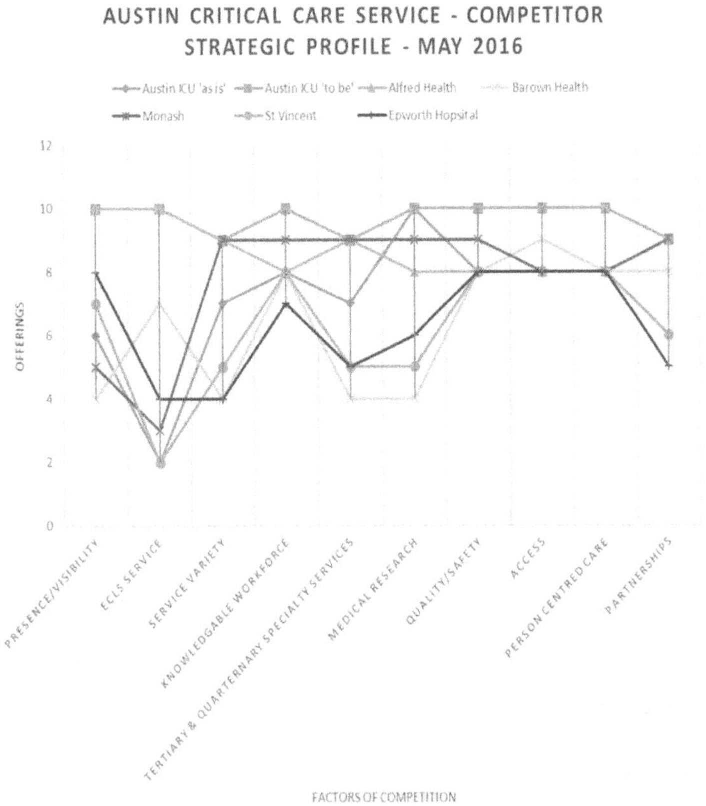

- (RAISE) CREATE an ECLS service
- RAISE Service Variety
- RAISE Knowledgeable Workforce
- RAISE Tertiary & Quaternary Specialty Services such as ECLS
- RAISE (Maintain) Medical Research
- RAISE Quality/Safety
- RAISE Access to ECLS
- RAISE Person Centred Care
- RAISE Partnerships with Centres of Excellence in critical care

By doing so, Austin's competitive advantage will increase.

Figure 9. Austin Strategic Profile

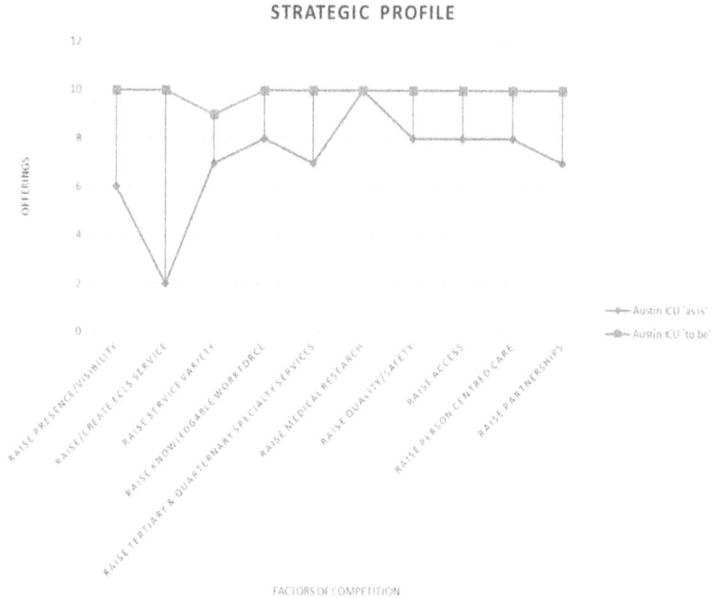

Market Analysis

Target Market Description

The following SWOT (Strengths, Weaknesses, Opportunities and Threats) analysis assesses the Market Attractiveness (Table 3 - Appendix 20) and the competitive (differential) advantage (Table 4 - Appendix 20) of the ECLS service. By quantitating external (opportunities and threats) and internal (strengths and weaknesses) factors, the actions in response to the SWOT analysis will aid Austin Health steering towards maximising value for its stakeholders (Appendix 20).

Step 1: Determining the Strategic Objective (Table 5)

The total weighted scores (Appendix 20) of both, average Threats & Opportunities (4.74) and Strengths & Weaknesses (3.89) have been plotted in to the Strategic Characterisation Matrix (SCM) (Table 2).

This allows the determination of the strategic objective and future projection. The analysis shows that the current ECLS service with its approximated market share of 5% is currently positioned in a growth area. As future demand for ECLS services has been forecasted, it can be confidently predicted that service growth is

Table 2. Assessing strategic options for the introduction of the ECLS Service at Austin Health utilising the Strategic Characterisation Matrix (SCM)

<table>
<tr><td rowspan="5">Threats & Opportunities</td><td rowspan="3">High 7
Med 3.5
Low 1</td><td>Divest/Growth</td><td>Growth
YES</td><td>Growth/Enter</td></tr>
<tr><td>Harvest</td><td>Maintain</td><td>Growth</td></tr>
<tr><td>Divest</td><td>Harvest</td><td>Maintain</td></tr>
<tr><td colspan="4">Differentiation Factors
Strengths & Weaknesses</td></tr>
<tr><td></td><td>1 Disadvantaged</td><td>3.5 Average</td><td>Advantaged 7</td></tr>
</table>

required. Consequently, the author recommends to support this valuable business opportunity by adjusting strategies and allocating further resources.

Following on from the analysis of market attractiveness and differential position, further analysis is required to determine (1) the value potential of the customer (patient/key stakeholders) and (2) the competitive potential of competitors (Appendix 18).

Step 2: Determining the Value Potential of the Customer (Patient/Key Stakeholders) for the ECLS Service

To determine the value potential of customers for the service, four criteria (strategic, significant, profitable, and loyal) were applied for the assessment on a scale from 1 (low) to 7 (high) for each of the segments. (Table 3).

The above analysis is indicative that the introduction of a fully integrated ECLS service stimulates significant customer value potential for Austin Health as a leading public health service provider. Segments such as the patients themselves, Cardiac Surgery, Cardiac Catheterisation Laboratory, Respiratory Medicine and Intensive Care Services will greatly benefit from an integrated ECLS service. As funding is activity based and occurs via WIES, the service is profitable. Calculations have shown that since July 2009, $6,132,500 in WIES funding was generated, covering 116% of the cost.

Therefore, the addition of an ECLS service for AH to deliver tertiary services should be promoted.

BUSINESS MODEL OVERVIEW

Business Model Canvas Strategyzer, 2016

An in-depth analysis of the above business model canvas can be found in Appendix 21.

Table 3. Value potential of for ECLS customers (patient / key stakeholders)

Segment	Strategic	Significant	Profitable	Loyal	Average
Patients/Families	7	7	2	5	5.25
Cardiac Surgery	7	7	6	7	6.75
Anaesthetics	3	4	6	3	4.0
Respiratory Medicine	7	7	6	7	6.75
Cardiac Catheterisation Laboratory	7	7	6	7	6.75
Intensive Care	7	7	6	7	6.75
Intensive Care Workforce	7	7	6	5	6.25
Clinical Perfusionist Services	7	7	1	6	5.25
Austin Health	7	7	6	5	6.25

Rating 1 – 7; 1 = low 7 = high

Technical Feasibility

There is sufficient academic and clinical expertise within the Intensive Care to teach, assess, accredit and sustain an ECLS service at Austin Health. Perfusionist Services already are fully operational and have two ECMO devices for cardiac theatres.

The cost for development is outlined in the financial feasibility section below.

Marketing Plan

A marketing plan including external advertising and promotion is not required for this project as it is an internal initiative and all key stakeholders are involved.

Information about the service however will be communicated to the Department of Health and also to ELSO when registering.

Management Feasibility

As this is a service addition to a fully established organisation, all legal structures, human resources and management resources are already in place. So are internal management teams and capabilities relevant to the business.

Operating Plan

The physical location is already present. Facilities, inventory and most equipment are covered by sunk costs. Additional equipment costs are included in the financial feasibility section below.

The workforce is already present. There is a requirement to acquire and maintain additional skill sets. This is outlined in the financial feasibility section below.

The supplier, Maquet, is already under contract with different equipment.

Financial Feasibility

Calculations have shown that median marginal cost for each ECLS episode is covered by median marginal revenue (government funding) by 116%.

Median WIES Revenue equals 126,239 and Median cost equal 108,362 based on 2009-2016 data. That means that WIES revenue covers 116% of the total cost (Figure 11).

Based on those calculations, forecasting, incorporating growth shows a total profit of $500, 000 over 5 years. This includes all training and equipment costs.

Excluded from the cost benefit analysis are: Consumables and Sunk Costs (salary/wages/rent). Economies of scale apply and the service becomes more profitable as throughput increases.

Figure 10. Revenue versus cost

wiesrev		cost	
Min.	: 25308	Min.	: 7664
1st Qu.	: 67568	1st Qu.	: 66053
Median	:126239	Median	:108382
Mean	:132621	Mean	:139375
3rd Qu.	:159426	3rd Qu.	:195376
Max.	:361571	Max.	:529656

Figure 11. ECMO cost analysis

```
> summary(ecmo)
       fy             e                        dd               ur                      wip            d_cnt
 2009-10:10   IP02328198: 1   2009-07-20 13:41:00: 1   099770 : 1   Crosses Fin years: 2   Min.   :1
 2010-11: 6   IP02330072: 1   2009-07-30 13:45:00: 1   194980 : 1   Within Fin year  :42   1st Qu.:1
 2011-12: 5   IP02333527: 1   2009-08-04 15:55:00: 1   2005076: 1                          Median :1
 2012-13: 4   IP02337641: 1   2009-08-24 11:05:00: 1   200985 : 1                          Mean   :1
 2013-14: 8   IP02343855: 1   2009-09-22 16:12:00: 1   2011864: 1                          3rd Qu.:1
 2014-15: 8   IP02345905: 1   2009-11-27 02:52:00: 1   2024195: 1                          Max.   :1
 2015-16: 3   (Other)   :38   (Other)            :38   (Other):38
      los             icuhr            mvhr             wies            wiesrev            cost
 Min.   :  1.00   Min.   :  7.0   Min.   :  6.0   Min.   :  5.96   Min.   : 25308   Min.   :  7664
 1st Qu.:  7.00   1st Qu.:130.0   1st Qu.: 93.0   1st Qu.: 18.11   1st Qu.: 67568   1st Qu.: 66053
 Median : 20.00   Median :247.5   Median :191.0   Median : 33.97   Median :126239   Median :108382
 Mean   : 28.36   Mean   :282.3   Mean   :256.3   Mean   : 35.71   Mean   :132621   Mean   :139375
 3rd Qu.: 38.25   3rd Qu.:425.5   3rd Qu.:339.0   3rd Qu.: 46.84   3rd Qu.:159426   3rd Qu.:195376
 Max.   :167.00   Max.   :944.0   Max.   :950.0   Max.   :100.44   Max.   :361571   Max.   :529656
```

Table 4. Excluded costs

	Year 1	Year 2	Year 3	Year 4	Year 5
	2016-17	2017-18	2018-19	2019-20	2020-21
Excluded	-195, 000	-210, 000	-240, 000	-256, 000	-272, 000
Sunk Costs (salary/wages/ rent)	x	x	x	x	x

Figure 12. Cost benefit analysis 2016-17 part 1

	Year 1 2016/17	Year 2 2017/18	Year 3 2018/19	Year 4 2019/20	Year 5 2021/22
Median Marginal Costs per episode (increase 2% annually)	-$ 108,362	-$ 110,529	-$ 112,740	-$ 114,995	-$ 117,295
Estimated Episodes (Annual Average)	13	14	15	16	17
Total Marginal Cost (Average) per all Episodes Annually	-$ 1,408,706	-$ 1,547,409	-$ 1,691,097	-$ 1,839,914	-$ 1,994,007
Capital Invest	-$ 220,000	$ -	$ -	$ -	$ -
Training Medical	-$ 20,000	-$ 5,000	-$ 5,000	-$ 5,000	-$ 5,000
Training Nursing	-$ 18,240	-$ 26,144	-$ 29,360	-$ 31,824	-$ 34,320
Backfill Nursing	-$ 31,920	-$ 28,728	-$ 32,105	-$ 34,726	-$ 37,346
ECMO Coordinator	-$ 7,904	-$ 8,112	-$ 8,320	-$ 17,056	-$ 17,472
Annual Simulation Fees	-$ 3,300	-$ 3,400	-$ 3,500	-$ 3,600	-$ 3,700
Service Agreement		-$ 2,000	-$ 2,000	-$ 2,800	-$ 2,800
Median Marginal Revenue in WIES/Episode (increase 2% annually)	$ 126,239	$ 128,764	$ 131,339	$ 133,966	$ 136,645
Median Marginal Revenue in WIES Annual Average (increase 2% annually)	$ 1,641,107	$ 1,802,693	$ 1,970,086	$ 2,143,453	$ 2,322,968
Total Profit	-$ 37,043	$ 210,628	$ 230,808	$ 243,259	$ 265,669

Figure 13. Cost benefit analysis part 2

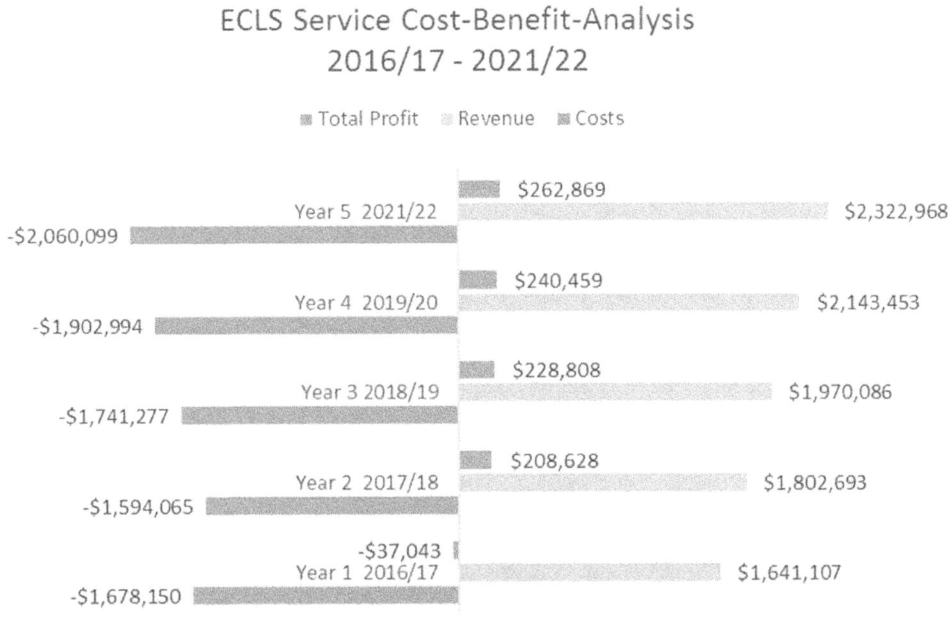

Table 5. Accumulative profit 5-year forecast

	Year 1	Year 2	Year 3	Year 4	Year 5
	2016-17	2017-18	2018-19	2019-20	2020-21
5-year accumulative total profit	-$ 37,043	$ 171,585	$ 437,436	$ 469,268	$ 503,328

Avoiding associated marginal costs from locum CP services ($51'000), consultant overtime ($25'000) and loss of opportunity costs for cardiac case cancellation ($34'000), additional savings of $110'000 could have been made during the first six months of 2015/16 alone.

Marginal Costs and Loss of Opportunity Costs Equated to $110'000 for July – January 2015/16

Marginal Costs

Locum clinical perfusionists: 2015/16 (July – January) = $51K
Consultant overtime approx. $25K

Figure 14. Total profit forecast

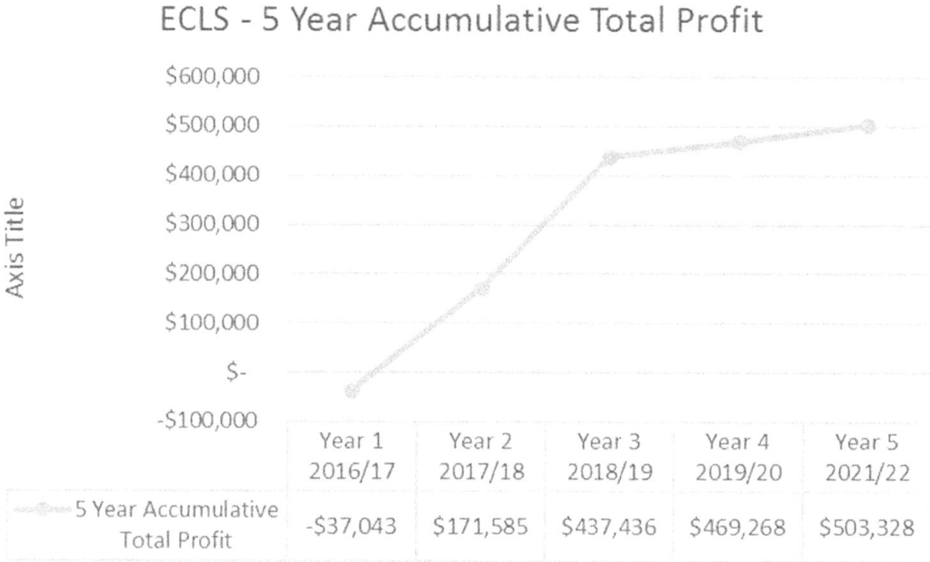

Loss of Opportunity Costs

$34K – cardiac cancellation

Exit and Growth Strategy

Forecasting demonstrates that demand for future ECLS episodes will increase annually by one episode. Formal training (refresher) requirements will reduce with greater exposure to ECLS therapy.

With research also advancing, new, game changing therapies, such as liver or brain ECLS, might be introduced in the future.

An exit strategy is not required as the service is activity based funded. If demand decreases, costs will also decrease. Training costs can be absorbed in to the overall budget for some time.

CONCLUSION

ECLS therapy instatement in the critically ill patient with reversible cardio/respiratory failure who is refractory to conventional treatment optimises patient outcome. Due to the nature of government activity based funding (Appendix 2, Appendix 3), a fully integrated ECLS service with accredited staff is a valuable addition to Austin's critical care services, meeting the need of the community and strengthening the Austin Brand. The integration of the service is increasing Austin's reputation and aids the recruitment and retention of a high performing workforce, preparing Austin Health for future growth.

It is therefore recommended to fund the introduction of an ECLS service at Austin Health.

KEY TERMS AND DEFINITIONS

CP: Clinical perfusionist
CSU: Clinical service unit
DRG: Diagnostic Related Groups
DoH: Department of Health
DHHS: Department of Health and Human Services
EBA: Enterprise Bargain Agreement
ECLS: Extra Corporeal Life Support
ECMO: Extra Corporeal Membrane Oxygenation
ELSO: Extra Corporeal Support Organisation
ERRC: Eliminate – Reduce – Raise – Create
ICU: Intensive Care Unit
IHPA: Independent Hospital Pricing Authority
SIG: Special Interest Group
SWOT: Strength – Weaknesses – Opportunity – Threats

WIES: Weighted Inlier Equivalent Separation. The Weighted Inlier Equivalent Separation (WIES) is a cost weight (W) that is adjusted for time spent in hospital (IES), and represents a relative measure of resource use for each episode of care in a DGR. WIES allocated to an episode depends upon the episode's DRG, the amount of time spent in hospital and the episode's eligibility for WIES co-payments.

Victorian WIES Cost Weights: Victorian cost weights are developed each year using the costs of treating patients as reported to the Department of Health & Human Services by public hospitals. The department pays a price per unit of WIES. WIES prices vary between hospitals to account for differences in specialisation, economies of scale and levels of remoteness.

APPENDIX 1

Victorian Wies Funding for Ecmo 2015 - 16 (Figure 15)

APPENDIX 2

ECMO Cost by Episode Austin 2009 – 2016 (Figure 16)

APPENDIX 3

ECMO Wies Revenue by Episode Austin 2009- 2016 (Figure 17)

APPENDIX 4

ECMO Patient ICU Admission Hours per FY 2009 – 2016 (Figure 18)

APPENDIX 5

ECMO Patient Mechanical Ventilation Hours per FY (Figure 19)

APPENDIX 6

Indications For ECLS Therapy (Table 6)

Figure 15. Victorian WIES funding for ECMO 2015-16

2.21.2 WIES22 2015–16 Victorian cost weights

Victorian AR-DRG 7.0 Code	Label	Mech.Vent. Copayment	Other Copayment	Inlier Low	Boundary High	Average Inlier Stay	Same/One Day DRG	Same Day Weight	One Day Weight	Multi-Day Low Outlier per Diem	Inlier Weight	High Outlier per Diem	HITH Outlier per Diem
A40A	ECMO W Tracheostomy	4		33	76	49.6		6.6971	7.3864	1.3367	51.4990	0.3621	0.2897
A40B	ECMO W/O Tracheostomy	4		15	35	22.2		3.8655	4.6080	1.3860	25.3973	0.3621	0.2897

Figure 16. ECMO cost by episode Austin 2009-2016

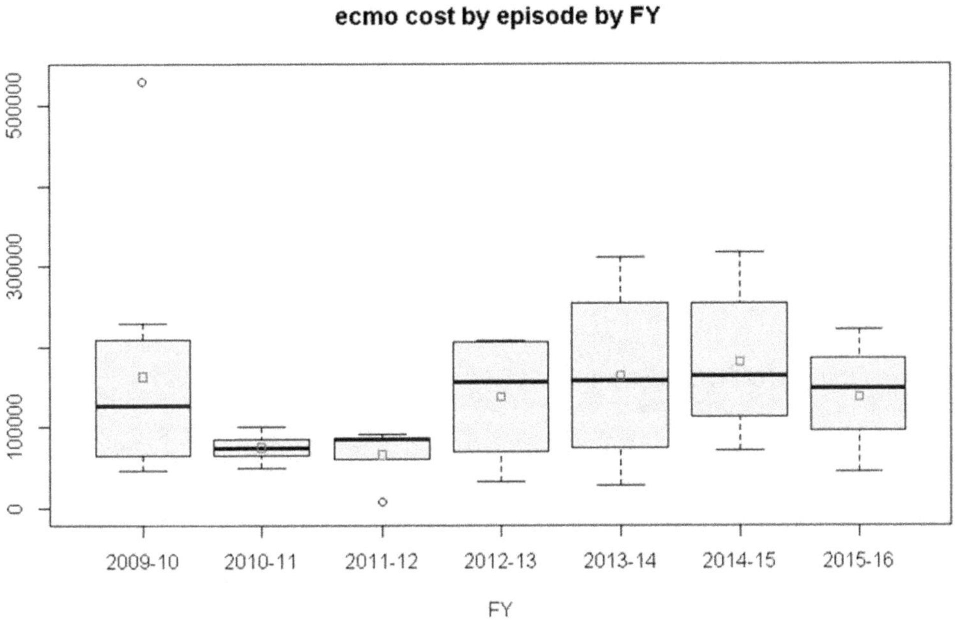

Figure 17. ECMO WIES revenue by episode Austin 2009 – 2016

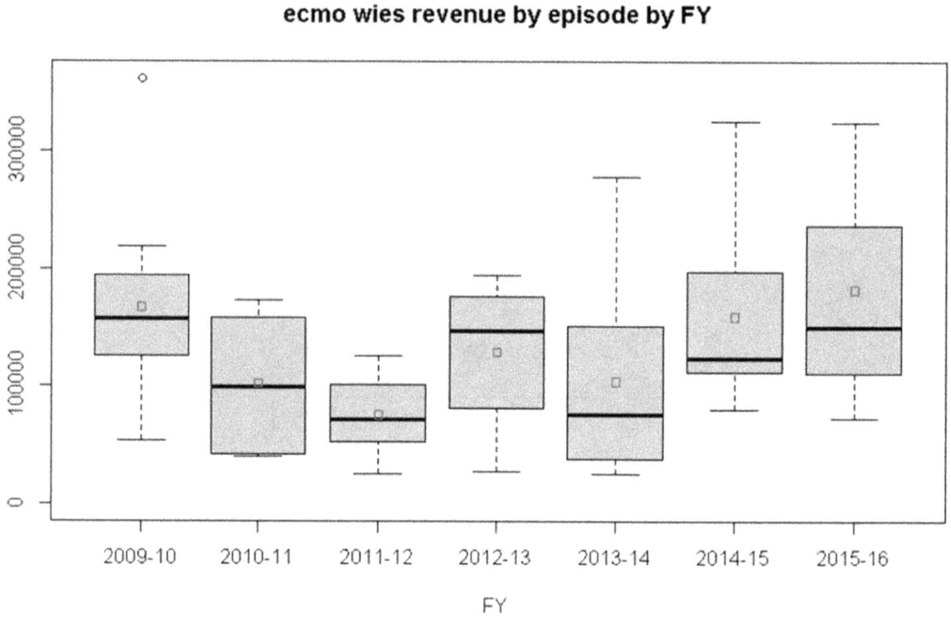

Figure 18. ECMO ICU admission

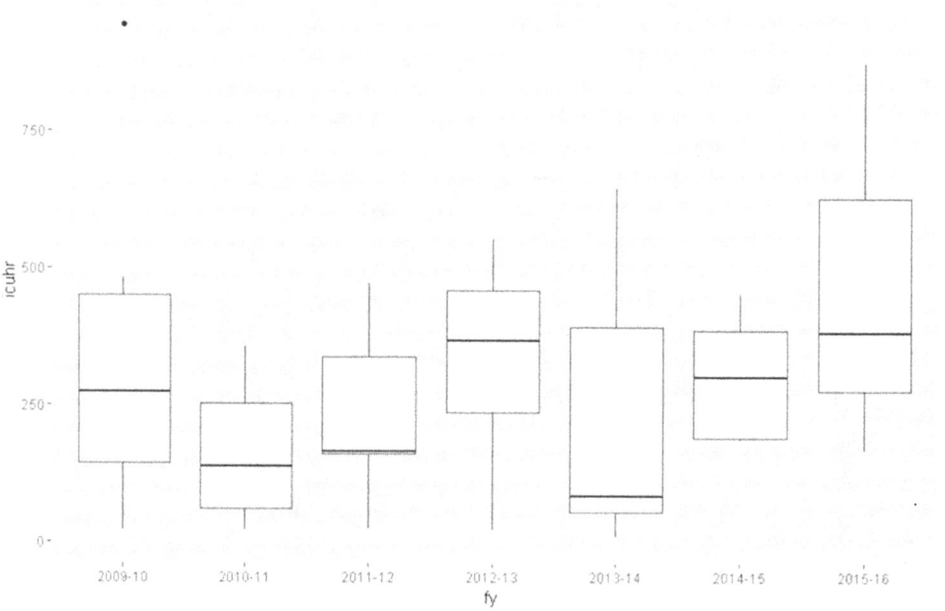

Figure 19. ECMO mechanical ventilation

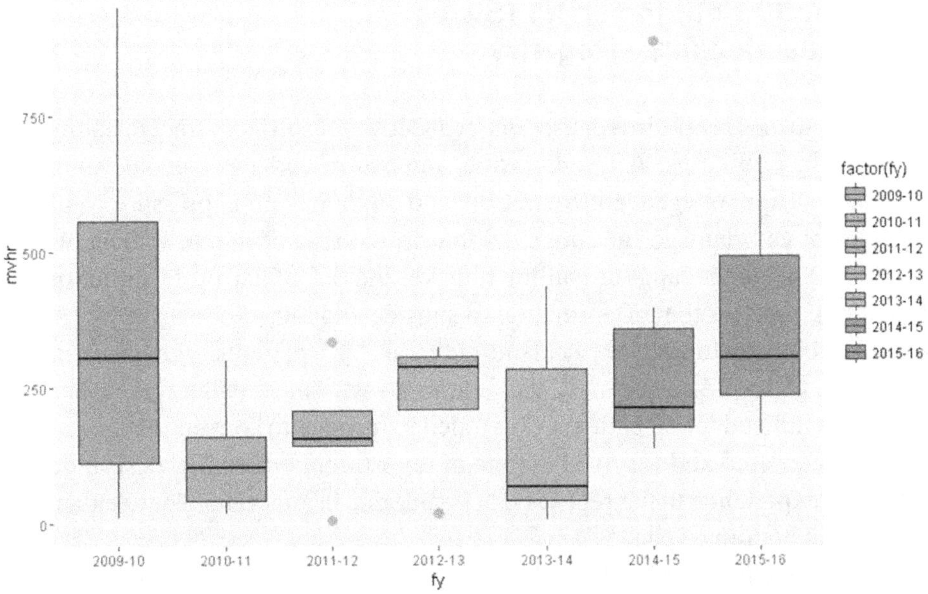

Table 6. Indications for ECLS

Heart	Lungs
Cardiogenic shock Cardiomyopathy myocarditis	ARDS (Adult Respiratory Distress Syndrome) Pneumonia Pulmonary hypertension Acute respiratory failure Pulmonary embolism

APPENDIX 7

Information About the H1N1 (Swine FLU) Epidemic 2009 - Registry

Infection with the H1N1 virus causes upper and lower respiratory tract inflammation and fever. In rare cases, ICU admission, intubation and mechanical ventilation is required. High oxygen concentration and high inflating pressure ventilator management can damage the lungs, adding to the risk of dying. Patient support with ECMO while the lungs are failing removes the risk of harmful ventilation, and allows more time for the inflammation to subside and lungs to recover.

In the 2009 Australia/New Zealand outbreak, 201 patients with confirmed or suspected H1N1 were treated in ECMO centres. Most of these patients recovered, but ECMO was utilized for 68 patients who failed to respond to conventional measures, with 79% recovered and survived at time of reporting. For detailed descriptions of the ECMO experience in the recent H1N1 epidemic in Australia/New Zealand, see references at bottom of page.

ECMO is the use of a modified heart-lung machine to take over the function of the heart and lungs for days or weeks in patients with acute or severe, heart or lung failure. ECMO has been used in over 40,000 patients of all ages. Because ECMO has potential complications, it is only used in patients who have high risk of dying. ECMO is complicated and used only in experienced centres. The limiting factor is not equipment, but people with the expertise in the technique. The outcome depends on whether the heart or lungs can recover with continuing time and treatment. Recovery and survival when ECMO is utilized in adult respiratory failure is currently about 50%. There are 160 ECMO centres in the Extracorporeal Life Support Organization (ELSO); 126 are in North America.

ECMO is a complex technique and requires thorough preparation, appropriate equipment, institutional commitment, practice and a dedicated team. If you are considering ECMO for a critically ill H1N1 patient and your centre is not prepared, it is better to refer the patient and not attempt ECMO until your centre is well-trained and prepared to do it. If transport is not possible, continue optimal conventional therapy. If the patient is dying despite optimal therapy and your centre is attempting ECMO anyway, additional support and advice should be sought from nearby ELSO centres.

APPENDIX 8

A Day in the Life

The Clinical Perfusionist Team

Peter is the head of the Clinical Perfusionist (CP) Team, overseeing 3 CPs. The ICU team calls and requests urgent support for ECMO instatement in a young female patient. The cardiac surgeons and the clinical perfusionists are busy in the operating theatres for several hours to come and cannot be of immediate assistance. ICU calls back a few hours later, stating that they have now put the patient on ECMO, requiring a perfusionist. The clinical perfusionist, who has assisted two cases in the operating theatre during the day, is now allocated by Peter to the ICU to operate the ECMO machine overnight. She is tired and wants to go home, yet another 12 hours are ahead. She is trying to keep upbeat and professional for Ria's family. It is a long night. Unsuccessful attempts are made by Peter and the Divisional Director to employ a locum perfusionist (at high cost). None can be found for several days as there are only a small number of CPs covering Victoria and as competition with private hospitals (which pay more attractive rates to the perfusionists) is high. Peter's team grows dangerously sleep deprived by working days assisting in the operating theatre and at night operating the ECMO in the ICU. At some point, the ECMO is only supported externally over a 5-hour period as Peter has been ordered to call back the perfusionist to the operating theatre to assist in a cardiac case and to provide 'remote' support only to the ICU team. Everyone is stressed and tired. Peter feels increasingly frustrated as this situation repeats itself with each ECMO episode. Peter's team members start calling in sick. Luckily, one of the medical ICU consultants, the only one who is accredited to operate the device, offers to cover the next night. A locum perfusionist is found on day 4 and charges $100/hour. Peter feels relief when Ria is retrieved to The Alfred on day 5.

The Nursing Team

None of the nursing staff are ECMO accredited and only a few are familiar with the concept. The nursing team is keen to assist but is stressed, feeling out of depth and fearing for Ria's life. Attempts are made to hide this from Ria's family, who repeatedly asks questions about the delayed initiation of the ECMO therapy. When ECMO is finally instated but then unassisted within the ICU, the nursing team grows irate and complaints are made to the ICU Nurse Unit Manager. The ICU nurses are very stressed and unhappy, which is obvious to Ria's family. Anxiety levels are at maximum height by all involved. Everybody is relieved when Ria is finally retrieved by The Alfred.

The Medical Team

Early on, the ICU medical team contemplates instating Ria on ECLS and is asking support from the cardiac surgical team and the clinical perfusionist service. The teams are held up in theatres. The ICU medical team hesitates, as only one senior medical staff is confident performing the procedure (cannulation) and to operate the ECMO machine. The nearest ECLS referral centre is contacted. Their busy ICU is unable to accommodate any additional patients for at least another 24 hours. To optimise Ria's chances of survival and recovery, the team decides to instate ECLS immediately. The experienced ICU consultant is called in. By the time he arrives, another 4 hours have passed. ECMO is instated and the medical consultant stays with the patient, operating the ECMO machine. The next day, the ECLS referral centre still has no bed for Ria. The ICU consultant is called back in from his days off to operate the ECMO machine in the ICU. He is a 3-hour drive away. Eventually, on day 5, Ria is accepted and retrieved by the ECLS referral centre (at $8000 thousand-dollar expenditure). The medical team lodges a complaint for negligence in patient care via the internal risk reporting system.

The Cardiac Patient on the Surgical Waitlist

Mr Rogers, a patient, scheduled for a cardiac bypass operation, was given a lift from the country side by his daughter the night before. It is a 4-hour drive and both stayed at a nearby hotel and presented to the hospital as planned at 6am. By 9am, a manager informs them that the surgery had to be cancelled because of an emergency in the ICU. Due to lack of the perfusionist service in theatre, the patient has to start the long trip back home. The patient is distressed. So is his daughter as she had to take annual leave from work and organised child care for her children. Both make the return trip home, awaiting rescheduling.

The Head of Cardiac Surgery

When it becomes clear that another one of the scheduled cardiac cases has to be cancelled due to a lack of perfusionist services in the operating theatres, the head of cardiac surgery calls a meeting with the ICU Nurse Unit Manager (NUM) and Medical Director. At the meeting, he proposes for the unaccredited ICU nurses to look after the ECMO to free up the perfusionist. Both, the NUM and Medical Director, deny the request due a lack of workforce training and accreditation processes and associated safety concerns for the patient.

The ICU Nurse Unit Manager

When the head of cardiac surgery suggests for the ICU nurses to operate the ECMO device, she deems the request unreasonable as none of the nurses is accredited and denies the request. In addition, the Director of Nursing calls and questions the ICU Nurse Manger of why the ICU nurses do not operate an ECMO. The Nurse Unit Manager takes the unconventional step to unsuccessfully call other hospitals asking to 'borrow' an accredited ECMO nurse.

APPENDIX 9

Business Canvas Analysis

Key Partners

Internal

- **Accounting:** Providing accurate data over costs and revenue, balancing overall budget
- **Austin Executive:** Fully supportive of integrated ECLS Service, supporting the Austin Brand
- **Cardiac Catheterisation Laboratory:** Meeting demand, lowering threshold to instate ECMO at the possible earliest time for target patient population
- **Cardiac Services:** Meeting demand, lowering threshold to instate ECMO at the possible earliest time, preventing loss of opportunity costs when cancelling cardiac cases
- **Clinical Perfusionist Team:** Reduced overtime and reduced stress levels
- **Critical Care Services - Intensive Care Unit:** Economical approach to optimising patient outcome
- **Research Team:** Opportunity to advance in liver and brain ECMO
- **Respiratory Services:** Meeting demand, lowering threshold to instate ECMO at the possible earliest time for target patient population
- **Workforce:** Nurses & Doctors reduced stress levels, attraction and retention of high performing clinicians, job satisfaction by optimising patient outcome

External

- **Alfred Health:** Alfred Health offers a fully integrated ECLS service, provides education and resources, working closely will allow fast development of skill sets and accreditation amongst clinicians
- **Supplier:** Maquet, Cardiohelp and circuits, company also provides clinician training and education; Xenios-Ag

Key Activities

- **Patient Care:** Providing best possible care to all patients
- **Critical Care Provision:** Being global leaders in the field, providing highly efficient and advanced care to critically ill patients
- **Marketing and Promoting the Austin Brand:** Having a competitive edge or competitive advantage; growing for future demand; promoting the Austin Brand by practicing advanced, cutting edge medicine

Key Resources

- **Capital:** 2 ECMO devices
- **Workforce:** Accredited Nursing & Medical team, Clinical Perfusionist Team
- Finance – Upfront funding of $300, 000
- Operating Theatre – Most ECMO devices would be instated in the Operating Suite
- Intensive Care Unit – Patients receiving ECLS therapy will be treated in the Intensive care unit

Value Proposition

- Addressing Key stake holder's gain
- We offer a fully integrated, financially viable, nurse-led, clinical perfusionist independent ECLS service as a strategic priority with prospect of organic growth, optimising patient outcome and promoting The Austin Health Brand of being a global leader in care provision and research
- Identifying Key stakeholders' pains
- Clinicians' limited ability to treat patients in acute cardio and/or respiratory failure requiring ECLS treatment most effectively and to best industry practice standards leading to frustration
- Financially non-viable model due to increased marginal costs: CP locum service costs and medical consultant overtime rates incurred. In addition, the

loss of opportunity costs by cancelling cardiac cases adds to the marginal costs.

- Risk of adverse patient outcomes: Early instatement of ECLS is associated with better patient outcome
- Inability to attract and retain highly skilled field experts: If growth of the critical care services stagnates, high performing clinicians might not be attracted to Austin Health, or current career driven employees might choose to seek employment elsewhere to advance their careers
- High stress levels for all key stake holders with each episode: these episodes lead to clinician burn-out and to loss of trust towards Austin Leadership
- Damaging for the Austin Brand: ECLS is commonly offered across tertiary health care institutions across the globe. By Austin offering the service, this increase reputation and add intangible value strengthening the Brand Name
- Competitive Disadvantage: In light of considerations by the DoH to reduce cardiac service centres by one (this could not be confirmed at the time of writing); Austin is at some risk to lose its cardiac services. Growing its critical care services by increasing activity and cardiac throughput and the inclusion of an ECLS service will create a greater competitive advantage over other centres

Customer Relationships

- Highest Quality Clinical Care
- Highly Skilled Workforce
- Patient/Family trust the Austin Brand
- Specialty departments within Austin fully cooperate

Channels

- **Austin Health Website:** The service will be advertised on the Austin Health Website
- **Internal Referral System:** A referral system will be developed, allowing quick access to the critical care teams once the need arises for the service
- DoH website
- **ELSO:** Extracorporeal Life Support Organization is an international non-profit consortium of health care institutions; dedicated to the development and evaluation of novel therapies for support of failing organ systems; promotion of a broad multidisciplinary collaboration; mission is to maintain a registry of in active ELSO centres; registry data is to be used to support clinical research, support regulatory agencies, and support individual ELSO

centres; provides educational programs for active centres as well as for the broader medical and lay communities

Customer Segments

- Patients in severe cardio/respiratory failure with reversible cause will benefit from early instatement of ECLS optimising outcome
- Intensive Care Team: will feel highly valued to operate the service promoting best quality care and optimising patient outcome. Career orientated clinicians will fulfil their career aspirations
- Respiratory and Cardiac Services: optimising patient outcome
- Clinical Perfusionist Service: significant reduction in work related stressors
- Cardiac Catheterisation Laboratory: optimising patient outcome
- Research team: advancing in research leading to game changing therapies (i.e. liver and brain ECMO), strengthening the Austin Research segment

Cost Structure

- **Sunk Costs (Salary/Wages/Capital/Imaging/Pathology/Physiotherapy/Dietitian):** Sunk costs have been excluded from the report as they are costed already in day-to-day operations
- **Marginal Costs:** Accrual of Clinical Perfusionist Locum costs and overtime at Clinical Consultant rates, by establishing the service, these should no longer occur; Nursing backfill – see next point
- **Study Leave Backfill Nursing:** Nurses are guaranteed paid annual study leave of 5 days (pro rata for part time employees) as per their Industry EBA. However, clinical cover for the clinical activity during their study leave absence lies within the individual departments and therefore requires costing to cover additional marginal cost
- **Capital Invest:** 2 new ECMO machines are required allowing optimum response time
- **Service Agreement:** The supplier of the ECMO device charges an annual fee to service the devices in the second year, the first year is covered by warranty
- **Training Medical & Nursing:** Training and accreditation is required within a formalised and sustainable framework
- **Annual Training and Simulation Lab Fees:** In order to maintain skill sets, staff requires quarterly refresher training in the SIM lab

- **ECLS Coordinator:** Responsible for operating the program efficiently and in sustainable fashion, the Coordinator is required to schedule training, track accreditation status for the clinicians, collect data, network, benchmark and promote the service

Revenue Streams

DGR, – WIES Revenue provided by DoH: Each ECMO episode creates cost, this cost is activity funded and covered by WIES. On average, since 2009, all costs/ episode were covered 116% with WIES

- Seed' Funding: Requests by Hospital Executive for seed funding has been responded to with nursing staff willing to donate 2 days of their 5-day study leave entitlement to attend training.
- Fundraising: contact has been made with the Austin Fundraising department to contribute to the purchase of the 2 ECMO devices
- Donation Appeals: can be considered in cooperation with the fundraising department, the appeal can address training costs as well as capital investment

Compilation of References

ACSQHC. (2010). *Patient-centred care: Improving quality and safety by focusing care of patients and consumers*. Discussion Paper. Australian Commission on Safety and Quality in Health Care. Retrieved from https://www.safetyandquality.gov.au/wp-content/uploads/2012/01/PCCC-DiscussPaper.pdf

Agarwal, E., Ferguson, M., Banks, M., Bauer, J., Capra, S., & Isenring, E. (2015). Malnutrition coding shortfalls in Australian and New Zealand hospitals. *Nutrition & Dietetics: the Journal of the Dietitians Association of Australia*, *72*(1), 69–73. doi:10.1111/1747-0080.12116

Alexander, M., & Walkenbach, J. (2010). *Excel dashboards and reports*. New York, NY: Wiley. doi:10.1002/9781118257500

Andersen, H. V., Lawrie, G., & Savic, N. (2004). Effective quality management through third-generation balanced scorecard. *International Journal of Productivity and Performance Management*, *53*(7), 634–645. doi:10.1108/17410400410561259

Aparicio, M., & Costa, C. (2015). Data visualization. *Communication Design Quarterly Review*, *3*(1), 7–11. doi:10.1145/2721882.2721883

Armijo, D., McDonnell, C., & Werner, K. (2009). Evaluation and use case framework. *Electronic Health Record Usability, 9*. AHRQ Publication. Retrieved from https://healthit.ahrq.gov/sites/default/files/docs/citation/09-10-0091-1-EF.pdf

Authority, N. B. (2012). *Patient Blood Management Guidelines: Module 2 Perioperative*. Retrieved from https://www.blood.gov.au/system/files/documents/pbm-module-2.pdf

Baliga, R. R. (2012). *250 Cases in Clinical Medicine E-Book* (4th ed.). Elsevier Health Sciences.

Baptista, D. R., Wiens, A., Pontarolo, R., Regis, L., Reis, W. C., & Correr, C. J. (2016). The chronic care model for type 2 diabetes: A systematic review. *Diabetology & Metabolic Syndrome*, *8*(7). doi:10.118613098-015-0119-z PMID:26807158

Bartha, E., Davidson, T., Hommel, A., Thorngren, K. G., Carlsson, P., & Kalman, S. (2012). Cost-effectiveness analysis of goal-directed hemodynamic treatment of elderly hip fracture patients: Before clinical research starts. *Anesthesiology*, *117*(3), 519–530. doi:10.1097/ALN.0b013e3182655eb2 PMID:22814385

Bassi, C., Dervenis, C., Butturini, G., Fingerhut, A., Yeo, C., Izbicki, J., ... Buchler, M. (2005). Postoperative pancreatic fistula: An international study group (ISGPF) definition. *Surgery*, *138*(1), 8–13. doi:10.1016/j.surg.2005.05.001 PMID:16003309

Beller, M. J., & Barnett, A. (2009). *Next generation business analytics*. Retrieved May 9, 2017 from https://www.slideshare.net/LightshipPartners/next-generation-business-analytics-presentation

Bertsimas, D., Bjarnadottir, M. V., Kane, M. A., Kryder, J. C., Pandey, R., Vempala, S., & Wang, G. (2008). Algorithmic prediction of health-care costs. *Operations Research*, *56*(6), 1382–1392. doi:10.1287/opre.1080.0619

Bowman, S. (2013). *Impact of electronic health record systems on information integrity: Quality and safety implications*. Retrieved from http://perspectives.ahima.org/impact-of-electronic-health-record-systems-on-information-integrity-quality-and-safety-implications/

Bragg, S. (Producer). (2010). When should I update standard costs? *Cost Accounting*. Retrieved from http://www.accountingtools.com/questions-and-answers/when-should-i-update-standard-costs.html

Braveman, P., & Gottlieb, L. (2014). *The social determinants of health: It's time to consider the causes of the causes* (Vol. 129). Public Health Reports. Retrieved from https://www.ncbi.nlm.nih.gov/pmc/articles/PMC3863696/

Briggs, J. (2017). *Management reports & dashboard best practice*. Retrieved May 8, 2017 from https://www.targetdashboard.com/site/Dashboard-Best-Practice/Management-Report-and-Dashboard-best-practice-index.aspx

Brown, E. G., Yang, A., Canter, R. J., & Bold, R. J. (2014). Outcomes of pancreaticoduodenectomy: Where should we focus our efforts on improving outcomes? *JAMA Surgery*, *149*(7), 694–699. doi:10.1001/jamasurg.2014.151 PMID:24849180

Bunn, S., & Crane, J. (2016). *Electronic health records*. Parliamentary Office of Science and Technology (519). United Kingdom: Houses of Parliament. Retrieved from http://researchbriefings.parliament.uk/ResearchBriefing/Summary/POST-PN-0519

Burke, L. A., & Ryan, A. M. (2014). The complex relationship between cost and quality in US health care. *AMA Journal of Ethics*, *16*(2), 124–130. Retrieved from http://journalofethics.ama-assn.org/2014/02/pfor1-1402.html PMID:24553333

Bush, G. W. (2004). *Promoting innovation and competitiveness, President Bush's technology agenda*. The White House. Retrieved from https://georgewbush-whitehouse.archives.gov/infocus/technology/

Campbell, E. M., Sittig, D. F., Ash, J. S., Guappone, K. P., & Dykstra, R. H. (2006). Types of unintended consequences related to computerised provider order entry. *Journal of the American Medical Informatics Association*, *13*(5), 547–556. doi:10.1197/jamia.M2042 PMID:16799128

Casteneda, C., Nalley, K., Mannion, C., Bhattacharyya, P., Blake, P., Pecora, A., ... Suh, K. S. (2015). Clinical decision support systems for improving diagnostic accuracy and achieving precision medicine. *Journal of Clinical Bioinformatics*, *5*(4). doi:10.118613336-015-0019-3 PMID:25834725

Cecconi, M., Corredor, C., Arulkumaran, N., Abuella, G., Ball, J., Grounds, R. M., ... Rhodes, A. (2013). Clinical review: Goal-directed therapy-what is the evidence in surgical patients? The effect on different risk groups. *Critical Care (London, England)*, *17*(2), 209. doi:10.1186/cc11823 PMID:23672779

Chapko, M. K., Liu, C. F., Perkins, M., Li, Y. F., Fortney, J. C., & Maciejewski, M. L. (2009). Equivalence of two healthcare costing methods: Bottom-up and top-down. *Health Economics*, *18*(10), 1188–1201. doi:10.1002/hec.1422 PMID:19097041

Charles, D., Gabriel, M., & Searcy, T. (2015). *Adoption of electronic health record systems among U.S. non-federal acute care hospitals: 2008-2014.* ONC Data Brief. The Office of the National Coordinator for Health Information Technology. Retrieved from http://docplayer.net/4931694-Adoption-of-electronic-health-record-systems-among-u-s-non-federal-acute-care-hospitals-2008-2014.html

Chelniciuc, A. (2013). *Adapting the balanced scorecard for an academic hospitalist group*. Retrieved May 8, 2017 from http://www.performancemagazine.org/adapting-the-balanced-scorecard-for-an-academic-hospitalist-group/

Chirchi, V. R., Waghmare, L. M., & Chirchi, E. R. (2011). Iris biometric; Recognition for person identification in security systems. *International Journal of Computers and Applications*, *24*(9), 1–6. doi:10.5120/2986-4002

Church, J., & Erkan, A. (2016, August 3). Scope or scalpel? A matched study of the treatment of large colorectal polyps. *ANZ Journal of Surgery*.

Cios, K. J., & Moore, G. W. (2002). Uniqueness of data mining. *Artificial Intelligence in Medicine*, *26*(1-2), 1–24. doi:10.1016/S0933-3657(02)00049-0 PMID:12234714

Code of Federal Regulations. (2015). *Administrative safeguards*. Code of Federal Regulations. Retrieved from https://www.law.cornell.edu/cfr/text/45/164.308

Code of Federal Regulations. (2015). Stage 3 meaningful use objectives and measures for EPs, eligible hospitals: Cornell Law School. Retrieved from https://www.law.cornell.edu/cfr/text/42/495.24

Code of Federal Regulations. (2015). *Technical Safeguards*. Code of Federal Regulations. Retrieved from https://www.law.cornell.edu/cfr/text/45/164.312

Coker, F. (2014). *Pulse: Understanding the vital signs of your business*. Bellevue, WA: Ambient Light Publishing.

Coolsen, M. M., van Dam, R. M., van der Wilt, A. A., Slim, K., Lassen, K., & Dejong, C. H. (2013). Systematic review and meta-analysis of enhanced recovery after pancreatic surgery with particular emphasis on pancreaticoduodenectomies. *World Journal of Surgery*, *37*(8), 1909–1918. doi:10.100700268-013-2044-3 PMID:23568250

Copeland, G. P., Jones, D., & Walters, M. (1991). POSSUM: A scoring system for surgical audit. *British Journal of Surgery*, *78*(3), 355–360. doi:10.1002/bjs.1800780327 PMID:2021856

Corcoran, T., Rhodes, J. E., Clarke, S., Myles, P. S., & Ho, K. M. (2012). Perioperative fluid management strategies in major surgery: A stratified meta-analysis. *Anesthesia and Analgesia*, *114*(3), 640–651. doi:10.1213/ANE.0b013e318240d6eb PMID:22253274

Council of Australian Governments. (2011). *National health reform agreement*. Canberra, Australia: Council of Australian Governments.

Cullis, P. (2015). *The personalized medicine revolution; How diagnosing and treating disease are about to change forever.* Vancouver: Greystone Books. Retrieved from https://vpl.bibliocommons.com/item/show/4176435038_the_personalized_medicine_revolution

Cutler, D. M., & Lleras-Muney, A. (2006). *Education and health: evaluating theories and evidence.* National Bureau of Economic Research Working Paper. Retrieved from http://www.scirp.org/reference/ReferencesPapers.aspx?ReferenceID=1244315

D'Hoore, W., Bouckaert, A., & Tilquin, C. (1996). Practical considerations on the use of the Charlson comorbidity index with administrative data bases. *Journal of Clinical Epidemiology*, *49*(12), 1429–1433. doi:10.1016/S0895-4356(96)00271-5 PMID:8991959

Dalfino, L., Giglio, M. T., Puntillo, F., Marucci, M., & Brienza, N. (2011). Haemodynamic goal-directed therapy and postoperative infections: Earlier is better. A systematic review and meta-analysis. *Critical Care (London, England)*, *15*(3), R154. doi:10.1186/cc10284 PMID:21702945

Davies, S. J., & Wilson, R. J. (2004). Preoperative optimization of the high-risk surgical patient. *British Journal of Anaesthesia*, *93*(1), 121–128. doi:10.1093/bja/aeh164 PMID:15121729

De Blester, L., Depreitere, R., De Waele, K., Vanhaecht, K., Vlayed, J., Yen, J., & Sermeus, W. (2006). Defining Pathways. *Journal of Nursing Management*, *14*(7), 553–563. doi:10.1111/j.1365-2934.2006.00702.x PMID:17004966

De La Maisoneuve, C., & Martins, J. O. (2013). *Public spending on health and long-term care: A new set of projections* (OECD Economic Policy Papers. No.6. ed.). OECD Publishing. Retrieved from https://www.oecd.org/eco/growth/Health%20FINAL.pdf

Dedić, N., & Stanier, C. (2016). Measuring the Success of Changes to Existing Business Intelligence Solutions to Improve Business Intelligence Reporting. *Research and Practical Issues of Enterprise Information Systems: 10th IFIP WG 8.9 Working Conference, CONFENIS 2016, Proceedings*, *10*, 225–236.

Department of Health Victoria. (2016). *Victorian Cost Data Collection data request specification and business rules for reporting cost data*. Melbourne, Australia: Department of Health Victoria.

DesRoches, C. M., Charles, D., Furukawa, M. F., Maulik, S. J., Kralovec, P., & Mostashiari, F. (2013). Adoption of electronic health records grows rapidly, but fewer than half of US hospitals had at least a basic system in 2012 [abstract]. *Health Affairs*, *32*(8), 1478–1485. doi:10.1377/hlthaff.2013.0308 PMID:23840052

Dictionary of Engineering. (2017). *Report generator*. Retrieved May 8, 2017 from http://www.dictionaryofengineering.com/definition/report-generator.html

Dindo, D., Demartines, N., & Clavien, P. A. (2004). Classification of surgical complications: A new proposal with evaluation in a cohort of 6336 patients and results of a survey. *Annals of Surgery*, *240*(2), 205–213. doi:10.1097/01.sla.0000133083.54934.ae PMID:15273542

Drouin, J. P., Hediger, V., & Henke, N. (2008). *Health care costs: A market-based view. The McKinsey Quarterly*.

Druss, B. G., Marcus, S. C., & Olfson, M. (2001). *Comparing the national economic burden of five chronic conditions*. Retrieved from https://www.ncbi.nlm.nih.gov/pubmed/11816664

Dyche, J. (2000). *E-data: Turning data into information with data warehousing*. Reading, MA: Addison-Wesley.

Eggleton, M. (2017). *Data as the fuel of the future*. Retrieved from The Australian Financial Review: http://www.afr.com/news/special-reports/future-now-series/data-as-the-fuel-of-the-future-20170716-gxc4u1

eHealth Ireland. (2016). *eHealth strategy for Ireland*. Department of Health. Retrieved from http://www.ehealthireland.ie/

EHTEL Connect. (2013). *eHealth strategy and action plan of Finland in a European context.* Helsinki: ETHEL Connect. Retrieved from https://www.google.com.au/search?site=&source=hp&q=https%3A%2F%2Fwww.ehtel.eu%2Freferences-files%2Fehtelconnect-support-documentation%2FEHTELconnect-Finland-PeerReview-Public-Report-RAP2013_11.pdf&oq=https%3A%2F%2Fwww.ehtel.eu%2Freferences-files%2Fehtelco

Eisenberg, J. D., Rosato, E. L., Lavu, H., Yeo, C. J., & Winter, J. M. (2015). Delayed Gastric Emptying After Pancreaticoduodenectomy: An Analysis of Risk Factors and Cost. *Journal of Gastrointestinal Surgery*, *19*(9), 1572–1580. doi:10.100711605-015-2865-5 PMID:26170145

Elton, J., & O'Riordan, A. (2016). *Healthcare disrupted; Next generation business models and strategies*. John Wiley & Sons. Retrieved from http://au.wiley.com/WileyCDA/WileyTitle/productCd-1119171881.html

Enestvedt, C. K., Diggs, B. S., Cassera, M. A., Hammill, C., Hansen, P. D., & Wolf, R. F. (2012). Complications nearly double the cost of care after pancreaticoduodenectomy. *American Journal of Surgery*, *204*(3), 332–338. doi:10.1016/j.amjsurg.2011.10.019 PMID:22464011

Enomoto, L. M., Gusani, N. J., Dillon, P. W., & Hollenbeak, C. S. (2014). Impact of surgeon and hospital volume on mortality, length of stay, and cost of pancreaticoduodenectomy. *Journal of Gastrointestinal Surgery, 18*(4), 690–700. doi:10.100711605-013-2422-z PMID:24297652

Epstein, R., & Street, R. I. (2011). The values and value of patient-centered care. *Annals of Family Medicine, 9*(2), 100–103. doi:10.1370/afm.1239 PMID:21403134

Evans, D. B., Hsu, J., & Boerma, T. (2013). Universal health coverage and universal access. *Bulletin of the World Health Organization, 91*(8), 546–546A. doi:10.2471/BLT.13.125450 PMID:23940398

Evenson, K. R., Goto, M. M., & Furberg, R. D. (2015). Systematic review of the validity and reliability of consumer-wearable activity trackers. *The International Journal of Behavioral Nutrition and Physical Activity, 12*(159). doi:10.118612966-015-0314-1 PMID:26684758

Falon, S. (2016). EHR records in Sweden and what the future brings. *Salus Digital.* Retrieved from http://salusdigital.net/ehr-records-sweden-future-brings/

Fenwick, E., Wilson, J., Sculpher, M., & Claxton, K. (2002). Pre-operative optimisation employing dopexamine or adrenaline for patients undergoing major elective surgery: A cost-effectiveness analysis. *Intensive Care Medicine, 28*(5), 599–608. doi:10.100700134-002-1257-y PMID:12029409

Ferruci, D., Levas, A., Bagchi, S., Gondek, D., & Mueller, E. T. (2013). Watson: Beyond jeopardy. *Artificial Intelligence, 199-200*, 93–105. doi:10.1016/j.artint.2012.06.009

Few, S. (2004). *Eenie, meenie, minie, moe: Selecting the right graph for your message*. Retrieved May 8, 2017 from http://www.perceptualedge.com/articles/ie/the_right_graph.pdf

Fihn, S. D., Francis, J., Clancy, C., Nielson, C., Nelson, K., Rumsfeld, J., ... Graham, G. (2014). Insights from advanced analytics at the veterans health administration. *Health Affairs, 33*(7), 1203–1211. doi:10.1377/hlthaff.2014.0054 PMID:25006147

Fleischman, W., Lowry, T., & Shapiro, J. (2014). *The visit-data warehouse: Enabling novel secondary use of health information exchange data*. Academic Press. doi:10.13063/2327-9214.1099

Frank, R., & Bernanke, B. (2009). *Principles of microeconomics*. New York, NY: McGraw-Hill/Irwin.

Friendly, M. (2001). *Gallery of Data Visualization*. Retrieved May 8, 2017 from http://www.datavis.ca/gallery/

Garber, S., Gates, S. M., Keeler, E. B., Vaiana, M. E., Mulcahy, A. W., Lau, C., & Kellermann, A. L. (2014). *Redirecting spending in U.S. health care: Options to decrease spending and increase value*. Santa Monica, CA: Rand Corporation. Retrieved from https://www.rand.org/pubs/research_reports/RR308.html

Garrett, P., & Seidman, J. (n.d.). EMR vs EHR – What is the difference? *Health IT Buzz*. Retrieved from https://www.healthit.gov/buzz-blog/electronic-health-and-medical-records/emr-vs-ehr-difference/

Giglio, M. T., Marucci, M., Testini, M., & Brienza, N. (2009). Goal-directed haemodynamic therapy and gastrointestinal complications in major surgery: A meta-analysis of randomized controlled trials. *British Journal of Anaesthesia, 103*(5), 637–646. doi:10.1093/bja/aep279 PMID:19837807

Glennie, H. R. (1974). Proposals for health reform. *The New Zealand Medical Journal*, (79): 575–578. PMID:4522414

Glennie, H. R. (1992). Downsizing of Hospitals with Effective Community Care. *The New Zealand Medical Journal*, *105*, 202–203. PMID:1625828

Glennie, H. R. (2012). Delivering health care cost-effectively using available technology. In *Proceedings of the Global Telehealth Conference 2012*. Sydney: IOS Press.

Gouma, D. J., van Geenen, R. C., van Gulik, T. M., de Haan, R. J., de Wit, L. T., Busch, O. R., & Obertop, H. (2000). Rates of complications and death after pancreaticoduodenectomy: Risk factors and the impact of hospital volume. *Annals of Surgery*, *232*(6), 786–795. doi:10.1097/00000658-200012000-00007 PMID:11088073

Government, H. M. (2014). Using data and technology to transform outcomes for patients and citizens; A framework for action. *Personalised health and care 2020*. NHS. Retrieved from https://www.gov.uk/government/uploads/system/uploads/attachment_data/file/384650/NIB_Report.pdf

Goyert, N., Eeson, G., Kagedan, D. J., Behman, R., Lemke, M., Hallet, J., ... Coburn, N. G. (2017). Pasireotide for the prevention of pancreatic fistula following pancreaticoduodenectomy: A cost-effectiveness analysis. *Annals of Surgery*, *265*(1), 2–10. doi:10.1097/SLA.0000000000001889 PMID:27537539

Greenes, R. A., Pappalardo, A. N., Marble, C. W., & Barnett, G. O. (1969). Design and implementation of a clinical data management system. *Computers and Biomedical Research, an International Journal*, *2*(5), 469–485. doi:10.1016/0010-4809(69)90012-3 PMID:11697375

Gregg, H. (2014). 10 Things to know about epic. *Becker's Hospital Review*. Retrieved from http://www.beckershospitalreview.com/lists/10-things-to-know-about-epic.html

Guedon-Moreau, L., Mabo, P., & Kacet, S. (2013). Current clinical evidence for remote patient management. *Eurospace*, *15*(1suppl_1), i6–i10. doi:10.1093/europace/eut119 PMID:23737234

Gupta, P. (2004). *Six sigma business scorecard: Ensuring performance for profit*. New York, NY: McGraw-Hill Professional.

Gupta, P. K., Turaga, K. K., Miller, W. J., Loggie, B. W., & Foster, J. M. (2011). Determinants of outcomes in pancreatic surgery and use of hospital resources. *Journal of Surgical Oncology*, *104*(6), 634–640. doi:10.1002/jso.21923 PMID:21520092

Hamilton, M. A., Cecconi, M., & Rhodes, A. (2011). A systematic review and meta-analysis on the use of preemptive hemodynamic intervention to improve postoperative outcomes in moderate and high-risk surgical patients. *Anesthesia and Analgesia*, *112*(6), 1392–1402. doi:10.1213/ANE.0b013e3181eeaae5 PMID:20966436

Harman, L. B., Flite, C. A., & Bond, K. (2012). Electronic health records: Privacy, confidentiality and security. *AMA Journal of Ethics*, *14*(9), 712–719. Retrieved from http://journalofethics.ama-assn.org/2012/09/stas1-1209.html PMID:23351350

Health Financing & Insurance Department. (2013). *Costing standards version 1.0.2013. State of Qatar*. Supreme Council of Health.

Health, N. S. W. (2017). *Clinical Costing and Reporting Analyst*. Retrieved May 8, 2017 from https://nswhealth.erecruit.com.au/ViewPosition.aspx?id=228072

HealthConsult. (2016). *Mental health costing study*. Author.

HealthIT.gov. (2013). *Strategic health IT advanced research projects (SHARP); Secondary uses of EHR data*. Retrieved from https://www.healthit.gov/policy-researchers-implementers/secondary-use-ehr-data

HealthIT.gov. (2016). Benefits Of EHR. *What Is an electronic medical record (EMR)? Differences between electronic medical records and electronic health records*. Retrieved from Health IT.gov: https://www.healthit.gov/providers-professionals/electronic-medical-records-emr

Heckerman, D. (1997). Bayesian networks for data mining. *Data Mining and Knowledge Discovery*, *1*(1), 79–119. doi:10.1023/A:1009730122752

Hernandez, L. M., & Blazer, D. G. (2006). *Genes, behavior and the social environment: Moving beyond the nature/nurture debate*. National Academies Press (US). Retrieved from https://www.ncbi.nlm.nih.gov/books/NBK19929/

HIMSS Analytics. (2012). *Electronic Medical Record Adoption Model (EMRAM)*. Retrieved from http://www.himss.org/electonic-medical-record-adoption-model-emram

HIMSS Analytics. (2017). *Healthcare provider models; Adoption and maturity models to move your organization forward through technology*. Retrieved from http://www.himssanalytics.org/healthcare-provider-models/all

Hodson, R. (2016). Precision medicine. *Nature Outlook, 537*(49). doi:10.1038/537S49a PMID:27602738

Hoffman, S. (2016). Electronic health records and medical big data: Law and policy (Cambridge Bioethics and Law ed., Vol. 32). Cambridge University Press. doi:10.1017/9781316711149

Horan, P. (2018, April 4). [Revenue dataset].

Hsiao, C. J., & Hing, E. (2014). *Use and charactistics of electronic health record systems among office-based physician practices: United States, 2001-2012*. NCHS Data Brief. National Centre for Health Statistics. Retrieved from http://docplayer.net/2252607-Use-and-characteristics-of-electronic-health-record-systems-among-office-based-physician-practices-united-states-2001-2013.html

Huber, C. A., Schneeweiss, S., Signorell, A., & Reich, O. (2013). Improved prediction of medical expenditures and health care utilization using an updated chronic disease score and claims data. *Journal of Clinical Epidemiology, 66*(10), 1118–1127. doi:10.1016/j.jclinepi.2013.04.011 PMID:23845184

Hurst, J., & Siciliani, L. (2003). Tackling excessive waiting times for elective surgery: A comparison of policies in twelve OECD countries. In *OECD Health Working Papers* (Vol. 6). Paris: OECD Publishing. 10.1787/108471127058

Ibrahim, S. A. (2007). The Veterans Health Administration: A domestic model for a national health care system? *American Journal of Public Health, 97*(12), 2124–2126. doi:10.2105/AJPH.2007.125575 PMID:17971535

IHPA. (2014). *Hospital Patient Costing Standards*. IHPA.

Institute of Medicine (US). (2011). *Patients charting the course* (L. Olsen, R. A. Saunders, & J. M. McGinnis, Eds.). Washington, DC: National Academies Press (US). Retrieved from https://www.ncbi.nlm.nih.gov/books/NBK91496/

Jackson, T. J., Michel, J. L., Roberts, R. F., Jorm, C. M., & Wakefield, J. G. (2009). A classification of hospital-acquired diagnoses for use with routine hospital data. *The Medical Journal of Australia, 191*(10), 544. PMID:19912086

Jackson, T., Nghiem, H. S., Rowell, D., Jorm, C., & Wakefield, J. (2011). Marginal costs of hospital-acquired conditions: Information for priority-setting for patient safety programmes and research. *Journal of Health Services Research & Policy, 16*(3), 141–146. doi:10.1258/jhsrp.2010.010050 PMID:21719478

Jena, A. B., Seabury, S., Lakdawalla, D., & Chandra, A. (2011). Malpractice Risk According to Physician Specialty. [PubMed]. *The New England Journal of Medicine, 365*(7), 629–636. doi:10.1056/NEJMsa1012370

Joubert, N., & Raeburn, J. (1998, September). Mental Health Promotion: People, Power and Passion. *The International Journal of Mental Health Promotion*, 15-22.

Kaplan, R. S., & Anderson, S. R. (2004, November). Time-driven activity-based costing. *Harvard Business Review*.

Kaplan, R. S., & Norton, D. P. (1992). The balanced scorecard—Measures that drive performance. *Harvard Business Review, 83*(7), 71–79. PMID:10119714

Kent, T. S., Sachs, T. E., Callery, M. P., & Vollmer, C. M. Jr. (2011). Readmission after major pancreatic resection: A necessary evil? *Journal of the American College of Surgeons, 213*(4), 515–523. doi:10.1016/j.jamcollsurg.2011.07.009 PMID:21840738

Kent, T. S., Sachs, T. E., Callery, M. P., & Vollmer, C. M. Jr. (2013). The burden of infection for elective pancreatic resections. *Surgery, 153*(1), 86–94. doi:10.1016/j.surg.2012.03.026 PMID:22698935

Khuri, S. F., Henderson, W. G., DePalma, R. G., Mosca, C., Healey, N. A., Kumbhani, D. J., & Participants in the V. A. N. S. Q. I. P. (2005). Determinants of long-term survival after major surgery and the adverse effect of postoperative complications. *Ann Surg, 242*(3), 326-341.

Kimball, R., & Ross, M. (2013). *The data warehouse toolkit: The definitive guide to dimensional modeling* (3rd ed.). New York, NY: Wiley.

Knechtle, W. S., Perez, S. D., Medbery, R. L., Gartland, B. D., Sullivan, P. S., Knechtle, S. J., ... Sweeney, J. F. (2015). The Association Between Hospital Finances and Complications After Complex Abdominal Surgery: Deficiencies in the Current Health Care Reimbursement System and Implications for the Future. *Annals of Surgery*, *262*(2), 273–279. doi:10.1097/SLA.0000000000001042 PMID:25405558

Koti, R. S., Gurusamy, K. S., Fusai, G., & Davidson, B. R. (2010). Meta-analysis of randomized controlled trials on the effectiveness of somatostatin analogues for pancreatic surgery: A Cochrane review. *HPB*, *12*(3), 155–165. doi:10.1111/j.1477-2574.2010.00157.x PMID:20590882

Kristensson, J., Modig, S., Midlov, P., Hallberg, I. R., & Jakobsson, U. (2010). Healthcare utilisation and knowledge concerning perscribed drugs among older people. *European Journal of Clinical Pharmacology*, *66*(10), 1047–1054. doi:10.100700228-010-0837-y PMID:20652233

Langreth, R. (2014). *Venter starts DNA-scanning company to boost longevity.* Retrieved from Health Freedom Alliance: http://www.healthfreedoms.org/venter-starts-dna-scanning-company-to-boost-longevity/

Llewellyn, S., Chambers, N., Ellwood, S., Begkos, C., & Wood, C. (2016). *Patient-level information and costing systems (PLICSs): A mixed-methods study of current practice and future potential for the NHS health economy*. Academic Press.

Lobo, S. M., Lobo, F. R., Polachini, C. A., Patini, D. S., Yamamoto, A. E., de Oliveira, N. E., ... Cunrath, G. S. (2006). Prospective, randomized trial comparing fluids and dobutamine optimization of oxygen delivery in high-risk surgical patients [ISRCTN42445141]. *Critical Care (London, England)*, *10*(3), R72. doi:10.1186/cc4913 PMID:16696864

Machado, N. O. (2012). Pancreatic fistula after pancreatectomy: Definitions, risk factors, preventive measures, and management-review. *International Journal of Surgical Oncology*, *602478*. doi:10.1155/2012/602478 PMID:22611494

Mandell, S. F. (1987). *Resistance to computerization. An examination of the relationship between resistance and the cognitive style of the clinician*. Retrieved from https://www.ncbi.nlm.nih.gov/pubmed/3668415

Manyika, J., Chui, M., Brown, B., Bughin, J., Dodds, R., Roxburgh, C., & Byers, A. H. (2012). *Big data: the next frontier for innovation, competition and productivity*. Retrieved from McKinsey & Company: http://www.mckinsey.com/business-functions/digital-mckinsey/our-insights/big-data-the-next-frontier-for-innovation

Ma, R. (2015). *From the margins to the mainstream: Clinical costing for clinical improvement*. Melbourne, Australia: IGI Global.

Ma, R. (2016). *From the margins to the mainstream: Clinical costing for clinical improvement. In J. Moon & M. P. Galea (Eds.), Improving Health Management through Clinical Decision Support Systems*. IGI Global. doi:10.4018/978-1-4666-9432-3.ch009

Marshall, S. M., & Flyvbjerg, M. (2006). Prevention and early detection of vascular complications of diabetes. *British Medical Journal*, *333*(7556), 475–480. doi:10.1136/bmj.38922.650521.80 PMID:16946335

Mathieson, S. A. (2015). Genomics big data compels IT to rediscover efficiency techniques. *Computer Weekly*. Retrieved from http://www.computerweekly.com/feature/Genomics-big-data-compels-IT-to-rediscover-efficiency-techniques

Mauney, J., Furlough, C., & Barnes, J. (2015). Developing a better clinical alert system in EHRs. *Proceedings of the International Symposium on Human Factors and Ergonomics in Health Care*, *4*(1), 29-36. doi:10.1177/2327857915041023

Melis, M., Marcon, F., Masi, A., Sarpel, U., Miller, G., Moore, H., ... Newman, E. (2012). Effect of intra-operative fluid volume on peri-operative outcomes after pancreaticoduodenectomy for pancreatic adenocarcinoma. *Journal of Surgical Oncology*, *105*(1), 81–84. doi:10.1002/jso.22048 PMID:21792977

Menachemi, N., & Collum, T. (2011). *Benefits and drawbacks of electronic health record systems*. Academic Press. doi:10.2147/RMHP.S12985

Morton, A., & Cornwell, J. (2009). What's the difference between a hospital and a bottling factory? *BMJ: British Medical Journal (Online), 339*.

Mujkic, S., & Marinkovic, V. (2017). *Critical appraisal of reimbursement list in Bosnia and Herzegovina.* Academic Press. doi:10.3389/fphar.2017.00129

New Zealand Government. (2017). *Digital Hospital. Ministry of Health New Zealand.* Retrieved from https://www.health.govt.nz/our-work/ehealth/digital-health-2020/digital-hospital

Nikfarjam, M., Weinberg, L., Low, N., Fink, M. A., Muralidharan, V., Houli, N., ... Christophi, C. (2013). A fast track recovery program significantly reduces hospital length of stay following uncomplicated pancreaticoduodenectomy. *JOP*, *14*(1), 63–70. doi:10.6092/1590-8577/1223 PMID:23306337

Norbeck, T. (2012). *Drivers of health care costs; A physicians foundation white paper.* The Physicians Foundation, Empowering Physicians, Improving Healthcare. Retrieved from http://www.physiciansfoundation.org/uploads/default/Drivers_of_Health_Care_Costs_-_November_2012.pdf

Obama's Speech on the Economy. (2009). Federal News Service. *New York Times.* Retrieved from http://www.nytimes.com/2009/01/08/us/politics/08text-obama.html

OECD. (2010). How much is too much? In *OECD Health Policy Studies - Value for Money in Health Spending* (pp. 21-42). OECD Publisher. Retrieved from http://www.oecd.org/els/health-systems/value-for-money-in-health-spending.htm

OECD. (2015). *Fiscal sustainability of health systems: Bridging health and finance perspectives.* Paris: OECD Publishing. doi:10.1787/9789264233386-

OECD. (2016). *Health at a Glance: Europe 2016; State of Health in the EU Cycle.* Paris: OECD Publishing. doi:10.1787/9789264265592-

Office of the National Coordinator for Health IT. (2016). *2016 interoperability Standards Advisory.* Office of the National Coordinator for Health IT. Retrieved from https://www.healthit.gov/sites/default/files/2016-interoperability-standards-advisory-final-508.pdf

Oliver, A. (2007). *The Veterans Health Administration: An American success story?* doi:10.1111/j.1468-0009.2007.00475.x

Ontario Medical Association. (n.d.). *Starting a practice; A guide for new physicians*. OMA. Retrieved from https://www.oma.org/wp-content/uploads/1_startingpractice.pdf

Pandit, J., Pandit, M., & Reynard, J. (2010). Understanding waiting lists as the matching of surgical capacity to demand: Are we wasting enough surgical time? *Anaesthesia*, *65*(6), 625–640. doi:10.1111/j.1365-2044.2010.06278.x PMID:20565395

Pareto, V. (1964). *Cours d'économie politique* (Vol. 1). Librairie Droz. doi:10.3917/droz.paret.1964.01

Patel, A. S., Bergman, A., Moore, B. W., & Haglund, U. (2013). The economic burden of complications occurring in major surgical procedures: A systematic review. *Applied Health Economics and Health Policy*, *11*(6), 577–592. doi:10.100740258-013-0060-y PMID:24166193

Pecorelli, N., Nobile, S., Partelli, S., Cardinali, L., Crippa, S., Balzano, G., ... Falconi, M. (2016). Enhanced recovery pathways in pancreatic surgery: State of the art. *World Journal of Gastroenterology*, *22*(28), 6456–6468. doi:10.3748/wjg.v22.i28.6456 PMID:27605881

Peplow, M. (2016). The 100000 Genomes Project. *BMJ (Clinical Research Ed.)*, *353*. doi:10.1136/bmj.i1757

Porter, M. (2015). An NHS under unsustainable pressure deserves a serious debate. *The Guardian*. Retrieved from https://www.theguardian.com/society/2015/jan/15/nhs-under-unsustainable-pressure-deserves-serious-debate

Power Health Solutions. (2017). *Power budgeting, forecasting and modelling; Business analytics functionality*. Adelaide, Australia: Power Health Solutions. Retrieved from http://www.powerhealthsolutions.com/budgeting

Pratt, W., Callery, M. P., & Vollmer, C. M. Jr. (2008). Optimal surgical performance attenuates physiologic risk in high-acuity operations. *Journal of the American College of Surgeons*, *207*(5), 717–730. doi:10.1016/j.jamcollsurg.2008.06.319 PMID:18954785

Pratt, W., Joseph, S., Callery, M. P., & Vollmer, C. M. Jr. (2008). POSSUM accurately predicts morbidity for pancreatic resection. *Surgery, 143*(1), 8–19. doi:10.1016/j.surg.2007.07.035 PMID:18154928

Press, G. (2013). *A very short history of data science*. Retrieved May 8, 2017 from https://www.forbes.com/sites/gilpress/2013/05/28/a-very-short-history-of-data-science/#6bea3ea555cf

Rahbari, N. N., Zimmermann, J. B., Schmidt, T., Koch, M., Weigand, M. A., & Weitz, J. (2009). Meta-analysis of standard, restrictive and supplemental fluid administration in colorectal surgery. *British Journal of Surgery, 96*(4), 331–341. doi:10.1002/bjs.6552 PMID:19283742

Rajarathinam, G., Kannan, D. G., Vimalraj, V., Amudhan, A., Rajendran, S., Jyotibasu, D., ... Surendran, R. (2008). Post pancreaticoduodenectomy haemorrhage: Outcome prediction based on new ISGPS Clinical severity grading. *HPB, 10*(5), 363–370. doi:10.1080/13651820802247086 PMID:18982153

Rennhackkamp, M. H., & Hart, G. (2016). Predicting unplanned hospital readmissions. *Proceedings of the Scientific Stream at the Health Data Analytics Conference*. Retrieved May 1, 2017 from http://ceur-ws.org/Vol-1683/

Rowland, C. (2014). Subsidies given for computerizing, but no reporting required when errors cause harm. Hazards tied to medical records rush. *The Boston Globe*. Retrieved from https://www.bostonglobe.com/news/nation/2014/07/19/obama-pushed-electronic-health-records-with-huge-taxpayer-subsidies-but-has-rebuffed-calls-for-hazards-monitoring-despite-evidence-harm/OV4njlT6JgLN67Fp1pZ01I/story.html

Rud, O. (2009). *Business intelligence success factors: Tools for aligning your business in the global economy*. Hoboken, NJ: Wiley & Sons.

Ryan, D. J., O'Regan, N. A., Caoimh, R. Ó., Clare, J., O'Connor, M., Leonard, M., ... Trzepacz, P. T. (2013). Delirium in an adult acute hospital population: Predictors, prevalence and detection. *BMJ Open, 3*(1), e001772. doi:10.1136/bmjopen-2012-001772 PMID:23299110

Safran, C., Bloomrosen, M., Hammond, W. E., Labkoff, S., Markel-Fox, S., Tang, P., & Detmer, D. E. (2007). Toward a framework for the secondary use of health data: An American medical informatics association white paper. *Journal of the American Medical Informatics Association*, *14*(1), 1–9. doi:10.1197/jamia.M2273 PMID:17077452

Santema, T. B., Visser, A., Busch, O. R., Dijkgraaf, M. G., Goslings, J. C., Gouma, D. J., & Ubbink, D. T. (2015). Hospital costs of complications after a pancreatoduodenectomy. *HPB*, *17*(8), 723–731. doi:10.1111/hpb.12440 PMID:26082095

Sarsfield, S. (2009). *The data governance imperative*. Ely, UK: IT Governance Publishing.

Schmidt, C. M., Turrini, O., Parikh, P., House, M. G., Zyromski, N. J., Nakeeb, A., ... Lillemoe, K. D. (2010). Effect of hospital volume, surgeon experience, and surgeon volume on patient outcomes after pancreaticoduodenectomy: A single-institution experience. *Archives of Surgery (Chicago, Ill.)*, *145*(7), 634–640. doi:10.1001/archsurg.2010.118 PMID:20644125

Schneeweiss, S., & Maclure, M. (2000). Use of comorbidity scores for control of confounding in studies using administrative databases. *International Journal of Epidemiology*, *29*(5), 891–898. doi:10.1093/ije/29.5.891 PMID:11034974

Scholl, M., Stine, K., Hash, J., Bowen, P., Johnson, A., Smith, C. D., & Steinberg, D. J. (2008). *An introductory resource guide for implementing the health insurance portability and accountability act (HIPAA) security rule*. National Institute of Standards and Technology, US Department of Commerce. Retrieved from http://nvlpubs.nist.gov/nistpubs/Legacy/SP/nistspecialpublication800-66r1.pdf

Shulkin, D. J. (2016). *Beyond the VA crisis: Becoming a high-performance network*. New England Medical Journal.

Silber, J. H., Kaestner, R., Even-Shoshan, O., Wang, Y., & Bressler, L. J. (2010). Aggressive treatment style and surgical outcomes. *Health Services Research*, *45*(6), 1872–1892. doi:10.1111/j.1475-6773.2010.01180.x PMID:20880043

Snyder, M. (2016). *Genomics and personalized medicine*. Oxford University Press. Retrieved from https://global.oup.com/academic/product/genomics-and-personalized-medicine-9780190234768?cc=us&lang=

Sowale, Y. (2017). Effectively using big data in healthcare. *Information Management*. Retrieved May 1, 2017 from https://www.information-management.com/opinion/effectively-using-big-data-in-healthcare

Stanton, M. A. (2006). The high concentration of U.S. health care expenditures. *Research in Action,* (19). Retrieved from https://archive.ahrq.gov/research/findings/factsheets/costs/expriach/

Steen, J. (c 1663). The Sick Woman. *Shutterstock*. Retrieved from www.shutterstock.com

Stephens, Z. D., Lee, S. V., Faghri, F., Campbell, R. H., Zhai, C., Efron, M. J., . . . Robinson, G. E. (2015). Big data: Astronomical or genomical? doi: 10.1371/journal.pbio.1002195

Stowers, M. D., Lemanu, D. P., & Hill, A. G. (2015). Health economics in Enhanced Recovery After Surgery programs. *Canadian Journal of Anaesthesia*, *62*(2), 219–230. doi:10.100712630-014-0272-0 PMID:25391739

Sukel, K. (2015). *Cerner, Qualcomm partner to advance remote home health monitoring*. Retrieved from Healthcare Informatics: https://www.healthcare-informatics.com/news-item/cerner-qualcomm-partner-advance-remote-home-health-monitoring

Taylor, C. A., Draney, M. T., Ku, J. P., Parker, D., Steele, B. N., Wang, K., & Zarins, C. K. (1999). Predictive pedicine: Computational techniques in therapeutic decision-making. *Computer Aided Surgery*, *4*(5), 231–247. doi:10.3109/10929089909148176 PMID:10581521

The Clinical Costing Standards Association of Australia. (2013). *Clinical costing standards: version 5.1.17*. Melbourne, Australia: The Clinical Costing Standards Association of Australia.

The Guardian. (2014). The NHS could be 'overwhelmed' by people with long-term medical conditions. *The Guardian*. Retrieved from https://www.theguardian.com/society/2014/jan/03/nhs-overwhelmed-long-term-medical-conditions

The Independent Hospital Pricing Authority. (2014). *The Australian Hospital Patient Costing Standards, version 3.1*. Sydney, Australia: The Independent Hospital Pricing Authority.

The Office of the National Coordinator for Health Information Technology. (2015). *Connecting health and care for the nation; A shared nationwide interoperability roadmap*. The Office of the National Coordinator for Health Information Technology.

The Parliament of Victoria. (2014). *Mental Health Act 2014*. Melbourne: The Parliament of Victoria.

The Victorian Government. (2016). *Department of Health and Human Services policy and funding guidelines 2016*. Melbourne, Australia: The Victorian Government.

Thomas, G. (2013). *The DGI data governance framework*. Retrieved May 1, 2017 from http://www.datagovernance.com/wp-content/uploads/2014/11/dgi_framework.pdf

Topal, B., Peeters, G., Vandeweyer, H., Aerts, R., & Penninckx, F. (2007). Hospital cost-categories of pancreaticoduodenectomy. *Acta Chirurgica Belgica*, *107*(4), 373–377. doi:10.1080/00015458.2007.11680078 PMID:17966528

Triggle, N. (2007). Blair's legacy: Health. *BBC News*. Retrieved from http://news.bbc.co.uk/2/hi/health/4555344.stm

Tufte, E. (1983). *The visual display of quantitative information*. Cheshire, CT: Graphics Press.

Turney, P. (2008). *Activity-based costing: An emerging foundation for performance management*. Cary, NC: SAS Institute Inc.

Vanounou, T., Pratt, W. B., Callery, M. P., & Vollmer, C. M. Jr. (2007). Selective administration of prophylactic octreotide during pancreaticoduodenectomy: A clinical and cost-benefit analysis in low- and high-risk glands. *Journal of the American College of Surgeons*, *205*(4), 546–557. doi:10.1016/j.jamcollsurg.2007.05.011 PMID:17903728

Veterans Affairs. (2016). Million veteran program. *Genomics*. US Department of Veterans Affairs. Retrieved from https://www.research.va.gov/topics/genomics.cfm#research2

Victoria Health. (2017). *Clinical costing and activity based funding*. Retrieved May 8, 2017 from https://www2.health.vic.gov.au/hospitals-and-health-services/funding-performance-accountability/activity-based-funding/clinical-costing

Victorian Department of Health. (2017a). *Department of Health and Human Services policy and funding guidelines 2017*. Melbourne: Department of Health and Human Services.

Victorian Department of Health. (2017b). *Victorian Admitted Episodes Dataset (VAED) manual*. Melbourne: Department of Health and Human Services.

Vollmer, C. M. Jr, Pratt, W., Vanounou, T., Maithel, S. K., & Callery, M. P. (2007). Quality assessment in high-acuity surgery: Volume and mortality are not enough. *Archives of Surgery (Chicago, Ill.)*, *142*(4), 371–380. doi:10.1001/archsurg.142.4.371 PMID:17438173

Vonlanthen, R., Slankamenac, K., Breitenstein, S., Puhan, M. A., Muller, M. K., Hahnloser, D., ... Clavien, P. A. (2011). The impact of complications on costs of major surgical procedures: A cost analysis of 1200 patients. *Annals of Surgery*, *254*(6), 907–913. doi:10.1097/SLA.0b013e31821d4a43 PMID:21562405

Wachter, R. (2015). *The digital doctor: Hope, hype, and harm at the dawn of medicine's computer age (business books)*. Amazon. Retrieved from https://www.amazon.com/Digital-Doctor-Hope-Medicines-Computer/dp/0071849467

Wagner, E. H., Austin, B. T., Davis, C., Hindmarsh, M., Schaefer, J., & Bonomi, A. (2001). Improving chronic illness care: Translating evidence into action. *Health Affairs*, *20*(6), 64–78. doi:10.1377/hlthaff.20.6.64 PMID:11816692

Wagner, E. H., Davis, C., Schaefer, J., Von Korff, M., & Austin, B. (1999). A survey of leading chronic disease management programs: Are they consistent with the literature? *Managed Care Quarterly*, *7*(3), 56–66. PMID:10620960

Warburton, D. E., Nicol, C. W., & Bredlin, S. S. (2006). Health benefits of physical activity: The evidence. *Canadian Medical Association Journal, 174*(6), 801–809. doi:10.1503/cmaj.051351 PMID:16534088

Warrillow, S. J., Weinberg, L., Parker, F., Calzavacca, P., Licari, E., Aly, A., ... Bellomo, R. (2010). Perioperative fluid prescription, complications and outcomes in major elective open gastrointestinal surgery. *Anaesthesia and Intensive Care, 38*(2), 259–265. PMID:20369757

Watzlaf, V. J., Zeng, X., Jarymowycz, C., & Firouzan, P. A. (2005). *Standards for the content of the electronic health record.* Retrieved from http://perspectives.ahima.org/standards-for-the-content-of-the-electronic-health-record/

Webb, P., & Bain, C. (2011). *Essential epidemiology: An introduction for students and health professionals* (2nd ed.). Cambridge, UK: Cambridge University Press.

Weinberg, L., Wong, D., Karalapillai, D., Pearce, B., Tan, C. O., Tay, S., ... Nikfarjam, M. (2014). The impact of fluid intervention on complications and length of hospital stay after pancreaticoduodenectomy (Whipple's procedure). *BMC Anesthesiology, 14*(1), 35. doi:10.1186/1471-2253-14-35 PMID:24839398

Welsch, T., Borm, M., Degrate, L., Hinz, U., Buchler, M. W., & Wente, M. N. (2010). Evaluation of the International Study Group of Pancreatic Surgery definition of delayed gastric emptying after pancreatoduodenectomy in a high-volume centre. *British Journal of Surgery, 97*(7), 1043–1050. doi:10.1002/bjs.7071 PMID:20632270

Wente, M. N., Bassi, C., Dervenis, C., Fingerhut, A., Gouma, D. J., Izbicki, J. R., ... Buchler, M. W. (2007). Delayed gastric emptying (DGE) after pancreatic surgery: A suggested definition by the International Study Group of Pancreatic Surgery (ISGPS). *Surgery, 142*(5), 761–768. doi:10.1016/j.surg.2007.05.005 PMID:17981197

Whipple, A. O., Parsons, W. B., & Mullins, C. R. (1935). Treatment of Carcinoma of the Ampulla of Vater. *Annals of Surgery, 102*(4), 763–779. doi:10.1097/00000658-193510000-00023 PMID:17856666

Widen, S., & Haseltine, W. A. (2015). *The Estonian eHealth and eGovernance system*. ACCESS Health International. Retrieved from http://accessh.org/resource/case-study-the-estonian-ehealth-and-egovernance-system/

Wright, G. P., Koehler, T. J., Davis, A. T., & Chung, M. H. (2014). The drowning whipple: Perioperative fluid balance and outcomes following pancreaticoduodenectomy. *Journal of Surgical Oncology*, *110*(4), 407–411. doi:10.1002/jso.23662 PMID:24861716

Yang, W., Dall, T. M., Halder, P., Gallo, P., Kowal, S. L., & Hogan, P. F. (2013). Economic costs of diabetes in the U.S. in 2012. *Diabetes Care*, *36*(4), 1033–1046. doi:10.2337/dc12-2625 PMID:23468086

Yoshioka, R., Yasunaga, H., Hasegawa, K., Horiguchi, H., Fushimi, K., Aoki, T., ... Kokudo, N. (2014). Impact of hospital volume on hospital mortality, length of stay and total costs after pancreaticoduodenectomy. *British Journal of Surgery*, *101*(5), 523–529. doi:10.1002/bjs.9420 PMID:24615349

Related References

To continue our tradition of advancing information science and technology research, we have compiled a list of recommended IGI Global readings. These references will provide additional information and guidance to further enrich your knowledge and assist you with your own research and future publications.

Abu Seman, S. A., & Ramayah, T. (2017). Are We Ready to App?: A Study on mHealth Apps, Its Future, and Trends in Malaysia Context. In J. Pelet (Ed.), *Mobile Platforms, Design, and Apps for Social Commerce* (pp. 69–83). Hershey, PA: IGI Global. doi:10.4018/978-1-5225-2469-4.ch005

Aggarwal, S., & Azad, V. (2017). A Hybrid System Based on FMM and MLP to Diagnose Heart Disease. In S. Bhattacharyya, S. De, I. Pan, & P. Dutta (Eds.), *Intelligent Multidimensional Data Clustering and Analysis* (pp. 293–325). Hershey, PA: IGI Global. doi:10.4018/978-1-5225-1776-4.ch011

Akaichi, J., & Mhadhbi, L. (2016). A Clinical Decision Support System: Ontology-Driven Approach for Effective Emergency Management. In J. Moon & M. Galea (Eds.), *Improving Health Management through Clinical Decision Support Systems* (pp. 270–294). Hershey, PA: IGI Global. doi:10.4018/978-1-4666-9432-3.ch013

Akerkar, R. (2016). Towards an Intelligent Integrated Approach for Clinical Decision Support. In A. Aggarwal (Ed.), *Managing Big Data Integration in the Public Sector* (pp. 187–205). Hershey, PA: IGI Global. doi:10.4018/978-1-4666-9649-5.ch011

Al-Busaidi, S. S. (2018). Interdisciplinary Relationships Between Medicine and Social Sciences. In M. Al-Suqri, A. Al-Kindi, S. AlKindi, & N. Saleem (Eds.), *Promoting Interdisciplinarity in Knowledge Generation and Problem Solving* (pp. 124–137). Hershey, PA: IGI Global. doi:10.4018/978-1-5225-3878-3.ch009

Al Kareh, T., & Thoumy, M. (2018). The Impact of Health Information Digitization on the Physiotherapist-Patient Relationship: A Pilot Study of the Lebanese Community. *International Journal of Healthcare Information Systems and Informatics, 13*(2), 29–53. doi:10.4018/IJHISI.2018040103

Alenzuela, R. (2017). Research, Leadership, and Resource-Sharing Initiatives: The Role of Local Library Consortia in Access to Medical Information. In S. Ram (Ed.), *Library and Information Services for Bioinformatics Education and Research* (pp. 199–211). Hershey, PA: IGI Global. doi:10.4018/978-1-5225-1871-6.ch012

Ameri, H., Alizadeh, S., & Noughabi, E. A. (2017). Application of Data Mining Techniques in Clinical Decision Making: A Literature Review and Classification. In E. Noughabi, B. Raahemi, A. Albadvi, & B. Far (Eds.), *Handbook of Research on Data Science for Effective Healthcare Practice and Administration* (pp. 257–295). Hershey, PA: IGI Global. doi:10.4018/978-1-5225-2515-8.ch012

Anand, S. (2017). Medical Image Enhancement Using Edge Information-Based Methods. In B. Singh (Ed.), *Computational Tools and Techniques for Biomedical Signal Processing* (pp. 123–148). Hershey, PA: IGI Global. doi:10.4018/978-1-5225-0660-7.ch006

Angjellari-Dajci, F., Sapienza, C., Lawless, W. F., & Kavanagh, K. (2016). Human Capital Accumulation in Medical Simulated Learning Environments: A Framework for Economic Evaluation. In M. Russ (Ed.), *Quantitative Multidisciplinary Approaches in Human Capital and Asset Management* (pp. 65–88). Hershey, PA: IGI Global. doi:10.4018/978-1-4666-9652-5.ch004

Anil, M., Ayyildiz-Tamis, D., Tasdemir, S., Sendemir-Urkmez, A., & Gulce-Iz, S. (2016). Bioinspired Materials and Biocompatibility. In M. Bououdina (Ed.), *Emerging Research on Bioinspired Materials Engineering* (pp. 294–322). Hershey, PA: IGI Global. doi:10.4018/978-1-4666-9811-6.ch011

Anton, J. L., Soriano, J. V., Martinez, M. I., & Garcia, F. B. (2018). Comprehensive E-Learning Appraisal System. In M. Khosrow-Pour, D.B.A. (Ed.), Encyclopedia of Information Science and Technology, Fourth Edition (pp. 5787-5799). Hershey, PA: IGI Global. doi:10.4018/978-1-5225-2255-3.ch503

Arabi, M. (2016). Redesigning the Organizational Structure to Reach Efficiency: The Case of Ministry of Health and Medical Education of Iran. In R. Gholipour & K. Rouzbehani (Eds.), *Social, Economic, and Political Perspectives on Public Health Policy-Making* (pp. 257–294). Hershey, PA: IGI Global. doi:10.4018/978-1-4666-9944-1.ch012

Assis-Hassid, S., Heart, T., Reychav, I., & Pliskin, J. S. (2016). Modelling Factors Affecting Patient-Doctor-Computer Communication in Primary Care. *International Journal of Reliable and Quality E-Healthcare, 5*(1), 1–17. doi:10.4018/IJRQEH.2016010101

Atzori, B., Hoffman, H. G., Vagnoli, L., Messeri, A., & Grotto, R. L. (2018). Virtual Reality as Distraction Technique for Pain Management in Children and Adolescents. In M. Khosrow-Pour, D.B.A. (Ed.), Encyclopedia of Information Science and Technology, Fourth Edition (pp. 5955-5965). Hershey, PA: IGI Global. doi:10.4018/978-1-5225-2255-3.ch518

Audibert, M., Mathonnat, J., Pélissier, A., & Huang, X. X. (2018). The Impact of the New Rural Cooperative Medical Scheme on Township Hospitals' Utilization and Income Structure in Weifang Prefecture, China. In I. Management Association (Ed.), Health Economics and Healthcare Reform: Breakthroughs in Research and Practice (pp. 109-121). Hershey, PA: IGI Global. doi:10.4018/978-1-5225-3168-5.ch007

Ayyachamy, S. (2016). Analysis and Comparison of Developed 2D Medical Image Database Design using Registration Scheme, Retrieval Scheme, and Bag-of-Visual-Words. In N. Dey & A. Ashour (Eds.), *Classification and Clustering in Biomedical Signal Processing* (pp. 149–168). Hershey, PA: IGI Global. doi:10.4018/978-1-5225-0140-4.ch007

Babalola, A. C. (2016). Literacy and Decision Making on Health Issues among Married Women in Southwest Nigeria. In V. Wang (Ed.), *Handbook of Research on Advancing Health Education through Technology* (pp. 191–212). Hershey, PA: IGI Global. doi:10.4018/978-1-4666-9494-1.ch009

Babu, A., & Ayyappan, S. (2017). A Methodological Evaluation of Crypto-Watermarking System for Medical Images. In C. Bhatt & S. Peddoju (Eds.), *Cloud Computing Systems and Applications in Healthcare* (pp. 189–217). Hershey, PA: IGI Global. doi:10.4018/978-1-5225-1002-4.ch010

Bakke, A. (2017). Ethos in E-Health: From Informational to Interactive Websites. In M. Folk & S. Apostel (Eds.), *Establishing and Evaluating Digital Ethos and Online Credibility* (pp. 85–103). Hershey, PA: IGI Global. doi:10.4018/978-1-5225-1072-7.ch005

Bali, S. (2018). Enhancing the Reach of Health Care Through Telemedicine: Status and New Possibilities in Developing Countries. In U. Pandey & V. Indrakanti (Eds.), *Open and Distance Learning Initiatives for Sustainable Development* (pp. 339–354). Hershey, PA: IGI Global. doi:10.4018/978-1-5225-2621-6.ch019

Barrett, T. E. (2018). Essentials for Education and Training for Tomorrow's Physicians. In C. Smith (Ed.), *Exploring the Pressures of Medical Education From a Mental Health and Wellness Perspective* (pp. 230–252). Hershey, PA: IGI Global. doi:10.4018/978-1-5225-2811-1.ch010

Barrett, T. J. (2016). Knowledge in Action: Fostering Health Education through Technology. In V. Wang (Ed.), *Handbook of Research on Advancing Health Education through Technology* (pp. 39–62). Hershey, PA: IGI Global. doi:10.4018/978-1-4666-9494-1.ch003

Berrahal, S., & Boudriga, N. (2017). The Risks of Wearable Technologies to Individuals and Organizations. In A. Marrington, D. Kerr, & J. Gammack (Eds.), *Managing Security Issues and the Hidden Dangers of Wearable Technologies* (pp. 18–46). Hershey, PA: IGI Global. doi:10.4018/978-1-5225-1016-1.ch002

Bhagat, A. P., & Atique, M. (2016). Medical Image Mining Using Fuzzy Connectedness Image Segmentation: Efficient Retrieval of Patients' Stored Images. In W. Karâa & N. Dey (Eds.), *Biomedical Image Analysis and Mining Techniques for Improved Health Outcomes* (pp. 184–209). Hershey, PA: IGI Global. doi:10.4018/978-1-4666-8811-7.ch009

Bhargava, P. (2018). Blended Learning: An Effective Application to Clinical Teaching. In S. Tang & C. Lim (Eds.), *Preparing the Next Generation of Teachers for 21st Century Education* (pp. 302–320). Hershey, PA: IGI Global. doi:10.4018/978-1-5225-4080-9.ch018

Binh, N. T., & Tuyet, V. T. (2016). The Combination of Adaptive Filters to Improve the Quality of Medical Images in New Wavelet Domain. In N. Dey & A. Ashour (Eds.), *Classification and Clustering in Biomedical Signal Processing* (pp. 46–76). Hershey, PA: IGI Global. doi:10.4018/978-1-5225-0140-4.ch003

Bird, J. L. (2017). Writing Healing Narratives. In V. Bryan & J. Bird (Eds.), *Healthcare Community Synergism between Patients, Practitioners, and Researchers* (pp. 1–28). Hershey, PA: IGI Global. doi:10.4018/978-1-5225-0640-9.ch001

Bottrighi, A., Leonardi, G., Piovesan, L., & Terenziani, P. (2016). Knowledge-Based Support to the Treatment of Exceptions in Computer Interpretable Clinical Guidelines. *International Journal of Knowledge-Based Organizations*, *6*(3), 1–27. doi:10.4018/IJKBO.2016070101

Bougoulias, K., Kouris, I., Prasinos, M., Giokas, K., & Koutsouris, D. (2017). Ob/Gyn EMR Software: A Solution for Obstetricians and Gynecologists. In A. Moumtzoglou (Ed.), *Design, Development, and Integration of Reliable Electronic Healthcare Platforms* (pp. 101–111). Hershey, PA: IGI Global. doi:10.4018/978-1-5225-1724-5.ch006

Bouslimi, R., Ayadi, M. G., & Akaichi, J. (2018). Medical Image Retrieval in Healthcare Social Networks. *International Journal of Healthcare Information Systems and Informatics*, *13*(2), 13–28. doi:10.4018/IJHISI.2018040102

Bouzaabia, O., Bouzaabia, R., & Mejri, K. (2017). Role of Internet in the Development of Medical Tourism Service in Tunisia. In A. Capatina & E. Rancati (Eds.), *Key Challenges and Opportunities in Web Entrepreneurship* (pp. 211–241). Hershey, PA: IGI Global. doi:10.4018/978-1-5225-2466-3.ch009

Briz-Ponce, L., Juanes-Méndez, J. A., & García-Peñalvo, F. J. (2016). The Role of Gender in Technology Acceptance for Medical Education. In M. Cruz-Cunha, I. Miranda, R. Martinho, & R. Rijo (Eds.), *Encyclopedia of E-Health and Telemedicine* (pp. 1013–1027). Hershey, PA: IGI Global. doi:10.4018/978-1-4666-9978-6.ch079

Briz-Ponce, L., Juanes-Méndez, J. A., & García-Peñalvo, F. J. (2016). A Research Contribution to the Analysis of Mobile Devices in Higher Education from Medical Students' Point of View. In L. Briz-Ponce, J. Juanes-Méndez, & F. García-Peñalvo (Eds.), *Handbook of Research on Mobile Devices and Applications in Higher Education Settings* (pp. 196–221). Hershey, PA: IGI Global. doi:10.4018/978-1-5225-0256-2.ch009

Brown-Jackson, K. L. (2018). Telemedicine and Telehealth: Academics Engaging the Community in a Call to Action. In S. Burton (Ed.), *Engaged Scholarship and Civic Responsibility in Higher Education* (pp. 166–193). Hershey, PA: IGI Global. doi:10.4018/978-1-5225-3649-9.ch008

Bwalya, K. J. (2017). Next Wave of Tele-Medicine: Virtual Presence of Medical Personnel. In K. Moahi, K. Bwalya, & P. Sebina (Eds.), *Health Information Systems and the Advancement of Medical Practice in Developing Countries* (pp. 168–180). Hershey, PA: IGI Global. doi:10.4018/978-1-5225-2262-1.ch010

Carlton, E. L., Holsinger, J. W. Jr, & Anunobi, N. (2016). Physician Engagement with Health Information Technology: Implications for Practice and Professionalism. *International Journal of Computers in Clinical Practice*, *1*(2), 51–73. doi:10.4018/IJCCP.2016070103

Castillo-Page, L., Eliason, J., Conrad, S. S., & Nivet, M. A. (2016). Diversity in Undergraduate Medical Education: An Examination of Organizational Culture and Climate in Medical Schools. In C. Scott & J. Sims (Eds.), *Developing Workforce Diversity Programs, Curriculum, and Degrees in Higher Education* (pp. 304–326). Hershey, PA: IGI Global. doi:10.4018/978-1-5225-0209-8.ch016

Cebeci, H. I., & Hiziroglu, A. (2016). Review of Business Intelligence and Intelligent Systems in Healthcare Domain. In N. Celebi (Ed.), *Intelligent Techniques for Data Analysis in Diverse Settings* (pp. 192–206). Hershey, PA: IGI Global. doi:10.4018/978-1-5225-0075-9.ch009

Celik, G. (2018). Determining Headache Diseases With Genetic Algorithm. In U. Kose, G. Guraksin, & O. Deperlioglu (Eds.), *Nature-Inspired Intelligent Techniques for Solving Biomedical Engineering Problems* (pp. 249–262). Hershey, PA: IGI Global. doi:10.4018/978-1-5225-4769-3.ch012

Chakraborty, C., Gupta, B., & Ghosh, S. K. (2016). Mobile Telemedicine Systems for Remote Patient's Chronic Wound Monitoring. In A. Moumtzoglou (Ed.), *M-Health Innovations for Patient-Centered Care* (pp. 213–239). Hershey, PA: IGI Global. doi:10.4018/978-1-4666-9861-1.ch011

Chakraborty, S., Chatterjee, S., Ashour, A. S., Mali, K., & Dey, N. (2018). Intelligent Computing in Medical Imaging: A Study. In N. Dey (Ed.), *Advancements in Applied Metaheuristic Computing* (pp. 143–163). Hershey, PA: IGI Global. doi:10.4018/978-1-5225-4151-6.ch006

Chavez, A., & Kovarik, C. (2017). Open Source Technology for Medical Practice in Developing Countries. In K. Moahi, K. Bwalya, & P. Sebina (Eds.), *Health Information Systems and the Advancement of Medical Practice in Developing Countries* (pp. 33–59). Hershey, PA: IGI Global. doi:10.4018/978-1-5225-2262-1.ch003

Chen, E. T. (2016). Examining the Influence of Information Technology on Modern Health Care. In P. Manolitzas, E. Grigoroudis, N. Matsatsinis, & D. Yannacopoulos (Eds.), *Effective Methods for Modern Healthcare Service Quality and Evaluation* (pp. 110–136). Hershey, PA: IGI Global. doi:10.4018/978-1-4666-9961-8.ch006

Chin, S. (2016). Surviving Sandy: Recovering Collections after a Natural Disaster. In E. Decker & J. Townes (Eds.), *Handbook of Research on Disaster Management and Contingency Planning in Modern Libraries* (pp. 366–388). Hershey, PA: IGI Global. doi:10.4018/978-1-4666-8624-3.ch016

Chojnacki, M., & Wójcik, A. (2016). Security and the Role of New Technologies and Innovation in Medical Ethics. In A. Rosiek & K. Leksowski (Eds.), *Organizational Culture and Ethics in Modern Medicine* (pp. 52–77). Hershey, PA: IGI Global. doi:10.4018/978-1-4666-9658-7.ch003

Cılız, N., Yıldırım, H., & Temizel, Ş. (2016). Structure Development for Effective Medical Waste and Hazardous Waste Management System. In U. Akkucuk (Ed.), *Handbook of Research on Waste Management Techniques for Sustainability* (pp. 303–327). Hershey, PA: IGI Global. doi:10.4018/978-1-4666-9723-2.ch016

Ciufudean, C. (2018). Innovative Formalism for Biological Data Analysis. In M. Khosrow-Pour, D.B.A. (Ed.), Encyclopedia of Information Science and Technology, Fourth Edition (pp. 1814-1824). Hershey, PA: IGI Global. doi:10.4018/978-1-5225-2255-3.ch158

Ciufudean, C., & Ciufudean, O. (2016). Tele-Monitoring for Medical Diagnosis Availability. In M. Cruz-Cunha, I. Miranda, R. Martinho, & R. Rijo (Eds.), *Encyclopedia of E-Health and Telemedicine* (pp. 401–411). Hershey, PA: IGI Global. doi:10.4018/978-1-4666-9978-6.ch032

Colaguori, R., & Danesi, M. (2017). Medical Semiotics: A Revisitation and an Exhortation. *International Journal of Semiotics and Visual Rhetoric*, *1*(1), 11–18. doi:10.4018/IJSVR.2017010102

Cole, A. W., & Salek, T. A. (2017). Adopting a Parasocial Connection to Overcome Professional Kakoethos in Online Health Information. In M. Folk & S. Apostel (Eds.), *Establishing and Evaluating Digital Ethos and Online Credibility* (pp. 104–120). Hershey, PA: IGI Global. doi:10.4018/978-1-5225-1072-7.ch006

Contreras, E. C., & Puente, G. J. (2016). How to Identify Rheumatic Diseases by General Physicians. In T. Gasmelseid (Ed.), *Advancing Pharmaceutical Processes and Tools for Improved Health Outcomes* (pp. 136–166). Hershey, PA: IGI Global. doi:10.4018/978-1-5225-0248-7.ch006

D'Andrea, A., Ferri, F., & Grifoni, P. (2016). RFID Technologies in Healthcare Setting: Applications and Future Perspectives. *International Journal of Computers in Clinical Practice*, *1*(1), 15–27. doi:10.4018/IJCCP.2016010102

Damianakis, A., Kallonis, P., Loudos, G., Tsatsos, D., & Tsoukalis, A. (2016). Exploiting 3D Medical Equipment Simulations to Support Biomedical Engineering Academic Courses: Design Methodology and Implementation in a Small Scale National Project. In B. Khan (Ed.), *Revolutionizing Modern Education through Meaningful E-Learning Implementation* (pp. 277–295). Hershey, PA: IGI Global. doi:10.4018/978-1-5225-0466-5.ch015

Demiroz, E. (2016). Principles of Instructional Design for E-Learning and Online Learning Practices: Implications for Medical Education. In V. Wang (Ed.), *Handbook of Research on Advancing Health Education through Technology* (pp. 419–451). Hershey, PA: IGI Global. doi:10.4018/978-1-4666-9494-1.ch018

Deperlioglu, O. (2018). Intelligent Techniques Inspired by Nature and Used in Biomedical Engineering. In U. Kose, G. Guraksin, & O. Deperlioglu (Eds.), *Nature-Inspired Intelligent Techniques for Solving Biomedical Engineering Problems* (pp. 51–77). Hershey, PA: IGI Global. doi:10.4018/978-1-5225-4769-3.ch003

Dey, N., & Ashour, A. S. (2018). Meta-Heuristic Algorithms in Medical Image Segmentation: A Review. In N. Dey (Ed.), *Advancements in Applied Metaheuristic Computing* (pp. 185–203). Hershey, PA: IGI Global. doi:10.4018/978-1-5225-4151-6.ch008

Dey, N., Ashour, A. S., & Althoupety, A. S. (2017). Thermal Imaging in Medical Science. In V. Santhi (Ed.), *Recent Advances in Applied Thermal Imaging for Industrial Applications* (pp. 87–117). Hershey, PA: IGI Global. doi:10.4018/978-1-5225-2423-6.ch004

Di Virgilio, F., Camillo, A. A., & Camillo, I. C. (2017). The Impact of Social Network on Italian Users' Behavioural Intention for the Choice of a Medical Tourist Destination. *International Journal of Tourism and Hospitality Management in the Digital Age, 1*(1), 36–49. doi:10.4018/IJTHMDA.2017010103

Dias, C. M., Ribeiro, A. G., & Furtado, S. F. (2016). An Overview about the Use of Healthcare Applications on Mobile Devices. In M. Cruz-Cunha, I. Miranda, R. Martinho, & R. Rijo (Eds.), *Encyclopedia of E-Health and Telemedicine* (pp. 285–298). Hershey, PA: IGI Global. doi:10.4018/978-1-4666-9978-6.ch024

Dogra, A. K., & Dogra, P. (2017). The Medical Tourism Industry in the BRIC Nations: An Indian Analysis. In M. Dhiman (Ed.), *Opportunities and Challenges for Tourism and Hospitality in the BRIC Nations* (pp. 320–336). Hershey, PA: IGI Global. doi:10.4018/978-1-5225-0708-6.ch020

Drowos, J. L., & Wood, S. K. (2017). Preparing Future Physicians to Adapt to the Changing Health Care System: Promoting Humanism through Curricular Design. In V. Bryan & J. Bird (Eds.), *Healthcare Community Synergism between Patients, Practitioners, and Researchers* (pp. 106–125). Hershey, PA: IGI Global. doi:10.4018/978-1-5225-0640-9.ch006

Dulam, K. (2017). Medical Patents and Impact on Availability and Affordability of Essential Medicines in India. In R. Aggarwal & R. Kaur (Eds.), *Patent Law and Intellectual Property in the Medical Field* (pp. 41–57). Hershey, PA: IGI Global. doi:10.4018/978-1-5225-2414-4.ch003

Dutta, P. (2017). Decision Making in Medical Diagnosis via Distance Measures on Interval Valued Fuzzy Sets. *International Journal of System Dynamics Applications*, *6*(4), 63–83. doi:10.4018/IJSDA.2017100104

Edoh, T. O., Pawar, P. A., Brügge, B., & Teege, G. (2016). A Multidisciplinary Remote Healthcare Delivery System to Increase Health Care Access, Pathology Screening, and Treatment in Developing Countries: The Case of Benin. *International Journal of Healthcare Information Systems and Informatics*, *11*(4), 1–31. doi:10.4018/IJHISI.2016100101

El Guemhioui, K., & Demurjian, S. A. (2017). Semantic Reconciliation of Electronic Health Records Using Semantic Web Technologies. *International Journal of Information Technology and Web Engineering*, *12*(2), 26–48. doi:10.4018/IJITWE.2017040102

Ellouze, N., Rekhis, S., & Boudriga, N. (2016). Forensic Investigation of Digital Crimes in Healthcare Applications. In O. Isafiade & A. Bagula (Eds.), *Data Mining Trends and Applications in Criminal Science and Investigations* (pp. 169–210). Hershey, PA: IGI Global. doi:10.4018/978-1-5225-0463-4.ch007

Eneanya, A. N. (2016). Health Policy Implementation and Its Barriers: The Case Study of US Health System. In R. Gholipour & K. Rouzbehani (Eds.), *Social, Economic, and Political Perspectives on Public Health Policy-Making* (pp. 42–63). Hershey, PA: IGI Global. doi:10.4018/978-1-4666-9944-1.ch003

Entico, G. J. (2016). Knowledge Management and the Medical Health Librarians: A Perception Study. In J. Yap, M. Perez, M. Ayson, & G. Entico (Eds.), *Special Library Administration, Standardization and Technological Integration* (pp. 52–77). Hershey, PA: IGI Global. doi:10.4018/978-1-4666-9542-9.ch003

Ferradji, M. A., & Zidani, A. (2016). Collaborative Environment for Remote Clinical Reasoning Learning. *International Journal of E-Health and Medical Communications*, *7*(4), 62–81. doi:10.4018/IJEHMC.2016100104

Fisher, J. (2018). Sociological Perspectives on Improving Medical Diagnosis Emphasizing CAD. In M. Khosrow-Pour, D.B.A. (Ed.), Encyclopedia of Information Science and Technology, Fourth Edition (pp. 1017-1024). Hershey, PA: IGI Global. doi:10.4018/978-1-5225-2255-3.ch088

Flores, C. D., Respício, A., Coelho, H., Bez, M. R., & Fonseca, J. M. (2016). Simulation for Medical Training. In M. Cruz-Cunha, I. Miranda, R. Martinho, & R. Rijo (Eds.), *Encyclopedia of E-Health and Telemedicine* (pp. 827–842). Hershey, PA: IGI Global. doi:10.4018/978-1-4666-9978-6.ch064

Frank, E. M. (2018). Healthcare Education: Integrating Simulation Technologies. In V. Bryan, A. Musgrove, & J. Powers (Eds.), *Handbook of Research on Human Development in the Digital Age* (pp. 163–182). Hershey, PA: IGI Global. doi:10.4018/978-1-5225-2838-8.ch008

Garner, G. (2018). Foundations for Yoga Practice in Rehabilitation. In S. Telles & N. Singh (Eds.), *Research-Based Perspectives on the Psychophysiology of Yoga* (pp. 263–307). Hershey, PA: IGI Global. doi:10.4018/978-1-5225-2788-6.ch015

Gasmelseid, T. M. (2016). Improving Pharmaceutical Care through the Use of Intelligent Pharmacoinformatics. In T. Gasmelseid (Ed.), *Advancing Pharmaceutical Processes and Tools for Improved Health Outcomes* (pp. 167–188). Hershey, PA: IGI Global. doi:10.4018/978-1-5225-0248-7.ch007

Gavurová, B., Kováč, V., & Šoltés, M. (2018). Medical Equipment and Economic Determinants of Its Structure and Regulation in the Slovak Republic. In M. Khosrow-Pour, D.B.A. (Ed.), Encyclopedia of Information Science and Technology, Fourth Edition (pp. 5841-5852). Hershey, PA: IGI Global. doi:10.4018/978-1-5225-2255-3.ch508

Ge, X., Wang, Q., Huang, K., Law, V., & Thomas, D. C. (2017). Designing Simulated Learning Environments and Facilitating Authentic Learning Experiences in Medical Education. In J. Stefaniak (Ed.), *Advancing Medical Education Through Strategic Instructional Design* (pp. 77–100). Hershey, PA: IGI Global. doi:10.4018/978-1-5225-2098-6.ch004

Gewald, H., & Gewald, C. (2018). Inhibitors of Physicians' Use of Mandatory Hospital Information Systems (HIS). *International Journal of Healthcare Information Systems and Informatics, 13*(1), 29–44. doi:10.4018/IJHISI.2018010103

Ghosh, D., & Dinda, S. (2017). Health Infrastructure and Economic Development in India. In R. Das (Ed.), *Social, Health, and Environmental Infrastructures for Economic Growth* (pp. 99–119). Hershey, PA: IGI Global. doi:10.4018/978-1-5225-2364-2.ch006

Ghosh, K., & Sen, K. C. (2017). The Potential of Crowdsourcing in the Health Care Industry. In N. Wickramasinghe (Ed.), *Handbook of Research on Healthcare Administration and Management* (pp. 418–427). Hershey, PA: IGI Global. doi:10.4018/978-1-5225-0920-2.ch024

Ghrab, S., & Saad, I. (2016). Identifying Crucial Know-How and Knowing-That for Medical Decision Support. *International Journal of Decision Support System Technology, 8*(4), 14–33. doi:10.4018/IJDSST.2016100102

Giokas, K., Tsirmpas, C., Anastasiou, A., Iliopoulou, D., Costarides, V., & Koutsouris, D. (2016). Contemporary Heart Failure Treatment Based on Improved Knowledge and Personalized Care of Comorbidities. In D. Fotiadis (Ed.), *Handbook of Research on Trends in the Diagnosis and Treatment of Chronic Conditions* (pp. 301–314). Hershey, PA: IGI Global. doi:10.4018/978-1-4666-8828-5.ch014

Gopalan, V., Chan, E., & Ho, D. T. (2018). Deliberate Self-Harm and Suicide Ideology in Medical Students. In C. Smith (Ed.), *Exploring the Pressures of Medical Education From a Mental Health and Wellness Perspective* (pp. 122–143). Hershey, PA: IGI Global. doi:10.4018/978-1-5225-2811-1.ch005

Goswami, S., Dey, U., Roy, P., Ashour, A., & Dey, N. (2017). Medical Video Processing: Concept and Applications. In N. Dey, A. Ashour, & P. Patra (Eds.), *Feature Detectors and Motion Detection in Video Processing* (pp. 1–17). Hershey, PA: IGI Global. doi:10.4018/978-1-5225-1025-3.ch001

Goswami, S., Mahanta, K., Goswami, S., Jigdung, T., & Devi, T. P. (2018). Ageing and Cancer: The Epigenetic Basis, Alternative Treatment, and Care. In B. Prasad & S. Akbar (Eds.), *Handbook of Research on Geriatric Health, Treatment, and Care* (pp. 206–235). Hershey, PA: IGI Global. doi:10.4018/978-1-5225-3480-8.ch012

Gouva, M. I. (2017). The Psychological Impact of Medical Error on Patients, Family Members, and Health Professionals. In M. Riga (Ed.), *Impact of Medical Errors and Malpractice on Health Economics, Quality, and Patient Safety* (pp. 171–196). Hershey, PA: IGI Global. doi:10.4018/978-1-5225-2337-6.ch007

Gürcü, M., & Tengilimoğlu, D. (2017). Health Tourism-Based Destination Marketing. In A. Bayraktar & C. Uslay (Eds.), *Strategic Place Branding Methodologies and Theory for Tourist Attraction* (pp. 308–331). Hershey, PA: IGI Global. doi:10.4018/978-1-5225-0579-2.ch015

Gürsel, G. (2016). Mobility in Healthcare: M-Health. In A. Panagopoulos (Ed.), *Handbook of Research on Next Generation Mobile Communication Systems* (pp. 485–511). Hershey, PA: IGI Global. doi:10.4018/978-1-4666-8732-5.ch019

Gürsel, G. (2017). For Better Healthcare Mining Health Data. In S. Bhattacharyya, S. De, I. Pan, & P. Dutta (Eds.), *Intelligent Multidimensional Data Clustering and Analysis* (pp. 135–158). Hershey, PA: IGI Global. doi:10.4018/978-1-5225-1776-4.ch006

Guzman-Lugo, G., Lopez-Martinez, M., Lopez-Ramirez, B., & Avila-Vazquez, D. (2016). City-Driven Approach to Determine Health Services Based on Current User Location and Collaborative Information. *International Journal of Knowledge Society Research*, *7*(1), 53–62. doi:10.4018/IJKSR.2016010104

Gyaase, P. O., Darko-Lartey, R., William, H., & Borkloe, F. (2017). Towards an Integrated Electronic Medical Records System for Quality Healthcare in Ghana: An Exploratory Factor Analysis. *International Journal of Computers in Clinical Practice*, *2*(2), 38–55. doi:10.4018/IJCCP.2017070103

Handayani, P. W., Sandhyaduhita, P. I., Hidayanto, A. N., Pinem, A. A., Fajrina, H. R., Junus, K. M., ... Ayuningtyas, D. (2016). Integrated Hospital Information System Architecture Design in Indonesia. In T. Iyamu & A. Tatnall (Eds.), *Maximizing Healthcare Delivery and Management through Technology Integration* (pp. 207–236). Hershey, PA: IGI Global. doi:10.4018/978-1-4666-9446-0.ch013

Hanel, P. (2017). Is China Catching Up?: Health-Related Applications of Biotechnology. In T. Bas & J. Zhao (Eds.), *Comparative Approaches to Biotechnology Development and Use in Developed and Emerging Nations* (pp. 465–520). Hershey, PA: IGI Global. doi:10.4018/978-1-5225-1040-6.ch016

Harmsen, C. A., & Royle, R. N. (2016). St. Stephen's Hospital Hervey Bay: Study of Developing a Digital Hospital. In J. Moon & M. Galea (Eds.), *Improving Health Management through Clinical Decision Support Systems* (pp. 127–153). Hershey, PA: IGI Global. doi:10.4018/978-1-4666-9432-3.ch006

Harp, D., Shim, R. S., Johnson, J., Harp, J. A., Wilcox, W. C., & Wilcox, J. K. (2016). Race and Gender Inequalities in Medicine and Biomedical Research. In U. Thomas & J. Drake (Eds.), *Critical Research on Sexism and Racism in STEM Fields* (pp. 115–134). Hershey, PA: IGI Global. doi:10.4018/978-1-5225-0174-9.ch006

Hartman, A., & Brown, S. (2017). Synergism through Therapeutic Visual Arts. In V. Bryan & J. Bird (Eds.), *Healthcare Community Synergism between Patients, Practitioners, and Researchers* (pp. 29–48). Hershey, PA: IGI Global. doi:10.4018/978-1-5225-0640-9.ch002

Hazra, J., Chowdhury, A. R., & Dutta, P. (2016). Cluster Based Medical Image Registration Using Optimized Neural Network. In S. Bhattacharyya, P. Banerjee, D. Majumdar, & P. Dutta (Eds.), *Handbook of Research on Advanced Hybrid Intelligent Techniques and Applications* (pp. 551–581). Hershey, PA: IGI Global. doi:10.4018/978-1-4666-9474-3.ch018

Hung, S., Huang, W., Yen, D. C., Chang, S., & Lu, C. (2016). Effect of Information Service Competence and Contextual Factors on the Effectiveness of Strategic Information Systems Planning in Hospitals. *Journal of Global Information Management, 24*(1), 14–36. doi:10.4018/JGIM.2016010102

Iltchev, P., Śliwczyński, A., Szynkiewicz, P., & Marczak, M. (2016). Mobile Health Applications Assisting Patients with Chronic Diseases: Examples from Asthma Care. In A. Moumtzoglou (Ed.), *M-Health Innovations for Patient-Centered Care* (pp. 170–196). Hershey, PA: IGI Global. doi:10.4018/978-1-4666-9861-1.ch009

Iqbal, S., Ahmad, S., & Willis, I. (2017). Influencing Factors for Adopting Technology Enhanced Learning in the Medical Schools of Punjab, Pakistan. *International Journal of Information and Communication Technology Education, 13*(3), 27–39. doi:10.4018/IJICTE.2017070103

Jagan, J., Dalkiliç, Y., & Samui, P. (2016). Utilization of SVM, LSSVM and GP for Predicting the Medical Waste Generation. In G. Hua (Ed.), *Smart Cities as a Solution for Reducing Urban Waste and Pollution* (pp. 224–251). Hershey, PA: IGI Global. doi:10.4018/978-1-5225-0302-6.ch008

Jagiello, K., Sosnowska, A., Mikolajczyk, A., & Puzyn, T. (2017). Nanomaterials in Medical Devices: Regulations' Review and Future Perspectives. *Journal of Nanotoxicology and Nanomedicine, 2*(2), 1–11. doi:10.4018/JNN.2017070101

Jena, T. K. (2018). Skill Training Process in Medicine Through Distance Mode. In U. Pandey & V. Indrakanti (Eds.), *Optimizing Open and Distance Learning in Higher Education Institutions* (pp. 228–243). Hershey, PA: IGI Global. doi:10.4018/978-1-5225-2624-7.ch010

Jesus, Â., & Gomes, M. J. (2016). Web 2.0 Tools in Biomedical and Pharmaceutical Education: Updated Review and Commentary. In T. Gasmelseid (Ed.), *Advancing Pharmaceutical Processes and Tools for Improved Health Outcomes* (pp. 52–78). Hershey, PA: IGI Global. doi:10.4018/978-1-5225-0248-7.ch003

Joseph, V., & Miller, J. M. (2018). Medical Students' Perceived Stigma in Seeking Care: A Cultural Perspective. In C. Smith (Ed.), *Exploring the Pressures of Medical Education From a Mental Health and Wellness Perspective* (pp. 44–67). Hershey, PA: IGI Global. doi:10.4018/978-1-5225-2811-1.ch002

Joyce, B. L., & Swanberg, S. M. (2017). Using Backward Design for Competency-Based Undergraduate Medical Education. In J. Stefaniak (Ed.), *Advancing Medical Education Through Strategic Instructional Design* (pp. 53–76). Hershey, PA: IGI Global. doi:10.4018/978-1-5225-2098-6.ch003

Kaljo, K., & Jacques, L. (2018). Flipping the Medical School Classroom. In M. Khosrow-Pour, D.B.A. (Ed.), Encyclopedia of Information Science and Technology, Fourth Edition (pp. 5800-5809). Hershey, PA: IGI Global. doi:10.4018/978-1-5225-2255-3.ch504

Karon, R. (2016). Utilisation of Health Information Systems for Service Delivery in the Namibian Environment. In T. Iyamu & A. Tatnall (Eds.), *Maximizing Healthcare Delivery and Management through Technology Integration* (pp. 169–183). Hershey, PA: IGI Global. doi:10.4018/978-1-4666-9446-0.ch011

Kasina, H., Bahubalendruni, M. V., & Botcha, R. (2017). Robots in Medicine: Past, Present and Future. *International Journal of Manufacturing, Materials, and Mechanical Engineering*, *7*(4), 44–64. doi:10.4018/IJMMME.2017100104

Katehakis, D. G. (2018). Electronic Medical Record Implementation Challenges for the National Health System in Greece. *International Journal of Reliable and Quality E-Healthcare*, *7*(1), 16–30. doi:10.4018/IJRQEH.2018010102

Katz, A., & Shtub, A. (2016). Design and Build a Wizard of Oz (WOZ) Telemedicine Simulator Platform. In M. Cruz-Cunha, I. Miranda, R. Martinho, & R. Rijo (Eds.), *Encyclopedia of E-Health and Telemedicine* (pp. 128–141). Hershey, PA: IGI Global. doi:10.4018/978-1-4666-9978-6.ch011

Kaur, P. D., & Sharma, P. (2017). Success Dimensions of ICTs in Healthcare. In B. Singh (Ed.), *Computational Tools and Techniques for Biomedical Signal Processing* (pp. 149–173). Hershey, PA: IGI Global. doi:10.4018/978-1-5225-0660-7.ch007

Kaushik, P. (2018). Comorbidity of Medical and Psychiatric Disorders in Geriatric Population: Treatment and Care. In B. Prasad & S. Akbar (Eds.), *Handbook of Research on Geriatric Health, Treatment, and Care* (pp. 448–474). Hershey, PA: IGI Global. doi:10.4018/978-1-5225-3480-8.ch025

Khachane, M. Y. (2017). Organ-Based Medical Image Classification Using Support Vector Machine. *International Journal of Synthetic Emotions*, *8*(1), 18–30. doi:10.4018/IJSE.2017010102

Kirci, P. (2018). Intelligent Techniques for Analysis of Big Data About Healthcare and Medical Records. In N. Shah & M. Mittal (Eds.), *Handbook of Research on Promoting Business Process Improvement Through Inventory Control Techniques* (pp. 559–582). Hershey, PA: IGI Global. doi:10.4018/978-1-5225-3232-3.ch029

Kldiashvili, E. (2016). Cloud Computing as the Useful Resource for Application of the Medical Information System for Quality Assurance Purposes. *International Journal of Computers in Clinical Practice*, *1*(2), 1–23. doi:10.4018/IJCCP.2016070101

Kldiashvili, E. (2018). Cloud Approach for the Medical Information System: MIS on Cloud. In M. Khosrow-Pour (Ed.), *Incorporating Nature-Inspired Paradigms in Computational Applications* (pp. 238–261). Hershey, PA: IGI Global. doi:10.4018/978-1-5225-5020-4.ch008

Kldiashvili, E., Burduli, A., Ghortlishvili, G., & Sheklashvili, I. (2016). Georgian Experience in Telecytology. In M. Cruz-Cunha, I. Miranda, R. Martinho, & R. Rijo (Eds.), *Encyclopedia of E-Health and Telemedicine* (pp. 62–71). Hershey, PA: IGI Global. doi:10.4018/978-1-4666-9978-6.ch006

Ko, H., Mesicek, L., Choi, J., Choi, J., & Hwang, S. (2018). A Study on Secure Contents Strategies for Applications With DRM on Cloud Computing. *International Journal of Cloud Applications and Computing*, *8*(1), 143–153. doi:10.4018/IJCAC.2018010107

Komendziński, T., Dreszer-Drogorób, J., Mikołajewska, E., Mikołajewski, D., & Bałaj, B. (2016). Interdisciplinary Education for Research and Everyday Clinical Practice: Lessons Learned from InteRDoCTor Project. In A. Rosiek & K. Leksowski (Eds.), *Organizational Culture and Ethics in Modern Medicine* (pp. 78–110). Hershey, PA: IGI Global. doi:10.4018/978-1-4666-9658-7.ch004

Komendziński, T., Mikołajewska, E., & Mikołajewski, D. (2018). Cross-Cultural Decision-Making in Healthcare: Theory and Practical Application in Real Clinical Conditions. In A. Rosiek-Kryszewska & K. Leksowski (Eds.), *Healthcare Administration for Patient Safety and Engagement* (pp. 276–298). Hershey, PA: IGI Global. doi:10.4018/978-1-5225-3946-9.ch015

Konecny, L. T. (2018). Medical School Wellness Initiatives. In C. Smith (Ed.), *Exploring the Pressures of Medical Education From a Mental Health and Wellness Perspective* (pp. 209–228). Hershey, PA: IGI Global. doi:10.4018/978-1-5225-2811-1.ch009

Konieczna, A., & Słomkowski, P. (2016). Confrontation of Human Rights in Daily Clinical Situations. In A. Rosiek & K. Leksowski (Eds.), *Organizational Culture and Ethics in Modern Medicine* (pp. 255–281). Hershey, PA: IGI Global. doi:10.4018/978-1-4666-9658-7.ch011

Kromrei, H., Solomonson, W. L., & Juzych, M. S. (2017). Teaching Residents How to Teach. In J. Stefaniak (Ed.), *Advancing Medical Education Through Strategic Instructional Design* (pp. 164–185). Hershey, PA: IGI Global. doi:10.4018/978-1-5225-2098-6.ch008

Kulkarni, S., Savyanavar, A., Kulkarni, P., Stranieri, A., & Ghorpade, V. (2018). Framework for Integration of Medical Image and Text-Based Report Retrieval to Support Radiological Diagnosis. In M. Kolekar & V. Kumar (Eds.), *Biomedical Signal and Image Processing in Patient Care* (pp. 86–122). Hershey, PA: IGI Global. doi:10.4018/978-1-5225-2829-6.ch006

Kumar, A., & Sarkar, B. K. (2018). Performance Analysis of Nature-Inspired Algorithms-Based Bayesian Prediction Models for Medical Data Sets. In U. Singh, A. Tiwari, & R. Singh (Eds.), *Soft-Computing-Based Nonlinear Control Systems Design* (pp. 134–155). Hershey, PA: IGI Global. doi:10.4018/978-1-5225-3531-7.ch007

Kurtz, R. S. (2016). Fortitude: A Study of African Americans in Surgery in New York City. In U. Thomas & J. Drake (Eds.), *Critical Research on Sexism and Racism in STEM Fields* (pp. 153–169). Hershey, PA: IGI Global. doi:10.4018/978-1-5225-0174-9.ch009

Labbadi, W., & Akaichi, J. (2017). Efficient Algorithm for Answering Fuzzy Medical Requests in Pervasive Healthcare Information Systems. *International Journal of Healthcare Information Systems and Informatics*, *12*(2), 46–64. doi:10.4018/IJHISI.2017040103

Lagumdzija, A., & Swing, V. K. (2017). Health, Digitalization, and Individual Empowerment. In F. Topor (Ed.), *Handbook of Research on Individualism and Identity in the Globalized Digital Age* (pp. 380–402). Hershey, PA: IGI Global. doi:10.4018/978-1-5225-0522-8.ch017

Lamey, T. W., & Davidson-Shivers, G. V. (2017). Instructional Strategies and Sequencing. In J. Stefaniak (Ed.), *Advancing Medical Education Through Strategic Instructional Design* (pp. 30–52). Hershey, PA: IGI Global. doi:10.4018/978-1-5225-2098-6.ch002

Leon, G. (2017). The Role of Forensic Medicine in Medical Errors. In M. Riga (Ed.), *Impact of Medical Errors and Malpractice on Health Economics, Quality, and Patient Safety* (pp. 144–170). Hershey, PA: IGI Global. doi:10.4018/978-1-5225-2337-6.ch006

Lidia, B., Federica, G., & Maria, V. E. (2016). The Patient-Centered Medicine as the Theoretical Framework for Patient Engagement. In G. Graffigna (Ed.), *Promoting Patient Engagement and Participation for Effective Healthcare Reform* (pp. 25–39). Hershey, PA: IGI Global. doi:10.4018/978-1-4666-9992-2.ch002

Love, L., & McDowelle, D. (2018). Developing a Comprehensive Wellness Program for Medical Students. In C. Smith (Ed.), *Exploring the Pressures of Medical Education From a Mental Health and Wellness Perspective* (pp. 190–208). Hershey, PA: IGI Global. doi:10.4018/978-1-5225-2811-1.ch008

Lovell, K. L. (2017). Development and Evaluation of Neuroscience Computer-Based Modules for Medical Students: Instructional Design Principles and Effectiveness. In J. Stefaniak (Ed.), *Advancing Medical Education Through Strategic Instructional Design* (pp. 262–276). Hershey, PA: IGI Global. doi:10.4018/978-1-5225-2098-6.ch013

Lubin, R., & Hamlin, M. D. (2018). Medical Student Burnout: A Social Cognitive Learning Perspective on Medical Student Mental Health and Wellness. In C. Smith (Ed.), *Exploring the Pressures of Medical Education From a Mental Health and Wellness Perspective* (pp. 92–121). Hershey, PA: IGI Global. doi:10.4018/978-1-5225-2811-1.ch004

Luk, C. Y. (2018). Moving Towards Universal Health Coverage: Challenges for the Present and Future in China. In B. Fong, A. Ng, & P. Yuen (Eds.), *Sustainable Health and Long-Term Care Solutions for an Aging Population* (pp. 19–45). Hershey, PA: IGI Global. doi:10.4018/978-1-5225-2633-9.ch002

Mahat, M., & Pettigrew, A. (2017). The Regulatory Environment of Non-Profit Higher Education and Research Institutions and Its Implications for Managerial Strategy: The Case of Medical Education and Research. In L. West & A. Worthington (Eds.), *Handbook of Research on Emerging Business Models and Managerial Strategies in the Nonprofit Sector* (pp. 336–351). Hershey, PA: IGI Global. doi:10.4018/978-1-5225-2537-0.ch017

Maitra, I. K., & Bandhyopadhyaay, S. K. (2017). Adaptive Edge Detection Method towards Features Extraction from Diverse Medical Imaging Technologies. In S. Bhattacharyya, S. De, I. Pan, & P. Dutta (Eds.), *Intelligent Multidimensional Data Clustering and Analysis* (pp. 159–192). Hershey, PA: IGI Global. doi:10.4018/978-1-5225-1776-4.ch007

Mangu, V. P. (2017). Mobile Health Care: A Technology View. In C. Bhatt & S. Peddoju (Eds.), *Cloud Computing Systems and Applications in Healthcare* (pp. 1–18). Hershey, PA: IGI Global. doi:10.4018/978-1-5225-1002-4.ch001

Manirabona, A., Fourati, L. C., & Boudjit, S. (2017). Investigation on Healthcare Monitoring Systems: Innovative Services and Applications. *International Journal of E-Health and Medical Communications*, *8*(1), 1–18. doi:10.4018/IJEHMC.2017010101

Mannai, M. M., & Karâa, W. B. (2016). Biomedical Image Processing Overview. In W. Karâa & N. Dey (Eds.), *Biomedical Image Analysis and Mining Techniques for Improved Health Outcomes* (pp. 1–12). Hershey, PA: IGI Global. doi:10.4018/978-1-4666-8811-7.ch001

Manzoor, A. (2016). RFID in Health Care-Building Smart Hospitals for Quality Healthcare. *International Journal of User-Driven Healthcare, 6*(2), 21–45. doi:10.4018/IJUDH.2016070102

Marwan, M., Kartit, A., & Ouahmane, H. (2018). A Framework to Secure Medical Image Storage in Cloud Computing Environment. *Journal of Electronic Commerce in Organizations, 16*(1), 1–16. doi:10.4018/JECO.2018010101

Masoud, M. P., Nejad, M. K., Darebaghi, H., Chavoshi, M., & Farahani, M. (2018). The Decision Support System and Conventional Method of Telephone Triage by Nurses in Emergency Medical Services: A Comparative Investigation. *International Journal of E-Business Research, 14*(1), 77–88. doi:10.4018/IJEBR.2018010105

McDonald, W. G., Martin, M., & Salzberg, L. D. (2018). From Medical Student to Medical Resident: Graduate Medical Education and Mental Health in the United States. In C. Smith (Ed.), *Exploring the Pressures of Medical Education From a Mental Health and Wellness Perspective* (pp. 145–169). Hershey, PA: IGI Global. doi:10.4018/978-1-5225-2811-1.ch006

Medhekar, A. (2017). The Role of Social Media for Knowledge Dissemination in Medical Tourism: A Case of India. In R. Chugh (Ed.), *Harnessing Social Media as a Knowledge Management Tool* (pp. 25–54). Hershey, PA: IGI Global. doi:10.4018/978-1-5225-0495-5.ch002

Medhekar, A., & Haq, F. (2018). Urbanization and New Jobs Creation in Healthcare Services in India: Challenges and Opportunities. In U. Benna & I. Benna (Eds.), *Urbanization and Its Impact on Socio-Economic Growth in Developing Regions* (pp. 198–218). Hershey, PA: IGI Global. doi:10.4018/978-1-5225-2659-9.ch010

Mehta, G., Dutta, M. K., & Kim, P. S. (2016). An Efficient and Lossless Cryptosystem for Security in Tele-Ophthalmology Applications Using Chaotic Theory. *International Journal of E-Health and Medical Communications, 7*(4), 28–47. doi:10.4018/IJEHMC.2016100102

Mehta, P. (2017). Framework of Indian Healthcare System and its Challenges: An Insight. In V. Bryan & J. Bird (Eds.), *Healthcare Community Synergism between Patients, Practitioners, and Researchers* (pp. 247–271). Hershey, PA: IGI Global. doi:10.4018/978-1-5225-0640-9.ch011

Metelmann, B., & Metelmann, C. (2016). M-Health in Prehospital Emergency Medicine: Experiences from the EU funded Project LiveCity. In A. Moumtzoglou (Ed.), *M-Health Innovations for Patient-Centered Care* (pp. 197–212). Hershey, PA: IGI Global. doi:10.4018/978-1-4666-9861-1.ch010

Mi, M. (2017). Informal Learning in Medical Education. In J. Stefaniak (Ed.), *Advancing Medical Education Through Strategic Instructional Design* (pp. 225–244). Hershey, PA: IGI Global. doi:10.4018/978-1-5225-2098-6.ch011

Miglioretti, M., Mariani, F., & Vecchio, L. (2016). Could Patient Engagement Promote a Health System Free From Malpractice Litigation Risk? In G. Graffigna (Ed.), *Promoting Patient Engagement and Participation for Effective Healthcare Reform* (pp. 240–264). Hershey, PA: IGI Global. doi:10.4018/978-1-4666-9992-2.ch012

Misra, S. C., & Bisui, S. (2016). Feasibility of Large Scale Implementation of Personalized Medicine in the Current Scenario. *International Journal of E-Health and Medical Communications, 7*(2), 30–49. doi:10.4018/IJEHMC.2016040103

Misra, S. C., Bisui, S., & Fantazy, K. (2016). Identifying Critical Changes in Adoption of Personalized Medicine (PM) in Healthcare Management. *International Journal of E-Health and Medical Communications, 7*(3), 1–15. doi:10.4018/IJEHMC.2016070101

Mohammadian, M., Hatzinakos, D., Spachos, P., & Jentzsh, R. (2016). An Intelligent and Secure Framework for Wireless Information Technology in Healthcare for User and Data Classification in Hospitals. In V. Wang (Ed.), *Handbook of Research on Advancing Health Education through Technology* (pp. 452–479). Hershey, PA: IGI Global. doi:10.4018/978-1-4666-9494-1.ch019

Mokeddem, S., & Atmani, B. (2016). Assessment of Clinical Decision Support Systems for Predicting Coronary Heart Disease. *International Journal of Operations Research and Information Systems, 7*(3), 57–73. doi:10.4018/IJORIS.2016070104

Mokrzycka, A., & Kowalska-Bobko, I. (2016). Public Health Legislation and Patient's Rights: Health2020 Strategy, European Perspective. In A. Rosiek & K. Leksowski (Eds.), *Organizational Culture and Ethics in Modern Medicine* (pp. 298–322). Hershey, PA: IGI Global. doi:10.4018/978-1-4666-9658-7.ch013

Moon, J. D., & Galea, M. P. (2016). Overview of Clinical Decision Support Systems in Healthcare. In J. Moon & M. Galea (Eds.), *Improving Health Management through Clinical Decision Support Systems* (pp. 1–27). Hershey, PA: IGI Global. doi:10.4018/978-1-4666-9432-3.ch001

Mosadeghrad, A. M., & Woldemichael, A. (2017). Application of Quality Management in Promoting Patient Safety and Preventing Medical Errors. In M. Riga (Ed.), *Impact of Medical Errors and Malpractice on Health Economics, Quality, and Patient Safety* (pp. 91–112). Hershey, PA: IGI Global. doi:10.4018/978-1-5225-2337-6.ch004

Moumtzoglou, A. (2017). Digital Medicine: The Quality Standpoint. In A. Moumtzoglou (Ed.), *Design, Development, and Integration of Reliable Electronic Healthcare Platforms* (pp. 179–195). Hershey, PA: IGI Global. doi:10.4018/978-1-5225-1724-5.ch011

Moumtzoglou, A., & Pouliakis, A. (2018). Population Health Management and the Science of Individuality. *International Journal of Reliable and Quality E-Healthcare, 7*(2), 1–26. doi:10.4018/IJRQEH.2018040101

Mpofu, C. (2016). International Medical Experiences Outbound New Zealand: An Economic and Medical Workforce Strategy. In D. Velliaris & D. Coleman-George (Eds.), *Handbook of Research on Study Abroad Programs and Outbound Mobility* (pp. 446–469). Hershey, PA: IGI Global. doi:10.4018/978-1-5225-0169-5.ch018

Mukhtar, W. F., & Abuelyaman, E. S. (2017). Opportunities and Challenges of Big Data in Healthcare. In N. Wickramasinghe (Ed.), *Handbook of Research on Healthcare Administration and Management* (pp. 47–58). Hershey, PA: IGI Global. doi:10.4018/978-1-5225-0920-2.ch004

Munugala, S., Brar, G. K., Syed, A., Mohammad, A., & Halgamuge, M. N. (2018). The Much Needed Security and Data Reforms of Cloud Computing in Medical Data Storage. In M. Lytras & P. Papadopoulou (Eds.), *Applying Big Data Analytics in Bioinformatics and Medicine* (pp. 99–113). Hershey, PA: IGI Global. doi:10.4018/978-1-5225-2607-0.ch005

Narasimhamurthy, A. (2016). An Overview of Machine Learning in Medical Image Analysis: Trends in Health Informatics. In N. Dey & A. Ashour (Eds.), *Classification and Clustering in Biomedical Signal Processing* (pp. 23–45). Hershey, PA: IGI Global. doi:10.4018/978-1-5225-0140-4.ch002

Ngara, R. (2017). Multiple Voices, Multiple Paths: Towards Dialogue between Western and Indigenous Medical Knowledge Systems. In P. Ngulube (Ed.), *Handbook of Research on Theoretical Perspectives on Indigenous Knowledge Systems in Developing Countries* (pp. 332–358). Hershey, PA: IGI Global. doi:10.4018/978-1-5225-0833-5.ch015

O'Connor, Y., & Heavin, C. (2018). Defining and Characterising the Landscape of eHealth. In M. Khosrow-Pour, D.B.A. (Ed.), Encyclopedia of Information Science and Technology, Fourth Edition (pp. 5864-5875). Hershey, PA: IGI Global. doi:10.4018/978-1-5225-2255-3.ch510

Ochonogor, W. C., & Okite-Amughoro, F. A. (2018). Building an Effective Digital Library in a University Teaching Hospital (UTH) in Nigeria. In A. Tella & T. Kwanya (Eds.), *Handbook of Research on Managing Intellectual Property in Digital Libraries* (pp. 184–204). Hershey, PA: IGI Global. doi:10.4018/978-1-5225-3093-0.ch010

Olaniran, B. A. (2016). ICTs, E-health, and Multidisciplinary Healthcare Teams: Promises and Challenges. *International Journal of Privacy and Health Information Management*, *4*(2), 62–75. doi:10.4018/IJPHIM.2016070105

Olaniran, B. A. (2016). ICT Use and Multidisciplinary Healthcare Teams in the Age of e-Health. *International Journal of Reliable and Quality E-Healthcare*, *5*(1), 18–31. doi:10.4018/IJRQEH.2016010102

Olivares, S. L., Cruz, A. G., Cabrera, M. V., Regalado, A. I., & García, J. E. (2017). An Assessment Study of Quality Model for Medical Schools in Mexico. In S. Mukerji & P. Tripathi (Eds.), *Handbook of Research on Administration, Policy, and Leadership in Higher Education* (pp. 404–439). Hershey, PA: IGI Global. doi:10.4018/978-1-5225-0672-0.ch016

Omidoyin, E. O., Opeke, R. O., & Osagbemi, G. K. (2016). Utilization Pattern and Privacy Issues in the use of Health Records for Research Practice by Doctors: Selected Nigerian Teaching Hospitals as Case Study. *International Journal of Privacy and Health Information Management*, *4*(1), 1–11. doi:10.4018/IJPHIM.2016010101

Omoruyi, E. A., & Omidele, F. (2018). Resident Physician and Medical Academic Faculty Burnout: A Review of Current Literature. In C. Smith (Ed.), *Exploring the Pressures of Medical Education From a Mental Health and Wellness Perspective* (pp. 171–189). Hershey, PA: IGI Global. doi:10.4018/978-1-5225-2811-1.ch007

Osop, H., & Sahama, T. (2016). Data-Driven and Practice-Based Evidence: Design and Development of Efficient and Effective Clinical Decision Support System. In J. Moon & M. Galea (Eds.), *Improving Health Management through Clinical Decision Support Systems* (pp. 295–328). Hershey, PA: IGI Global. doi:10.4018/978-1-4666-9432-3.ch014

Ossowski, R., & Izdebski, P. (2016). Ethical Aspects of Talking to a Patient. In A. Rosiek & K. Leksowski (Eds.), *Organizational Culture and Ethics in Modern Medicine* (pp. 203–235). Hershey, PA: IGI Global. doi:10.4018/978-1-4666-9658-7.ch009

Pandian, P. S. (2016). An Overview of Telemedicine Technologies for Healthcare Applications. *International Journal of Biomedical and Clinical Engineering*, *5*(2), 29–52. doi:10.4018/IJBCE.2016070103

Papadopoulou, P., Lytras, M., & Marouli, C. (2018). Bioinformatics as Applied to Medicine: Challenges Faced Moving from Big Data to Smart Data to Wise Data. In M. Lytras & P. Papadopoulou (Eds.), *Applying Big Data Analytics in Bioinformatics and Medicine* (pp. 1–25). Hershey, PA: IGI Global. doi:10.4018/978-1-5225-2607-0.ch001

Paraskou, A., & George, B. P. (2018). An Overview of Reproductive Tourism. In *Legal and Economic Considerations Surrounding Reproductive Tourism: Emerging Research and Opportunities* (pp. 1–17). Hershey, PA: IGI Global. doi:10.4018/978-1-5225-2694-0.ch001

Park, S., & Moon, J. (2016). Strategic Approach towards Clinical Information Security. In J. Moon & M. Galea (Eds.), *Improving Health Management through Clinical Decision Support Systems* (pp. 329–359). Hershey, PA: IGI Global. doi:10.4018/978-1-4666-9432-3.ch015

Pereira, D., Castro, A., Gomes, P., Areias, J. C., Reis, Z. S., Coimbra, M. T., & Cruz-Correia, R. (2016). Digital Auscultation: Challenges and Perspectives. In M. Cruz-Cunha, I. Miranda, R. Martinho, & R. Rijo (Eds.), *Encyclopedia of E-Health and Telemedicine* (pp. 910–927). Hershey, PA: IGI Global. doi:10.4018/978-1-4666-9978-6.ch070

Peters, R. A., & Cruz, M. (2016). The States as Generators of Incremental Change in American Health Care Policy: 1935 to 1965. In R. Gholipour & K. Rouzbehani (Eds.), *Social, Economic, and Political Perspectives on Public Health Policy-Making* (pp. 86–114). Hershey, PA: IGI Global. doi:10.4018/978-1-4666-9944-1.ch005

Phuritsabam, B., & Devi, A. B. (2017). Information Seeking Behavior of Medical Scientists at Jawaharlal Nehru Institute of Medical Science: A Study. In S. Ram (Ed.), *Library and Information Services for Bioinformatics Education and Research* (pp. 177–187). Hershey, PA: IGI Global. doi:10.4018/978-1-5225-1871-6.ch010

Pieczka, B. (2018). Management of Risk and Adverse Events in Medical Entities. In A. Rosiek-Kryszewska & K. Leksowski (Eds.), *Healthcare Administration for Patient Safety and Engagement* (pp. 31–46). Hershey, PA: IGI Global. doi:10.4018/978-1-5225-3946-9.ch003

Poduval, J. (2016). Curriculum Development. In *Optimizing Medicine Residency Training Programs* (pp. 45–102). Hershey, PA: IGI Global. doi:10.4018/978-1-4666-9527-6.ch003

Poduval, J. (2016). Ethics and Professionalism. In *Optimizing Medicine Residency Training Programs* (pp. 103–133). Hershey, PA: IGI Global. doi:10.4018/978-1-4666-9527-6.ch004

Poduval, J. (2016). Management Skills and Leadership. In *Optimizing Medicine Residency Training Programs* (pp. 182–205). Hershey, PA: IGI Global. doi:10.4018/978-1-4666-9527-6.ch008

Poduval, J. (2016). Medicine Residency Training. In *Optimizing Medicine Residency Training Programs* (pp. 1–27). Hershey, PA: IGI Global. doi:10.4018/978-1-4666-9527-6.ch001

Poduval, J. (2016). Personal Issues. In *Optimizing Medicine Residency Training Programs* (pp. 206–221). Hershey, PA: IGI Global. doi:10.4018/978-1-4666-9527-6.ch009

Poduval, J. (2017). Medical Errors: Impact on Health Care Quality. In M. Riga (Ed.), *Impact of Medical Errors and Malpractice on Health Economics, Quality, and Patient Safety* (pp. 33–60). Hershey, PA: IGI Global. doi:10.4018/978-1-5225-2337-6.ch002

Politis, D., Stagiopoulos, P., Aidona, S., Kyriafinis, G., & Constantinidis, I. (2018). Autonomous Learning and Skill Accreditation: A Paradigm for Medical Studies. In A. Kumar (Ed.), *Optimizing Student Engagement in Online Learning Environments* (pp. 266–296). Hershey, PA: IGI Global. doi:10.4018/978-1-5225-3634-5.ch012

Pomares-Quimbaya, A., Gonzalez, R. A., Quintero, S., Muñoz, O. M., Bohórquez, W. R., García, O. M., & Londoño, D. (2016). A Review of Existing Applications and Techniques for Narrative Text Analysis in Electronic Medical Records. In M. Cruz-Cunha, I. Miranda, R. Martinho, & R. Rijo (Eds.), *Encyclopedia of E-Health and Telemedicine* (pp. 796–811). Hershey, PA: IGI Global. doi:10.4018/978-1-4666-9978-6.ch062

Pomares-Quimbaya, A., González, R. A., Sierra, A., Daza, J. C., Muñoz, O., García, A., ... Bohórquez, W. R. (2017). ICT for Enabling the Quality Evaluation of Health Care Services: A Case Study in a General Hospital. In A. Moumtzoglou (Ed.), *Design, Development, and Integration of Reliable Electronic Healthcare Platforms* (pp. 196–210). Hershey, PA: IGI Global. doi:10.4018/978-1-5225-1724-5.ch012

Pouliakis, A., Margari, N., Karakitsou, E., Archondakis, S., & Karakitsos, P. (2018). Emerging Technologies Serving Cytopathology: Big Data, the Cloud, and Mobile Computing. In I. El Naqa (Ed.), *Emerging Developments and Practices in Oncology* (pp. 114–152). Hershey, PA: IGI Global. doi:10.4018/978-1-5225-3085-5.ch005

Queirós, A., Silva, A. G., Ferreira, A., Caravau, H., Cerqueira, M., & Rocha, N. P. (2016). Assessing Mobile Applications Considered Medical Devices. In M. Cruz-Cunha, I. Miranda, R. Martinho, & R. Rijo (Eds.), *Encyclopedia of E-Health and Telemedicine* (pp. 111–127). Hershey, PA: IGI Global. doi:10.4018/978-1-4666-9978-6.ch010

Raffaeli, L., Spinsante, S., & Gambi, E. (2016). Integrated Smart TV-Based Personal e-Health System. *International Journal of E-Health and Medical Communications*, *7*(1), 48–64. doi:10.4018/IJEHMC.2016010103

Rai, A., Kothari, R., & Singh, D. P. (2017). Assessment of Available Technologies for Hospital Waste Management: A Need for Society. In R. Singh, A. Singh, & V. Srivastava (Eds.), *Environmental Issues Surrounding Human Overpopulation* (pp. 172–188). Hershey, PA: IGI Global. doi:10.4018/978-1-5225-1683-5.ch010

Ramamoorthy, S., & Sivasubramaniam, R. (2018). Image Processing Including Medical Liver Imaging: Medical Image Processing from Big Data Perspective, Ultrasound Liver Images, Challenges. In M. Lytras & P. Papadopoulou (Eds.), *Applying Big Data Analytics in Bioinformatics and Medicine* (pp. 380–392). Hershey, PA: IGI Global. doi:10.4018/978-1-5225-2607-0.ch016

Rathor, G. P., & Gupta, S. K. (2017). Improving Multimodality Image Fusion through Integrate AFL and Wavelet Transform. In V. Tiwari, B. Tiwari, R. Thakur, & S. Gupta (Eds.), *Pattern and Data Analysis in Healthcare Settings* (pp. 143–157). Hershey, PA: IGI Global. doi:10.4018/978-1-5225-0536-5.ch008

Rawat, D. B., & Bhattacharya, S. (2016). Wireless Body Area Network for Healthcare Applications. In N. Meghanathan (Ed.), *Advanced Methods for Complex Network Analysis* (pp. 343–358). Hershey, PA: IGI Global. doi:10.4018/978-1-4666-9964-9.ch014

Rea, P. M. (2016). Advances in Anatomical and Medical Visualisation. In M. Pinheiro & D. Simões (Eds.), *Handbook of Research on Engaging Digital Natives in Higher Education Settings* (pp. 244–264). Hershey, PA: IGI Global. doi:10.4018/978-1-5225-0039-1.ch011

Rexhepi, H., & Persson, A. (2017). Challenges to Implementing IT Support for Evidence Based Practice Among Nurses and Assistant Nurses: A Qualitative Study. *Journal of Electronic Commerce in Organizations*, *15*(2), 61–76. doi:10.4018/JECO.2017040105

Reychav, I., & Azuri, J. (2016). Including Elderly Patients in Decision Making via Electronic Health Literacy. In M. Cruz-Cunha, I. Miranda, R. Martinho, & R. Rijo (Eds.), *Encyclopedia of E-Health and Telemedicine* (pp. 241–249). Hershey, PA: IGI Global. doi:10.4018/978-1-4666-9978-6.ch020

Richards, D., & Caldwell, P. H. (2016). Gamification to Improve Adherence to Clinical Treatment Advice: Improving Adherence to Clinical Treatment. In D. Novák, B. Tulu, & H. Brendryen (Eds.), *Handbook of Research on Holistic Perspectives in Gamification for Clinical Practice* (pp. 47–77). Hershey, PA: IGI Global. doi:10.4018/978-1-4666-9522-1.ch004

Rissman, B. (2016). Medical Conditions Associated with NLD. In B. Rissman (Ed.), *Medical and Educational Perspectives on Nonverbal Learning Disability in Children and Young Adults* (pp. 27–66). Hershey, PA: IGI Global. doi:10.4018/978-1-4666-9539-9.ch002

Rosiek, A. (2018). The Assessment of Actions of the Environment and the Impact of Preventive Medicine for Public Health in Poland. In A. Rosiek-Kryszewska & K. Leksowski (Eds.), *Healthcare Administration for Patient Safety and Engagement* (pp. 106–119). Hershey, PA: IGI Global. doi:10.4018/978-1-5225-3946-9.ch006

Rosiek, A., Leksowski, K., Goch, A., Rosiek-Kryszewska, A., & Leksowski, Ł. (2016). Medical Treatment and Difficult Ethical Decisions in Interdisciplinary Hospital Teams. In A. Rosiek & K. Leksowski (Eds.), *Organizational Culture and Ethics in Modern Medicine* (pp. 121–153). Hershey, PA: IGI Global. doi:10.4018/978-1-4666-9658-7.ch006

Rosiek, A., & Rosiek-Kryszewska, A. (2018). Managed Healthcare: Doctor Life Satisfaction and Its Impact on the Process of Communicating With the Patient. In A. Rosiek-Kryszewska & K. Leksowski (Eds.), *Healthcare Administration for Patient Safety and Engagement* (pp. 244–261). Hershey, PA: IGI Global. doi:10.4018/978-1-5225-3946-9.ch013

Rosiek-Kryszewska, A., Leksowski, Ł., Rosiek, A., Leksowski, K., & Goch, A. (2016). Clinical Communication in the Aspect of Development of New Technologies and E-Health in the Doctor-Patient Relationship. In A. Rosiek & K. Leksowski (Eds.), *Organizational Culture and Ethics in Modern Medicine* (pp. 18–51). Hershey, PA: IGI Global. doi:10.4018/978-1-4666-9658-7.ch002

Rosiek-Kryszewska, A., & Rosiek, A. (2018). The Involvement of the Patient and his Perspective Evaluation of the Quality of Healthcare. In A. Rosiek-Kryszewska & K. Leksowski (Eds.), *Healthcare Administration for Patient Safety and Engagement* (pp. 121–144). Hershey, PA: IGI Global. doi:10.4018/978-1-5225-3946-9.ch007

Rosiek-Kryszewska, A., & Rosiek, A. (2018). The Impact of Management and Leadership Roles in Building Competitive Healthcare Units. In A. Rosiek-Kryszewska & K. Leksowski (Eds.), *Healthcare Administration for Patient Safety and Engagement* (pp. 13–30). Hershey, PA: IGI Global. doi:10.4018/978-1-5225-3946-9.ch002

Roşu, S. M., Păvăloiu, I. B., Dragoi, G., Apostol, C. G., & Munteanu, D. (2016). Telemedicine Based on LMDS in the Urban/Metropolitan Area: A Romanian Case Study. In M. Cruz-Cunha, I. Miranda, R. Martinho, & R. Rijo (Eds.), *Encyclopedia of E-Health and Telemedicine* (pp. 96–109). Hershey, PA: IGI Global. doi:10.4018/978-1-4666-9978-6.ch009

Rouzbehani, K. (2017). Health Policy Implementation: Moving Beyond Its Barriers in United States. In N. Wickramasinghe (Ed.), *Handbook of Research on Healthcare Administration and Management* (pp. 541–552). Hershey, PA: IGI Global. doi:10.4018/978-1-5225-0920-2.ch032

Ruiz, I. M., Cohen, D. S., & Marco, Á. M. (2016). ISO/IEEE11073 Family of Standards: Trends and Applications on E-Health Monitoring. In M. Cruz-Cunha, I. Miranda, R. Martinho, & R. Rijo (Eds.), *Encyclopedia of E-Health and Telemedicine* (pp. 646–660). Hershey, PA: IGI Global. doi:10.4018/978-1-4666-9978-6.ch050

Sam, S. (2017). Mobile Phones and Expanding Human Capabilities in Plural Health Systems. In K. Moahi, K. Bwalya, & P. Sebina (Eds.), *Health Information Systems and the Advancement of Medical Practice in Developing Countries* (pp. 93–114). Hershey, PA: IGI Global. doi:10.4018/978-1-5225-2262-1.ch006

Sankaranarayanan, S., & Ganesan, S. (2016). Applications of Intelligent Agents in Health Sector-A Review. *International Journal of E-Health and Medical Communications*, *7*(1), 1–30. doi:10.4018/IJEHMC.2016010101

Santos-Trigo, M., Suaste, E., & Figuerola, P. (2018). Technology Design and Routes for Tool Appropriation in Medical Practices. In M. Khosrow-Pour, D.B.A. (Ed.), Encyclopedia of Information Science and Technology, Fourth Edition (pp. 3794-3804). Hershey, PA: IGI Global. doi:10.4018/978-1-5225-2255-3.ch329

Sarivougioukas, J., Vagelatos, A., Parsopoulos, K. E., & Lagaris, I. E. (2018). Home UbiHealth. In M. Khosrow-Pour, D.B.A. (Ed.), Encyclopedia of Information Science and Technology, Fourth Edition (pp. 7765-7774). Hershey, PA: IGI Global. doi:10.4018/978-1-5225-2255-3.ch675

Sarkar, B. K. (2017). Big Data and Healthcare Data: A Survey. *International Journal of Knowledge-Based Organizations*, *7*(4), 50–77. doi:10.4018/IJKBO.2017100104

Saxena, K., & Banodha, U. (2017). An Essence of the SOA on Healthcare. In R. Bhadoria, N. Chaudhari, G. Tomar, & S. Singh (Eds.), *Exploring Enterprise Service Bus in the Service-Oriented Architecture Paradigm* (pp. 283–304). Hershey, PA: IGI Global. doi:10.4018/978-1-5225-2157-0.ch018

Schmeida, M., & McNeal, R. (2016). Consulting Online Healthcare Information: E-Caregivers as Knowledgeable Decision Makers. *International Journal of Computers in Clinical Practice, 1*(1), 42–52. doi:10.4018/IJCCP.2016010104

Sen, K., & Ghosh, K. (2018). Incorporating Global Medical Knowledge to Solve Healthcare Problems: A Framework for a Crowdsourcing System. *International Journal of Healthcare Information Systems and Informatics, 13*(1), 1–14. doi:10.4018/IJHISI.2018010101

Shakdher, A., & Pandey, K. (2017). REDAlert+: Medical/Fire Emergency and Warning System using Android Devices. *International Journal of E-Health and Medical Communications, 8*(1), 37–51. doi:10.4018/IJEHMC.2017010103

Shekarian, E., Abdul-Rashid, S. H., & Olugu, E. U. (2017). An Integrated Fuzzy VIKOR Method for Performance Management in Healthcare. In M. Tavana, K. Szabat, & K. Puranam (Eds.), *Organizational Productivity and Performance Measurements Using Predictive Modeling and Analytics* (pp. 40–61). Hershey, PA: IGI Global. doi:10.4018/978-1-5225-0654-6.ch003

Shi, J., Erdem, E., & Liu, H. (2016). Expanding Role of Telephone Systems in Healthcare: Developments and Opportunities. In A. Dwivedi (Ed.), *Reshaping Medical Practice and Care with Health Information Systems* (pp. 87–131). Hershey, PA: IGI Global. doi:10.4018/978-1-4666-9870-3.ch004

Shijina, V., & John, S. J. (2017). Multiple Relations and its Application in Medical Diagnosis. *International Journal of Fuzzy System Applications, 6*(4), 47–62. doi:10.4018/IJFSA.2017100104

Shipley, N., & Chakraborty, J. (2018). Big Data and mHealth: Increasing the Usability of Healthcare Through the Customization of Pinterest – Literary Perspective. In J. Machado, A. Abelha, M. Santos, & F. Portela (Eds.), *Next-Generation Mobile and Pervasive Healthcare Solutions* (pp. 46–66). Hershey, PA: IGI Global. doi:10.4018/978-1-5225-2851-7.ch004

Singh, A., & Dutta, M. K. (2017). A Reversible Data Hiding Scheme for Efficient Management of Tele-Ophthalmological Data. *International Journal of E-Health and Medical Communications, 8*(3), 38–54. doi:10.4018/IJEHMC.2017070103

Sivaji, A., Radjo, H. K., Amin, M., & Abu Hashim, M. A. (2016). Design of a Hospital Interactive Wayfinding System: Designing for Malaysian Users. In N. Mohamed, T. Mantoro, M. Ayu, & M. Mahmud (Eds.), *Critical Socio-Technical Issues Surrounding Mobile Computing* (pp. 88–123). Hershey, PA: IGI Global. doi:10.4018/978-1-4666-9438-5.ch005

Skourti, P. K., & Pavlakis, A. (2017). The Second Victim Phenomenon: The Way Out. In M. Riga (Ed.), *Impact of Medical Errors and Malpractice on Health Economics, Quality, and Patient Safety* (pp. 197–222). Hershey, PA: IGI Global. doi:10.4018/978-1-5225-2337-6.ch008

Smith, C. R. (2018). Medical Students' Quest Towards the Long White Coat: Impact on Mental Health and Well-Being. In C. Smith (Ed.), *Exploring the Pressures of Medical Education From a Mental Health and Wellness Perspective* (pp. 1–42). Hershey, PA: IGI Global. doi:10.4018/978-1-5225-2811-1.ch001

Smith, S. I., & Dandignac, M. (2018). Perfectionism: Addressing Lofty Expectations in Medical School. In C. Smith (Ed.), *Exploring the Pressures ofMedical Education From a Mental Health and Wellness Perspective* (pp. 68–91). Hershey, PA: IGI Global. doi:10.4018/978-1-5225-2811-1.ch003

Sobrinho, Á. A., Dias da Silva, L., Perkusich, A., Cunha, P., Pinheiro, M. E., & Melo de Medeiros, L. (2016). Towards Medical Systems to Aid the Detection and Treatment of Chronic Diseases. In D. Fotiadis (Ed.), *Handbook of Research on Trends in the Diagnosis and Treatment of Chronic Conditions* (pp. 50–69). Hershey, PA: IGI Global. doi:10.4018/978-1-4666-8828-5.ch003

Soczywko, J., & Rutkowska, D. (2018). The Patient/Provider Relationship in Emergency Medicine: Organization, Communication, and Understanding. In A. Rosiek-Kryszewska & K. Leksowski (Eds.), *Healthcare Administration for Patient Safety and Engagement* (pp. 74–105). Hershey, PA: IGI Global. doi:10.4018/978-1-5225-3946-9.ch005

Sołtysik-Piorunkiewicz, A., Furmankiewicz, M., & Ziuziański, P. (2016). Web Healthcare Applications in Poland: Trends, Standards, Barriers and Possibilities of Implementation and Usage of E-Health Systems. In I. Deliyannis, P. Kostagiolas, & C. Banou (Eds.), *Experimental Multimedia Systems for Interactivity and Strategic Innovation* (pp. 258–283). Hershey, PA: IGI Global. doi:10.4018/978-1-4666-8659-5.ch013

Soni, P. (2018). Implications of HIPAA and Subsequent Regulations on Information Technology. In M. Gupta, R. Sharman, J. Walp, & P. Mulgund (Eds.), *Information Technology Risk Management and Compliance in Modern Organizations* (pp. 71–98). Hershey, PA: IGI Global. doi:10.4018/978-1-5225-2604-9.ch004

Spinelli, R., & Benevolo, C. (2016). From Healthcare Services to E-Health Applications: A Delivery System-Based Taxonomy. In A. Dwivedi (Ed.), *Reshaping Medical Practice and Care with Health Information Systems* (pp. 205–245). Hershey, PA: IGI Global. doi:10.4018/978-1-4666-9870-3.ch007

Srivastava, A., & Aggarwal, A. K. (2018). Medical Image Fusion in Spatial and Transform Domain: A Comparative Analysis. In M. Anwar, A. Khosla, & R. Kapoor (Eds.), *Handbook of Research on Advanced Concepts in Real-Time Image and Video Processing* (pp. 281–300). Hershey, PA: IGI Global. doi:10.4018/978-1-5225-2848-7.ch011

Srivastava, S. K., & Roy, S. N. (2018). Recommendation System: A Potential Tool for Achieving Pervasive Health Care. In J. Machado, A. Abelha, M. Santos, & F. Portela (Eds.), *Next-Generation Mobile and Pervasive Healthcare Solutions* (pp. 111–127). Hershey, PA: IGI Global. doi:10.4018/978-1-5225-2851-7.ch008

Stancu, A. (2016). Correlations and Patterns of Food and Health Consumer Expenditure. In A. Jean-Vasile (Ed.), *Food Science, Production, and Engineering in Contemporary Economies* (pp. 44–101). Hershey, PA: IGI Global. doi:10.4018/978-1-5225-0341-5.ch003

Stanimirovic, D. (2017). Digitalization of Death Certification Model: Transformation Issues and Implementation Concerns. In S. Saeed, Y. Bamarouf, T. Ramayah, & S. Iqbal (Eds.), *Design Solutions for User-Centric Information Systems* (pp. 22–43). Hershey, PA: IGI Global. doi:10.4018/978-1-5225-1944-7.ch002

Stavros, A., Vavoulidis, E., & Nasioutziki, M. (2016). The Use of Mobile Health Applications for Quality Control and Accreditational Purposes in a Cytopathology Laboratory. In A. Moumtzoglou (Ed.), *M-Health Innovations for Patient-Centered Care* (pp. 262–283). Hershey, PA: IGI Global. doi:10.4018/978-1-4666-9861-1.ch013

Sukkird, V., & Shirahada, K. (2018). E-Health Service Model for Asian Developing Countries: A Case of Emergency Medical Service for Elderly People in Thailand. In M. Khosrow-Pour (Ed.), *Optimizing Current Practices in E-Services and Mobile Applications* (pp. 214–232). Hershey, PA: IGI Global. doi:10.4018/978-1-5225-5026-6.ch011

Sygit, B., & Wąsik, D. (2016). Patients' Rights and Medical Personnel Duties in the Field of Hospital Care. In A. Rosiek & K. Leksowski (Eds.), *Organizational Culture and Ethics in Modern Medicine* (pp. 282–297). Hershey, PA: IGI Global. doi:10.4018/978-1-4666-9658-7.ch012

Sygit, B., & Wąsik, D. (2016). The Idea of Human Rights in Conditions of Hospital Treatment. In A. Rosiek & K. Leksowski (Eds.), *Organizational Culture and Ethics in Modern Medicine* (pp. 236–254). Hershey, PA: IGI Global. doi:10.4018/978-1-4666-9658-7.ch010

Talbot, T. B. (2017). Making Lifelike Medical Games in the Age of Virtual Reality: An Update on "Playing Games with Biology" from 2013. In B. Dubbels (Ed.), *Transforming Gaming and Computer Simulation Technologies across Industries* (pp. 103–119). Hershey, PA: IGI Global. doi:10.4018/978-1-5225-1817-4.ch006

Tamposis, I., Pouliakis, A., Fezoulidis, I., & Karakitsos, P. (2016). Mobile Platforms Supporting Health Professionals: Need, Technical Requirements, and Applications. In A. Moumtzoglou (Ed.), *M-Health Innovations for Patient-Centered Care* (pp. 91–114). Hershey, PA: IGI Global. doi:10.4018/978-1-4666-9861-1.ch005

Tiago, M. T., Tiago, F., Amaral, F. E., & Silva, S. (2016). Healthy 3.0: Healthcare Digital Dimensions. In A. Dwivedi (Ed.), *Reshaping Medical Practice and Care with Health Information Systems* (pp. 287–322). Hershey, PA: IGI Global. doi:10.4018/978-1-4666-9870-3.ch010

Tripathy, B. (2016). Application of Rough Set Based Models in Medical Diagnosis. In S. Dash & B. Subudhi (Eds.), *Handbook of Research on Computational Intelligence Applications in Bioinformatics* (pp. 144–168). Hershey, PA: IGI Global. doi:10.4018/978-1-5225-0427-6.ch008

Turcu, C. E., & Turcu, C. O. (2017). Social Internet of Things in Healthcare: From Things to Social Things in Internet of Things. In C. Reis & M. Maximiano (Eds.), *Internet of Things and Advanced Application in Healthcare* (pp. 266–295). Hershey, PA: IGI Global. doi:10.4018/978-1-5225-1820-4.ch010

Unwin, D. W., Sanzogni, L., & Sandhu, K. (2017). Developing and Measuring the Business Case for Health Information Technology. In K. Moahi, K. Bwalya, & P. Sebina (Eds.), *Health Information Systems and the Advancement of Medical Practice in Developing Countries* (pp. 262–290). Hershey, PA: IGI Global. doi:10.4018/978-1-5225-2262-1.ch015

Urooj, S., & Singh, S. P. (2016). Wavelet Transform-Based Soft Computational Techniques and Applications in Medical Imaging. In P. Saxena, D. Singh, & M. Pant (Eds.), *Problem Solving and Uncertainty Modeling through Optimization and Soft Computing Applications* (pp. 339–363). Hershey, PA: IGI Global. doi:10.4018/978-1-4666-9885-7.ch016

Vasant, P. (2018). A General Medical Diagnosis System Formed by Artificial Neural Networks and Swarm Intelligence Techniques. In U. Kose, G. Guraksin, & O. Deperlioglu (Eds.), *Nature-Inspired Intelligent Techniques for Solving Biomedical Engineering Problems* (pp. 130–145). Hershey, PA: IGI Global. doi:10.4018/978-1-5225-4769-3.ch006

Waegemann, C. P. (2016). mHealth: History, Analysis, and Implementation. In A. Moumtzoglou (Ed.), M-Health Innovations for Patient-Centered Care (pp. 1-19). Hershey, PA: IGI Global. doi:10.4018/978-1-4666-9861-1.ch001

Watfa, M. K., Majeed, H., & Salahuddin, T. (2016). Computer Based E-Healthcare Clinical Systems: A Comprehensive Survey. *International Journal of Privacy and Health Information Management, 4*(1), 50–69. doi:10.4018/IJPHIM.2016010104

Wietholter, J. P., Coetzee, R., Nardella, B., Kincaid, S. E., & Slain, D. (2016). International Healthcare Experiences: Caring While Learning and Learning While Caring. In D. Velliaris & D. Coleman-George (Eds.), *Handbook of Research on Study Abroad Programs and Outbound Mobility* (pp. 470–496). Hershey, PA: IGI Global. doi:10.4018/978-1-5225-0169-5.ch019

Witzke, K., & Specht, O. (2017). M-Health Telemedicine and Telepresence in Oral and Maxillofacial Surgery: An Innovative Prehospital Healthcare Concept in Structurally Weak Areas. *International Journal of Reliable and Quality E-Healthcare, 6*(4), 37–48. doi:10.4018/IJRQEH.2017100105

Wójcik, A., & Chojnacki, M. (2016). Behavior and Ethical Problems in the Functioning of the Operating Theater (Case Study). In A. Rosiek & K. Leksowski (Eds.), *Organizational Culture and Ethics in Modern Medicine* (pp. 154–179). Hershey, PA: IGI Global. doi:10.4018/978-1-4666-9658-7.ch007

Wolk, K., & Marasek, K. P. (2016). Translation of Medical Texts using Neural Networks. *International Journal of Reliable and Quality E-Healthcare, 5*(4), 51–66. doi:10.4018/IJRQEH.2016100104

Wong, A. K., & Lo, M. F. (2018). Using Pervasive Computing for Sustainable Healthcare in an Aging Population. In B. Fong, A. Ng, & P. Yuen (Eds.), *Sustainable Health and Long-Term Care Solutions for an Aging Population* (pp. 187–202). Hershey, PA: IGI Global. doi:10.4018/978-1-5225-2633-9.ch010

Wu, W., Martin, B. C., & Ni, C. (2017). A Systematic Review of Competency-Based Education Effort in the Health Professions: Seeking Order Out of Chaos. In K. Rasmussen, P. Northrup, & R. Colson (Eds.), *Handbook of Research on Competency-Based Education in University Settings* (pp. 352–378). Hershey, PA: IGI Global. doi:10.4018/978-1-5225-0932-5.ch018

Yadav, N., Aliasgari, M., & Poellabauer, C. (2016). Mobile Healthcare in an Increasingly Connected Developing World. *International Journal of Privacy and Health Information Management*, *4*(2), 76–97. doi:10.4018/IJPHIM.2016070106

Yadav, S., Ekbal, A., Saha, S., Pathak, P. S., & Bhattacharyya, P. (2017). Patient Data De-Identification: A Conditional Random-Field-Based Supervised Approach. In S. Saha, A. Mandal, A. Narasimhamurthy, S. V, & S. Sangam (Eds.), Handbook of Research on Applied Cybernetics and Systems Science (pp. 234-253). Hershey, PA: IGI Global. doi:10.4018/978-1-5225-2498-4.ch011

Yu, B., Wijesekera, D., & Costa, P. C. (2017). Informed Consent in Healthcare: A Study Case of Genetic Services. In A. Moumtzoglou (Ed.), *Design, Development, and Integration of Reliable Electronic Healthcare Platforms* (pp. 211–242). Hershey, PA: IGI Global. doi:10.4018/978-1-5225-1724-5.ch013

Yu, B., Wijesekera, D., & Costa, P. C. (2017). Informed Consent in Electronic Medical Record Systems. In I. Management Association (Ed.), Healthcare Ethics and Training: Concepts, Methodologies, Tools, and Applications (pp. 1029-1049). Hershey, PA: IGI Global. doi:10.4018/978-1-5225-2237-9.ch049

Yu, M., Li, J., & Wang, W. (2017). Creative Life Experience among Students in Medical Education. In C. Zhou (Ed.), *Handbook of Research on Creative Problem-Solving Skill Development in Higher Education* (pp. 158–184). Hershey, PA: IGI Global. doi:10.4018/978-1-5225-0643-0.ch008

Zarour, K. (2017). Towards a Telehomecare in Algeria: Case of Diabetes Measurement and Remote Monitoring. *International Journal of E-Health and Medical Communications*, *8*(4), 61–80. doi:10.4018/IJEHMC.2017100104

Zavyalova, Y. V., Korzun, D. G., Meigal, A. Y., & Borodin, A. V. (2017). Towards the Development of Smart Spaces-Based Socio-Cyber-Medicine Systems. *International Journal of Embedded and Real-Time Communication Systems*, *8*(1), 45–63. doi:10.4018/IJERTCS.2017010104

Zeinali, A. A. (2018). Word Formation Study in Developing Naming Guidelines in the Translation of English Medical Terms Into Persian. In M. Khosrow-Pour, D.B.A. (Ed.), Encyclopedia of Information Science and Technology, Fourth Edition (pp. 5136-5147). Hershey, PA: IGI Global. doi:10.4018/978-1-5225-2255-3.ch446

Ziminski, T. B., Demurjian, S. A., Sanzi, E., & Agresta, T. (2016). Toward Integrating Healthcare Data and Systems: A Study of Architectural Alternatives. In T. Iyamu & A. Tatnall (Eds.), *Maximizing Healthcare Delivery and Management through Technology Integration* (pp. 270–304). Hershey, PA: IGI Global. doi:10.4018/978-1-4666-9446-0.ch016

Ziminski, T. B., Demurjian, S. A., Sanzi, E., Baihan, M., & Agresta, T. (2016). An Architectural Solution for Health Information Exchange. *International Journal of User-Driven Healthcare*, *6*(1), 65–103. doi:10.4018/IJUDH.2016010104

Zineldin, M., & Vasicheva, V. (2018). Reducing Medical Errors and Increasing Patient Safety: TRM and 5 Q's Approaches for Better Quality of Life. In *Technological Tools for Value-Based Sustainable Relationships in Health: Emerging Research and Opportunities* (pp. 87–115). Hershey, PA: IGI Global. doi:10.4018/978-1-5225-4091-5.ch005

About the Contributors

Ronald Ma graduated with Bachelor of Medicine and Bachelor of Surgery, and specialised in surgery. He graduated with Post-graduate Diploma and Master of Public Health with First Class Honours from The University of Auckland in 2004 following which he was awarded the Doctor of Philosophy at the School of Population Health. He is currently employed in the Austin Health. He writes and presents on the issues of Public Health, the Participatory Action Research approaches to promote the well-being of ethnic minorities, and Health Economics including Clinical Costing.

* * *

Yvonne Ballueer is Nurse Unit Manager, Austin Health Intensive Care Unit, Melbourne, Australia.

Harry Chiam is commercial analyst for Boston Scientific. He has broad experience in hospitals and healthcare and has good understanding of models in the activity based funding regime. He is currently completing a graduate certificate in health economics. Harry has a bachelor's degree from Cornell University USA and is a qualified CPA.

Stephen Cole has worked for over 35 years in healthcare and has more than 20 years of experience with casemix and Activity Based Funding (ABF). He has experience in the development of ABF classification, counting, costing and funding models in multiple jurisdictions. Originally a diagnostic radiographer, Stephen has subsequently developed hospital information systems designed for casemix requirements during its introduction into Australia in the early 1990s. As casemix has developed, he has implemented and managed systems in hospitals to capture ABF information, managing the transition to an ABF funding environment. He has also worked with state health departments developing and refining monitoring and management systems for use with ABF. In England he was consultant to the NHS Information Centre for the revision of HRG4 (Healthcare Resource Groupings). On returning to Queensland, he developed the peer group weights forming the initial Queensland Health ABF model. At Gold Coast Hospital & Health Service, he designed and implemented an Activity Based Budget extension to the Activity Based Costing system (PPM) to support the annual budget process.

Henry Glennie is a Consultant Otolaryngologist-Head and Neck Surgeon (ear, nose and throat specialist). He holds two surgical fellowships, a science degree and master's degrees in business administration and public policy. Henry has written various publications on otolaryngology-head and neck surgery, healthcare delivery and reform. He is the senior medical advisor for Medilink Australia and has particular expertise in the development of innovations in the health sector to effectively monitor delivery systems, improve outcomes and quality of care. He resides in Cairns, North Queensland but travels to Sydney each week for various clinical and administrative projects.

Graeme Hart is Associate Professor Health and Biomedical Informatics Centre (HaBIC), University of Melbourne as well as Senior Staff Specialist, Dept of Intensive Care, Austin Health, Melbourne, Australia.

Martin Rennhackkamp has 30 years' experience focussing on data and information strategy, as well as technical- and information architectures. He considers data, information, insight and knowledge sharing as critical elements to business success. His current interests include data management and modern data architectures that covers big data, business analytics and information visualisation. Martin has consulted to telecommunications, insurance, financial services, retail and healthcare clients in Australia, UK and all over Africa. He was the lead of the Health Insights Challenge, a collaborative project between PBT, Austin Health, Deakin University, EntityThree and the Australian Centre for Health Innovation, that developed an analytics model for Austin Health that predicts the likelihood of patients having unplanned hospital readmissions within 30 days of discharge. He was a key member on teams that developed data strategies for Direct Axis and MTN, and was responsible for the BI strategy for Epworth Healthcare. He lectures at Deakin and La Trobe universities in their Masters of Business Analytics programs, and his blog is at www.MartInSights.com.

Jason Wang received his B-BMED from the University of Melbourne in 2013, and will receive his MD from the University of Melbourne in 2017. He is interested in anaesthesia, surgery and health economic research.

Index

E

F

G

H

I

L

M

N

O

P

www.ingramcontent.com/pod-product-compliance
Lightning Source LLC
LaVergne TN
LVHW061538290926
849162LV00004B/830
* 9 7 8 1 5 2 2 5 5 0 8 2 2 *